Wheeling in Good Hands

Wheeling in Good Hands

HOLISTIC MASSAGE FOR WHEELCHAIR USERS

Christine Sutherland, RMT

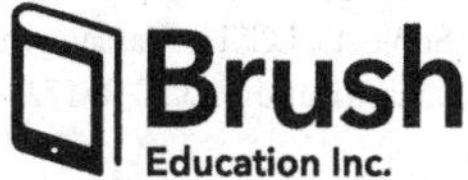

23 24 25 26 27 5 4 3 2 1

Printed and manufactured in Canada

This book is available in print, PDF, and Global Certified Acessible™ EPUB formats.

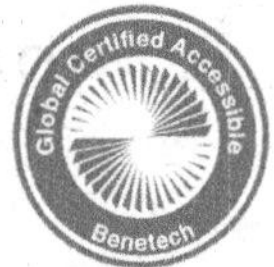

Brush Education Inc.
www.brusheducation.ca
contact@brusheducation.ca

Brush Education is located in amiskwaciwâskahikan, Edmonton, Alberta, within Treaty 6 territory and Métis Nation of Alberta Region 4, and on the traditional and ancestral territories of the Nêhiyawak, Denesuliné, Nakota Sioux, and Saulteaux Peoples.

Copyediting: Lynn Zwicky
Cover and interior design: Carol Dragich, Dragich Design
Indexing: Alexandra Peace
Photo Credits: Photo on p. 2 (caption: "A caregiver…"), 2.27B, 3.2A, 3.2F, 3.2H, 3.2K, 3.3B, 3.3C, 3.14A by James Munroe of SerpMedia. Photo of Warren Ming-Sun and his children on p. 6 by Lorrie Ming-Sun. Photos in chapter 6 and 13.2A by Chelsey Farquhar. Photo of Mary-Jo Fetterly on p. 173, credit Mary-Jo Fetterly, www.mary-jo.com. Other photos by Sussi Dorrell, Crystal Anielewicz, Will Anielewicz, Peter Schramm, Peter McCory, Jill Stewart, and Halley Roback.
Illustration Credits: 2.14B, 3.10C, 3.10D, 3.10E, 3.22, 3.34A by Brandon Besharah, RMT, illustrator. 4.2–4.7E, 4.9A–4.9G, 4.10A–4.12B, 4.14A–4.15A, 4.19A–4.31, 4.33, 4.34A, 4.37–4.39R by Chao Yu, Vancouver. All other illustrations by Barbara Brown, Raven Creations.

Disclaimer

The publisher, authors, contributors, and editors bring substantial expertise to this reference and have made their best efforts to ensure that it is useful, accurate, safe, and reliable.

Nonetheless, practitioners must always rely on their own experience, knowledge, and judgment when consulting any of the information contained in this reference or employing it in patient care. When using any of this information, they should remain conscious of their responsibility for their own safety and the safety of others, and for the best interests of those in their care.

To the fullest extent of the law, neither the publishers, the authors, the contributors, nor the editors assume any liability for injury or damage to persons or property from any use of information or ideas contained in this reference.

Library and Archives Canada Cataloguing in Publication

Title: Wheeling in good hands : holistic massage for wheelchair users / Christine Sutherland, RMT.
Names: Sutherland, Christine, 1951- author.
Description: Includes bibliographical references and index.
Identifiers: Canadiana (print) 2023049871X | Canadiana (ebook) 20230498744 | ISBN 9781550599367 (softcover) | ISBN 9781550599374 (PDF) | ISBN 9781550599381 (EPUB)
Subjects: LCSH: Massage therapy. | LCSH: People with disabilities. | LCSH: Wheelchairs.
Classification: LCC RM721 .S885 2023 | DDC 615.8/220873—dc23

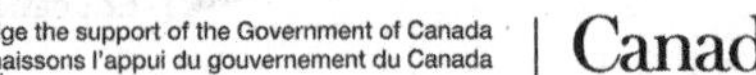
We acknowledge the support of the Government of Canada
Nous reconnaissons l'appui du gouvernement du Canada | Canada

This book is dedicated to my first wheelchair massage superstars,

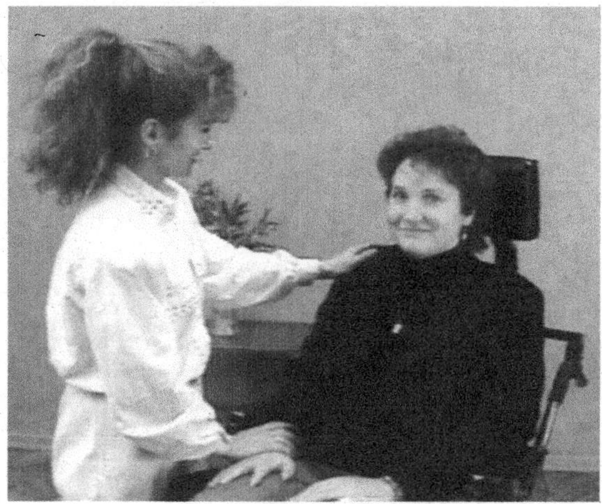

Barbara Turnbull

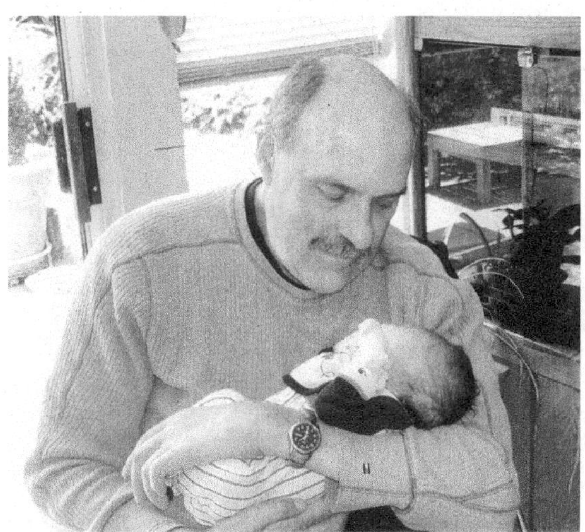

and Dennis Cherenko.

Contents

Contents

PREFACE

I realized how much the ancient medical art of massage had been rediscovered in contemporary society, and particularly within the sports community, when I attended the international wheelchair rugby finals in Pretoria, South Africa, years ago. All five teams in the finals were using massage as part of their therapeutic protocol. I was even able to offer some new techniques and include a teaching component that I labeled "How to massage your family from your wheelchair." It is important that people on the receiving end of caregiving have a way to physically give back with reciprocal massages. But mostly, I was excited that they were using massage therapeutically to make them better players with quicker rehab times.

My introduction to massage therapy happened in 1970, when I was a young resident at the Sorrento Anglican Lay Training Centre. There I met Don Grayston, an Anglican priest, and his wife Ginger, who were to become lifelong friends and huge influences in my life. It was Don and Ginger who persuaded me to go with them to a spa, insisting that I try a professional massage. Don laughingly called it another type of "spiritual" experience. Little did he know how right he was and what a profound experience it would be for me. It was enlightening: for the first time in my life, I understood the power of touch. Don became my most intimate departure partner when I lived with him for the last four months of his life at Cottage Hospice in Vancouver, BC. We were able to teach together, laugh together, and share the most powerful wheelchair experience in his final 48 hours! Don's story is the final story in this book.

In the early seventies, there were only three massage therapy schools in Canada. Each offered a one-year diploma program. In those days, massage therapy was often perceived by the public as a service occupation—a vocation, not a profession. It was not taken seriously as a healing art or as part of the medical and health-care industry. I knew massage was healing; I had experienced it myself. I also knew it was important and it clearly had unexplored medical applications. I felt there was so much potential for growth and so much missing in how massage was being taught. After graduating, I was lucky enough to be asked to teach in a reputable new massage school in Toronto (3HO School of Massage Therapy). It was there that I got my teacher training, making all my mistakes with the best of students. It was there that I met Grace Chan, one of the best of the best!

Grace and I began talking about starting a new massage school. We were on the same page. We both believed strongly that massage was an important healing art and professional therapy that was largely unrecognized by the medical community. We envisioned a program that would take massage therapy seriously and return it, as a profession, to the health-care field where it belonged. We saw and understood the gaps in our own training and felt that, by expanding the curriculum and giving students more hands-on experience in outreach settings and clinics, we could make a difference.

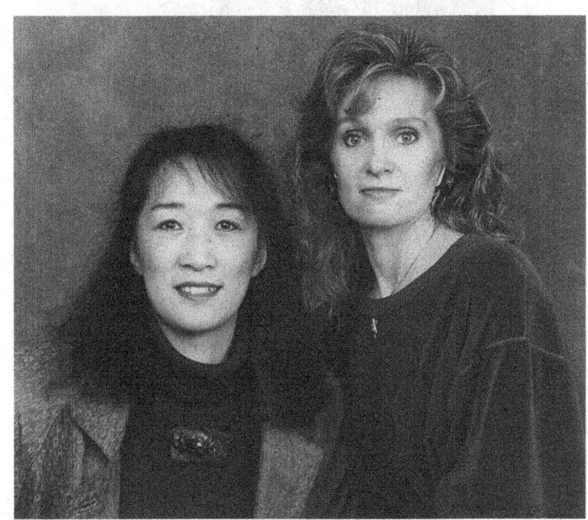

Grace Chan and me in the 1970s.

Our dreams were translated into action in January, 1978, when we opened our own school, the Sutherland-Chan School and Teaching Clinic. We had fourteen students, a dream, and much optimism. Sutherland-Chan has thrived, and is now one of the oldest and most successful free-standing massage therapy schools in Canada. We were the first school in Canada to offer a two-year program in massage therapy and this led to a change in the standards in Canada and throughout North America.

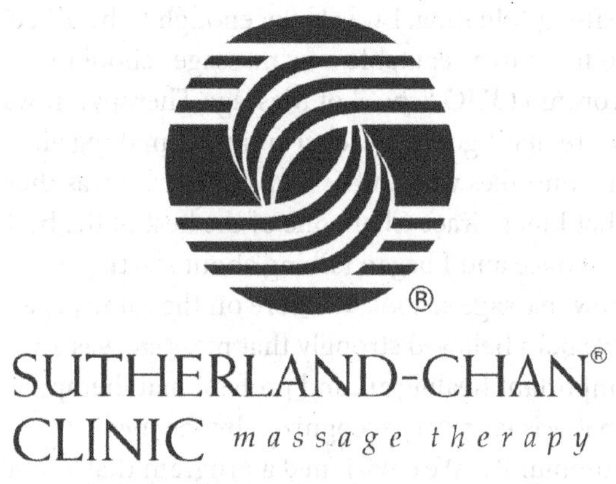

The Sutherland-Chan Clinic is one of the oldest freestanding massage therapy schools in Canada.

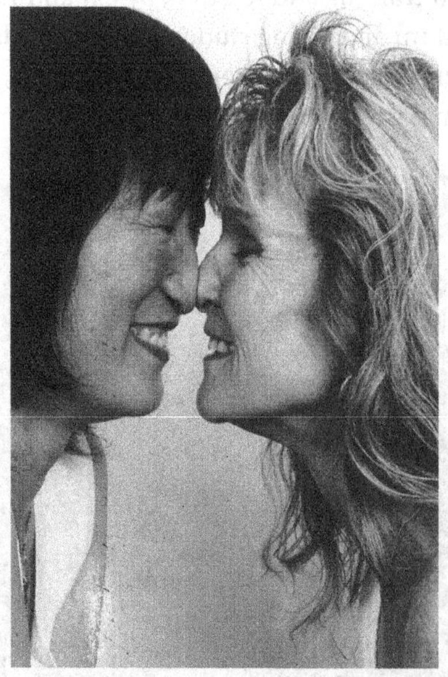

Grace and I were on the same page: returning massage therapy, as a profession, to the field of health care.

The dream that Grace and I had has come to fruition. There are now more than forty massage therapy programs in Ontario alone and many more across Canada. The one-year vocational program of the 1970s has become a two- and three-year professional program that is being recognized and integrated into the health-care system. There are now an estimated ten thousand massage therapists in Canada; it is considered a rising profession. More importantly, scientific research has begun to back up what we understood and talked about as young therapists entering the field.

While the word *massage* will always conjure up ideas of relaxation and well-being—that certainly is part of the magic of massage—the profession itself is much broader, with direct physical and medical applications. For example, massage therapists are trained to work with a wide range of medical disorders and conditions. You can, in increasing numbers, find massage therapists working in hospitals, pain clinics, long-term care facilities, postsurgical and chronic care facilities, in palliative care, and in sports arenas all over the world. Their patients can be people in wheelchairs, with spinal cord injuries, strokes, neurological disorders, Parkinson's disease, cancer, mobility issues, and a multitude of other medical conditions. The world of wheelchair massage is very big when it comes to chronic disabilities, but wheelchair massage is also at the center of wheelchair sports, from local teams to Paralympic athletes.

The strongest support for massage therapy in recent years has come through medical science. The 1971 book, *Touching: The Human Significance of the Skin* by Ashley Montagu, a medical anthropologist, humanist, and scientist, was my bible of organized research about the power of touch. Dr. Montagu cited hundreds of studies about the importance of touch in human and animal development. Since then, research on touch has expanded, and has moved from developmental science into medical science and into the health-care field.

We have come full circle with massage therapy. I thank Tiffany Field, Director of the Touch Research Institute, for her dedicated work about the power of touch. The earliest anthropological evidence of massage as an integral part of healing practice was alive and well in ancient India and China between six to eight thousand years ago. Over 2,600 years ago, Hippocrates, the Greek "Father of Medicine" wrote: "Anyone wishing to study medicine must master the art of massage." And we now have research departments in universities and schools of medicine that are dedicated to studying and proving that therapeutic massage is a natural and effective means of alleviating pain, and of aiding bodily functions in our circulatory, digestive, and respiratory systems, and it appears to have benefits, as the Greeks thought so many years ago, in preventing and healing illness.

Through this book, I will teach you the basics of wheelchair massage in and out of the chair, starting with the head, neck, and shoulders, and moving down the body. I will include the important ways for wheelchair people to massage their caregivers, family, fellow athletes, and kids. I have had the opportunity to learn from so many wheelchair folks over the years, and it is my pleasure to pass along their secret successes and make them public for all of you to benefit from today.

If you have read any of my books, watched my films and videos, or taken my courses, you understand that I am a passionate advocate for massage therapy in all phases of life's arrivals and departures.

It would be good for us all to have an opportunity to assist someone close to us as they navigate wheelchair life. Or we may be in a wheelchair ourselves. With the techniques outlined in this book, we can wheel together in good hands.

The Chapters and Stories in this Book

The **Introduction** begins with a look at the power of touch for everyone, including people in wheelchairs. It also introduces non-wheelers who will be massaging wheelchair users to the importance of getting first-hand experience of what it's like to be in a wheelchair. **Chapters 1 to 4** present the basics of massaging people who use wheelchairs: common problems stemming from wheelchair use; basic massage strokes; steps for massaging someone sitting in a wheelchair; and massage routines for specific issues. **Chapter 5** is about the benefits of underwater massage for wheelchair users, and includes a section on transferring people in wheelchairs to other locations, such as pools—and also cars, so you can take them to the pool! If you can't get to a pool, you can provide underwater massage in a bathtub. The chapter includes routines for tub massage and how to transfer to a tub. **Chapter 6** focuses on massage for wheelchair athletes, including routines before, during, and after competition, and long-term maintenance routines. **Chapters 7 to 12** focus on the particular needs of particular wheelchair users, including people recovering from stroke and spinal cord injuries, people with chronic neurological conditions, people who are elderly, people in palliative care, and pregnant people. **Chapter 13** finishes the book with ways for wheelchair users to give back by massaging others from the chair.

Throughout the book, I have profiled people in my care who have used wheelchairs. I have learned so much from so many people during my career as a massage therapist, and these are some of them. Wheelchairs are part of their stories, but their stories are about more than that. I have shared their stories with details beyond wheelchair massage, to show you the individuals I came to know: their courage and generosity, and their connection to family, friends, and caregivers, including me.

VIDEO LIBRARY

I encourage you to visit the online classroom I've prepared for many of the chapters of this book. You will find a list of videos at the end of most chapters and can see the full list of videos available by visiting www.brusheducation.ca/wheeling-in-good-hands. The videos are arranged according to chapter and were specifically created to help readers understand the techniques and concepts in this book.

The Power of Touch

Dr. Matt Hertenstein teaches in the psychology department at DePauw University and studies, among other things, how touch is used in communication.

In a 2013 interview in *Psychology Today*, he talked about giving his son a back rub every evening at bedtime. It was a bonding opportunity. "Oxytocin levels go up, heart rates go down, all these wonderful things that you can't see." While he was giving the back rub, he also benefited: "You can't touch without being touched. A lot of those same beneficial physiological consequences happen to me, the person doing the touching."[1]

The interesting part about touch is that it is a two-way street. When you give a massage, you too are being touched. We have conversations through the skin.

Those conversations are so important to people and mammals of all kinds. For people in wheelchairs, touch may be less easily given and received than for others. The wheelchair often becomes a visual barrier to simple touch, like easy hugging. So, it is especially important to learn to massage these folks—not waiting for transfers to more traditional massage locations like the bed or couch. A wheelchair head, neck, and shoulder massage can make all the difference between lonely and well loved.

Therapeutic touch is healing on all levels, including emotional relationships among friends and family. Many people become wheelchair users after serious injury, and when newly injured, touch helps them and their loved ones navigate the startling new reality that confronts them. I have been part of many caring teams for newly injured folks, and I always encourage them to have their kids and their spouses climb carefully into their hospital beds, and curl up around them, reading, sleeping, or watching TV together. The levels of oxygen uptake and the heart rate are changed with these measures.

Touch is a great equalizer, including for people who use wheelchairs and the people who love them. It brings families and friends comfort and connection.

The Importance of Massage Teams

I strongly advocate building and working with teams to increase the number of massages and the number of people giving the massages. The more people you teach to do wheelchair massage, the more comfortable the person in the chair will be, and the more connected.

When you are massaging, you are being touched, and when you are teaching, you are being taught. All of these processes are ways of communicating and transmitting information.

A person living in a wheelchair belongs to other people—friends and family. Friends and family want to help them. Depending on the situation and depending on the family or friendship group, learning basic massage and learning about wheelchairs can be a big step. It is important to invite the family and friends into the circle of care. Invite them to massage along in tandem with you.

Teaching Massage to Build Teams

I usually teach massage in teams of two. This tandem method of teaching is simple. The massaging pair mirror each other, doing identical strokes with identical rhythm, pressure, and speed. Team members can see how easy it is to pass along the hands-on procedures, how fast they can learn in the tutorial.

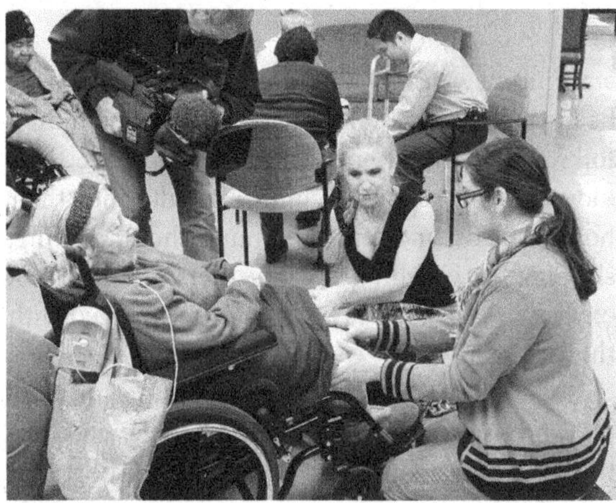

Tandem massage: a caregiver mirrors what I do, stroke by stroke.

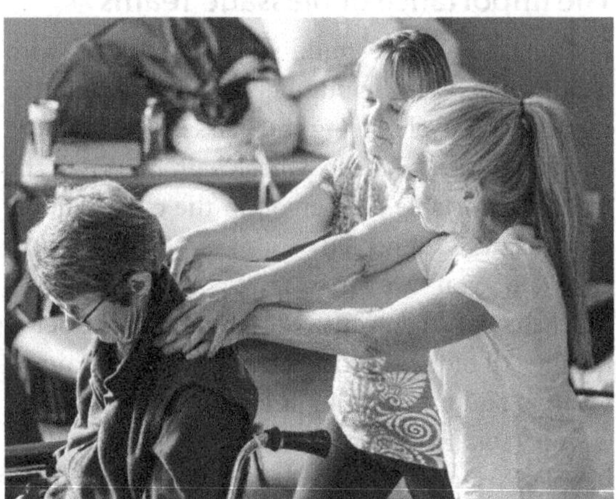

A caregiver places her hands on my hands to get a "feel" for shoulder massage!

Triads and bigger groups also work. I like to organize teams on each side of the wheelchair for the back massage, each with a leg or arm for the extremities, and one person for the tummy and another person massaging the face. It seems like a mob scene, but with the right music and rhythm everyone can be effleuraging together in a thoughtful manner! Three people can also work out a balance: the simplest is with two people on the extremities and someone on the shoulders or face.

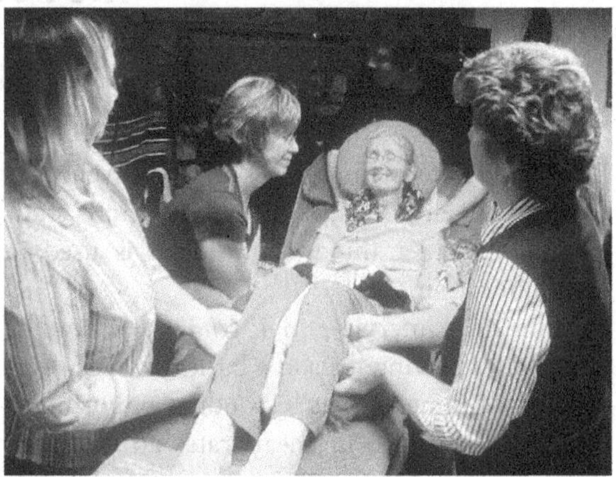

Mary Coletti's team. You can read about the Coletti family in the story about George, on page 81.

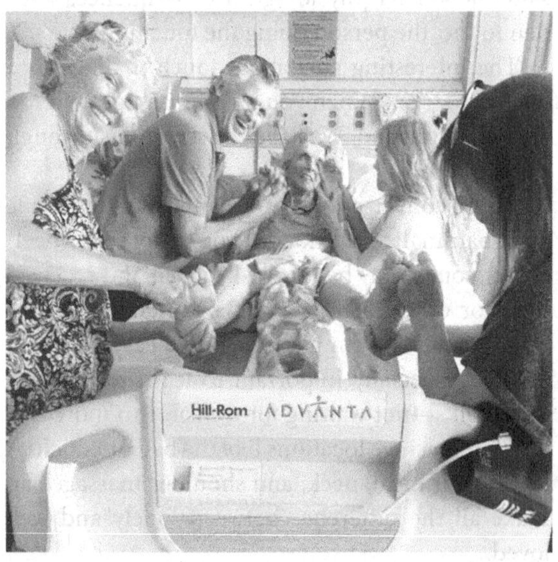

Doady Patton's family, working as a team. Doady's story is in chapter 7.

My favorite job has been teaching wheelchair massage teams. I have given tutorials in ICU, where people had new spinal cord injuries. I also love teaching in chronic care facilities, where families can often feel helpless or inadequate in the daily care of their aging loved ones. Even if the need for a wheelchair is short term—for example, in some cases of palliative care and maternity care, or in recovery from hip surgery—every situation is a valuable opportunity to teach wheelchair massage.

No two teams are alike. Recruit the willing—so many want to join in! Some teams include everyone in the family, some include teammates, some include young children. Children are great team members! My daughter loved massaging her grandmother (my mum) when she became confined to a wheelchair in the last weeks before she died. Learning wheelchair massage is a great way to demystify trauma and to teach young people that they can help. It empowers everyone.

Remember that visitors during your massage session are perfect tandem massage partners who might want to learn this life skill for immediate and practical application. If I arrive to do massage and find a visitor with my client, I include them in my massage routine immediately. They massage along with me and learn stroke by stroke. If someone is popping in for a short visit, then I include them for a short time. They just have to wash their hands and they are ready to go. You are the one to invite them in.

Some examples of the ways that I ask for help are:

> "Would you be able to help me for five minutes to do the other leg while I do this leg?"
>
> "Just follow me and then I've got more time to devote to Bo's arms!"
>
> "Can you hold this sheet for me?"
>
> "Can you pass me the massage oil?"
>
> "Can you help me with this lower leg massage?"

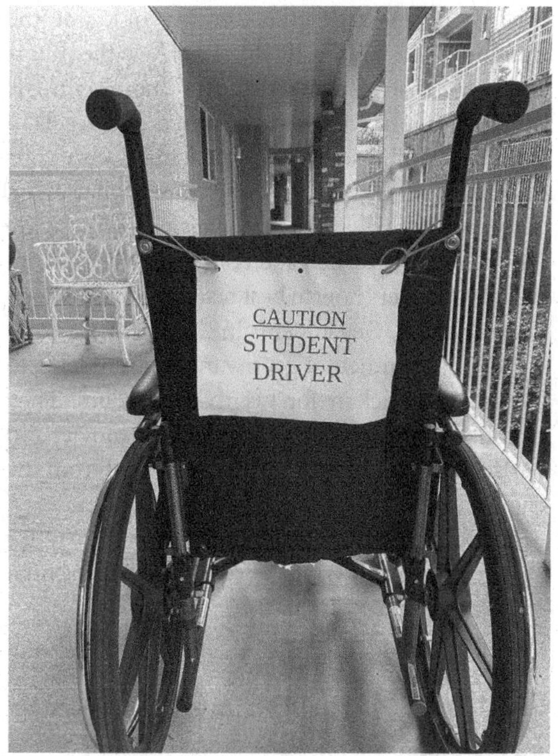

A wheelchair ready for one of my students. Experience has shown the value of this sign!

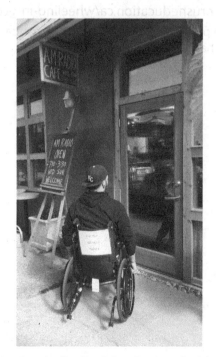

A student learning first-hand about barriers wheelchair users face.

The Importance of the Wheelchair POV

I not only teach massage to teams of family and friends, I also teach students who want to become professional massage therapists, like me.

My style of teaching wheelchair massage to my students follows that of Ashley Montagu's quote: "In teaching, it is the method and not the content that is the message…the drawing out, not the pumping in." This astutely describes the interactive style of teaching that I promote with my potential instructors; learn to teach and teach to learn is my philosophy. Experiencing twenty-four hours in a wheelchair, teaching from a wheelchair, and receiving massages in a wheelchair: these are all ways I have learned and continue to learn from wheelchair users how to best teach students wheelchair massage. Get students in wheelchairs!

As an assignment, I get my massage students to live in a wheelchair for twenty-four hours. They negotiate downtown, go for a meal or movie, and participate in our classroom activities, all from the chair.

I've been teaching in this experiential way for over forty years. I wish it were mandatory for high school students to spend twenty-four hours in a wheelchair before they were allowed to graduate.

I always remind my students that being on the receiving end is the best teaching tool for many things in life. The 24-hour wheelchair experience helps my students understand the benefits of wheelchair massage. The best way to learn wheelchair massage is to receive a wheelchair massage. This kind of life skill and awareness is far-reaching.

Only by experiencing a wheelchair do you start to acquire the special point of view of wheelchair users. So, if you're a caregiver, try the wheelchair out yourself. The learnings can be practical or philosophical, but you will acquire a different point of view, and it will make you a better wheelchair massage therapist.

VIDEO LIBRARY

Visit brusheducation.ca/wheeling-in-good-hands to watch this video:

The power of touch: Molly and Fernanda share their experiences of massage

Warren

I met Warren Ming-Sun in ICU. He was on support systems to keep him breathing. He was surrounded by family and friends all eager to be taught how to massage him.

Warren had broken his neck in a hockey game at the age of thirty-eight. At the time, he was married with two boys, working for Sirius XM Canada in Toronto.

Warren's parents became my most eager students. They learned to massage Warren with all his tubes and life-support machines buzzing around them. His parents massaged him in the morning, afternoon, and evening. I also taught them to massage each other.

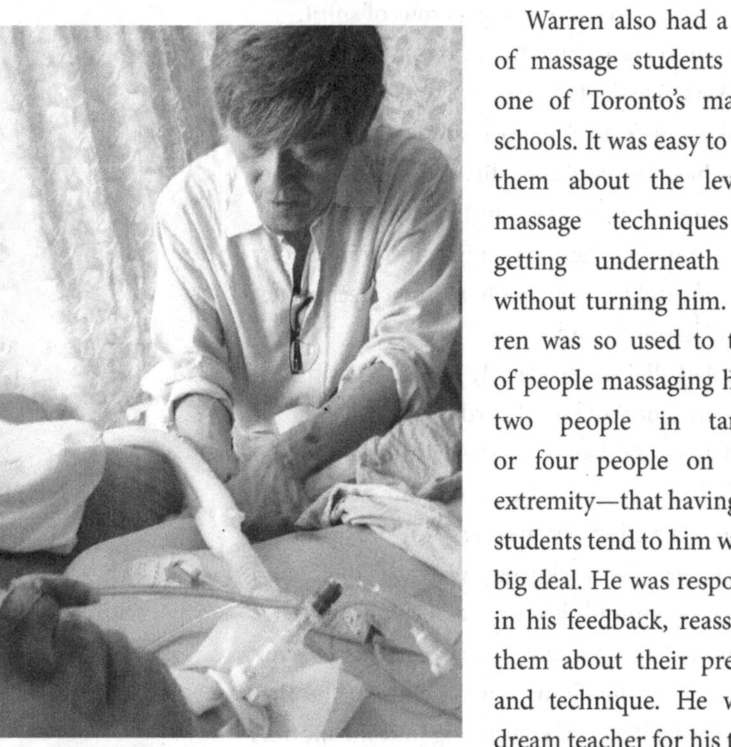

Warren's father was my best student.

At the same time, I taught all of Warren's hockey buddies and friends to do everything, including the most elaborate respiratory massage. They became rib-raking experts!

Warren's sister and her husband were a welcome addition to our family massage team. This family was my dream team working around the clock to help keep Warren's lungs clear of the life-threatening congestion that was continuously building up. We pumped those lungs like I had never pumped before!

Warren also had a team of massage students from one of Toronto's massage schools. It was easy to teach them about the levering massage techniques for getting underneath him without turning him. Warren was so used to teams of people massaging him—two people in tandem or four people on every extremity—that having four students tend to him was no big deal. He was responsive in his feedback, reassuring them about their pressure and technique. He was a dream teacher for his team!

The staff in the spinal cord injury department loved the student teaching sessions because we always ended with a care-for-the-caregiver head, neck, and shoulders routine. All of Warren's hospital staff got rubbed the right way!

I had never worked with a patient who was self-suctioning. Warren had been outfitted with a suction tube strapped to his arm at just the right length to reach inside his mouth. He was able to suction himself as we pumped his chest and created positive expectoration. I had also never been as aggressive as I was taught in Sunnybrook Hospital when helping to aid Warren in producing such exciting results. It became common for me to teach Warren's friends and family this same powerful expectoration procedure. When I see the film clips today, I don't think that I have been in such an ideal massage scenario since Warren's trip to the ICU.

Warren was the ideal patient—proactive and positive, eager to learn, and generous of spirit.

His family renovated their house to accommodate Warren's adapted bedroom and have his two kids sleep over. In the years since Warren's accident, I have taken classes directly to his home to teach wheelchair massage and to "pay back" Warren's family for their ongoing education of my skills, not only in hands-on massage techniques but also in other ways.

Most of all, Warren's family brought new meaning to my world of spinal cord injury. I had never experienced the hands-on strength of family and friends so eager to massage around the clock. His parents learned every massage skill for preventing pressure sores, clearing Warren's lungs, and massaging around his upper respiratory tubes and drains. The amount of massage that Warren received from his family and friends in his first weeks in the ICU and continuing into the months following his ICU step-down was beyond my wildest dreams!

His friends were a team of fast tactile learners with huge amounts of humor. Just like Warren's family, they were full of enthusiasm that made Warren smile through all his challenges, aches, and pains.

Beyond Canada, Warren's parents helped me teach in South Africa. They organized their close friends in Johannesburg to keep me safe throughout my teaching in that country, including taking me to the wheelchair rugby world championship on my final day.

Thank you Warren, David, Lorrie, and Karen for including me and my students on the Ming-Sun Team!

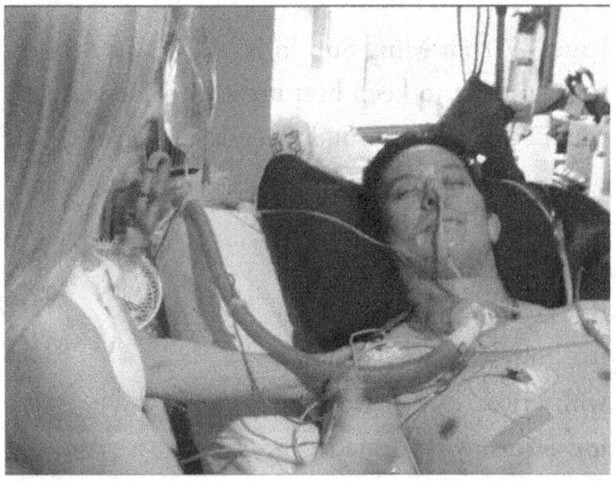

I met Warren in ICU massaging him through his life-support hoses, tubes, and electrodes.

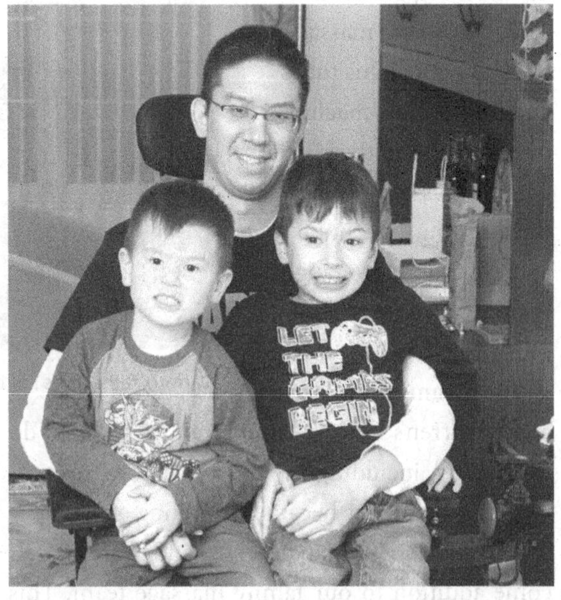

Wheeling with the boys — Warren's happy family.

1

Massage Needs of All Wheelchair Users

Part of my interest in wheelchair massage is literally the massage challenge it presents. There is much that is unpredictable about it. The patient can be young or old. The reason they are in a wheelchair can be infirmity, an accident, or a medical condition. The wheelchair can be a permanent or temporary solution. Each case is different.

Because wheelchair massage covers such a broad spectrum of people and conditions, it often requires creativity to solve problems. There is no one size fits all. I can't stress this enough. This makes wheelchair massage challenging. It forces you to be inventive, flexible, and adaptable. It may require you to alter your techniques or invent new ones. And sometimes the wheelchair itself presents a problem.

However, the massage needs of wheelchair users are universal. These needs are governed by one condition: immobility. They are also governed by one physical reality: a wheelchair.

You may be massaging wheelchair users in or out of their chairs, but the focus of massage for these folks is on the issues created by prolonged sitting.

Issues Arising from Immobility

Wheelchairs help people with impaired mobility, which can occur for many reasons. Common examples include amputation, cerebral palsy, MS, Parkinson's disease, ALS, spinal cord injury, geriatric conditions, maternity complications, postsurgical recovery, and palliative care.

No matter why a person is in a wheelchair, the primary conditions you will be addressing as a massage therapist result from immobility. We all know what can happen when a person is sedentary or immobilized: the three main systems of the body—digestive, respiratory, and circulatory—function less effectively. This can lead to serious medical conditions, and in some cases, premature death. Therapeutic massage can and does address many of the problems that arise from immobility.

Digestion is compromised when people spend a lot of time with their tummy flexed in a seated position and with their hips not moving. The daily application of massage for the digestive system helps with constipation and other digestive complaints to either calm or stimulate the small and large intestines.

Respiration always needs stimulation for people who are immobilized. Massage can ease breathing, promote bigger breaths, and make exercises in deep breathing more effective.

Circulatory and musculoskeletal issues are chronic problems with prolonged sitting in a wheelchair. Typical challenges include hip problems, sciatica, contracted iliotibial band, knee problems, leg cramping, and foot problems (flat feet from loss of arches or foot contractures causing the ankle to fix).

Knee problems arise because the knees are bent most of the time in a seated position. So, the hamstring muscles in the back of the thigh become shortened and the popliteal fossa (the back of the knee) becomes congested with shortened tendinous attachments from the thigh and the lower leg converging into this space. The gastrocnemius (calf muscle) is also shortened, so it is important to focus on the tendinous attachments on either side of the back of the knee and at the heel of the foot, where the Achilles tendon attaches into the calcaneus (heel bone). There's lots to do to massage the back of the leg from where the hamstrings attach into the ischial tuberosity at the bottom of the rear end down the back of the leg to the heel of the foot.

Hip problems arise because the seated position cramps and shortens muscles in the front of the hip where the abdomen meets the lower body.

The axial skeleton can also become compromised from lack of muscle tone and strength, which can lead to looseness of the spine and hyperflexibility: some people develop scoliotic lateral curves to the spine, where the spine deviates to the side and the vertebrae twist, causing simple or compound spinal curves. This is especially true in people who are completely immobilized and need assistance to wheel their chairs.

Swelling in the extremities is another common problem, especially for assisted wheelers, and especially in the lower legs. Inactivity and lack of leg flexing result in swelling. For folks who are immobilized from the neck down, you will find the same symptoms of swelling in the arms due to immobility. Lymphedema is a particularly dangerous outcome, leading to infection and amputation. Massage is important for helping circulation and preventing complications.

Pressure sores happen when people can't shift their position, and an area of their body is compressed against a surface for extended periods. The compression compromises circulation and skin integrity. Pressure sores are dangerous if they get started, because over time they become more and more resistant to healing. Massage to common pressures sites, and to ulcerated tissue, can improve circulation and prevent or help heal sores.

People who wheel their own chairs can have issues directly linked to how they get around. Some people only have the use of their arms.

FIGURE 1.1. **Typical Pressure Points from Wheelchair Use**

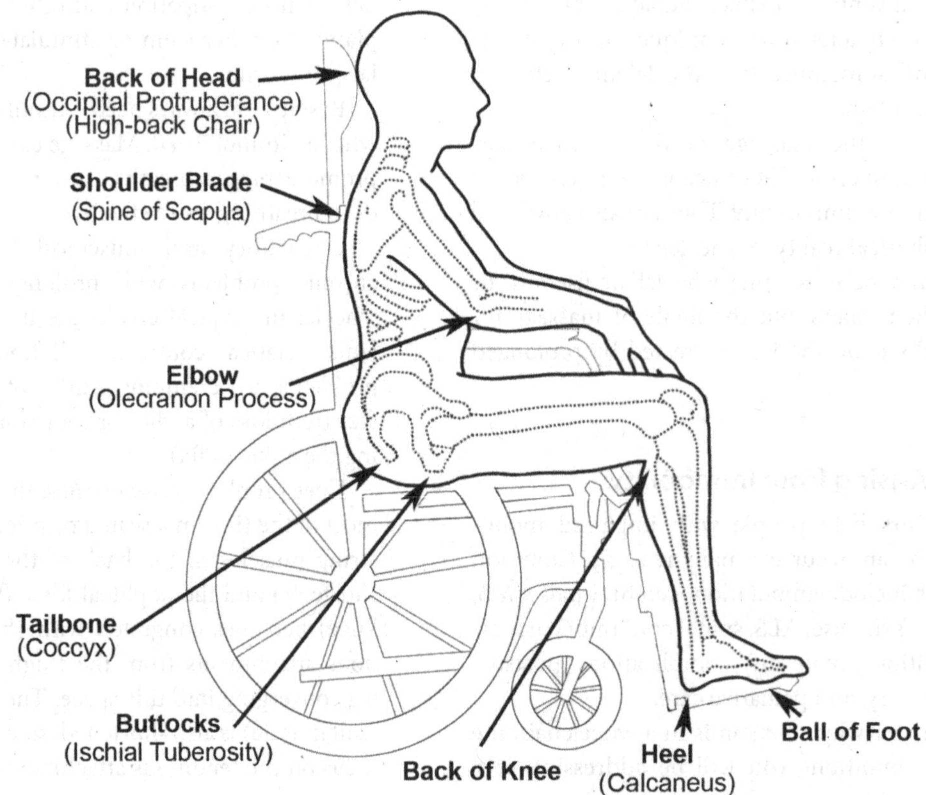

Others have the use of both their arms and legs and can push or pull themselves in the chair. Issues for self-wheelers can include headaches, neck and shoulder issues, elbow overuse conditions similar to tennis elbow and golfer's elbow, carpal tunnel syndrome in the wrist, Dupuytren's contracture in the hands, and sprains and strains. For them, it's all about muscles that are overused and muscles that are underused.

The iliotibial band is a particular area of concern. It is a band of fascia extending down the outside of the leg from the ilium (or pelvis) to the tibial attachment at the top of the outer side of the knee and lower leg. This band is almost always tight, but a serious case of contracted iliotibial band is painful and restricts movement, and this structure becomes inflexible with time in a wheelchair.

Types of Wheelchairs and Massage

Getting a wheelchair that meets each person's individual needs is very important. The right wheelchair, whether manual or electric, sitting or standing, tilting or fully reclining, will be the one that offers the best opportunities for comfort, independence, and mobility.

From a massage point of view, high-backed electric wheelchairs can present the most challenges. Each chair has customized support for the user, and is molded to the person's back. This can leave little access room for massaging people in the chair. Learning how to gain access from the side, and under and behind the person, and to use a levering technique against the chair, takes practice.

Some wheelchairs allow a variety of sitting and leg positions. These include tilt wheelchairs, which tip back. Some reclining chairs go completely flat. The ability to change body positions is a great advantage in a wheelchair, because it can ease pressure points for the user, and because it allows different access to parts of the body for massage. The abdomen, in particular, is much easier to access if a person is lying back versus sitting up.

Some people who are immobilized have standing wheelchairs that allow them to become completely vertical. This gives great access for massage, so if you have a client with this kind of chair, take full advantage of it!

When I started massaging people in wheelchairs, there was not as much variety available, and I didn't see a standing wheelchair for the first thirty years of working with wheelchair users. When I saw my first standing wheelchair, about twenty years ago, it was an eye opener. Now standing frames are commonplace and affordable.

Chairs that allow people to stretch out or stand while supported are my crusade items for anyone who needs a wheelchair. Rigid wheelchair designs, however, are still common, and make the problems associated with prolonged sitting more pronounced. Most of our focus in this book is related to the complications arising from sitting in one position.

VIDEO LIBRARY

Visit brusheducation.ca/wheeling-in-good-hands to watch this video:

Massaging wheelchair users: Seated therapist, chair-to-chair with Molly and Kyrie

2

Basic Strokes for Massaging Wheelchair Users

"Anyone wishing to study medicine must master the art of massage."

– Hippocrates, 460–377 BCE, Father of Modern Medicine

As a massage therapist, you may be massaging wheelchair users in or out of their chairs, taking care of the issues that arise from wheelchair use, especially from prolonged sitting.

The setting of massage is not the focus here. In this chapter, I will be talking about basic strokes useful for everyone, highlighting those that are particularly useful for wheelchair users.

If you are familiar with my books *Birthing in Good Hands* and *Dying in Good Hands*, you will be familiar with much of this chapter.

The Importance of Communication

When I start with a new client, whether in a wheelchair or not, I always begin with a case history. I use body diagrams for the person to identify problem and pain areas. It is also important to know what medications your patient is taking and their side effects, and your patient's history of new and old injuries.

During the treatment, I rely on their feedback to guide me. I check all along the way: I need to know if I am firm enough or too firm, whether I am hitting all the right spots or missing some. I rely on their feedback to guide me.

Communication is essential in all massage. I call it the "f-word": feedback feedback, feedback.

Sometimes it feels like you can read the reactions of clients without asking for feedback, but I am constantly surprised how asking for feedback provides accurate information that I didn't get from my own radar.

Getting feedback will enhance your own intuition about how things are going. You are giving the massage, but you need to get their reactive instruction. The person on the receiving end of your massage is your teacher!

One of the first questions I ask is about pressure. Remember that the person on the receiving end of the massage always has the right answer about pressure. Sometimes what the person needs seems counterintuitive. My dad was built like a football player, but he couldn't tolerate firm pressure; he didn't even want me using my thumbs! By contrast, I have a patient who is tiny; she has severe spasticity and takes bulldozer pressure. So, you can't tell about pressure tolerance from the outside: you have to ask.

But you have to ask the right questions to get the right answers. Checking in about pressure sounds like, "Should I be lighter or firmer?" If you ask "How's it going?" you will get a general answer of "great" and not the directive you need to make it the best wheelchair massage.

Getting people in chairs to ask to be massaged is not an easy task, so learn to make it easier for them to approach you. I always use a "coming back" phrase when leaving, such as, "See you next Monday, Mary!" It's a built-in promise of continuing connection and communication.

I also communicate with the next therapist by leaving notes, telling them who I massaged and who was on the team, along with documentation on the massage itself. Log books are another way of keeping the massage team connected. Those little notes and logbook entries work magic. They make a record of what works best for individual wheelchair users, and what works best in general. I hope you will pass on your latest and greatest wheelchair massage techniques so I can expand my own repertoire of strokes!

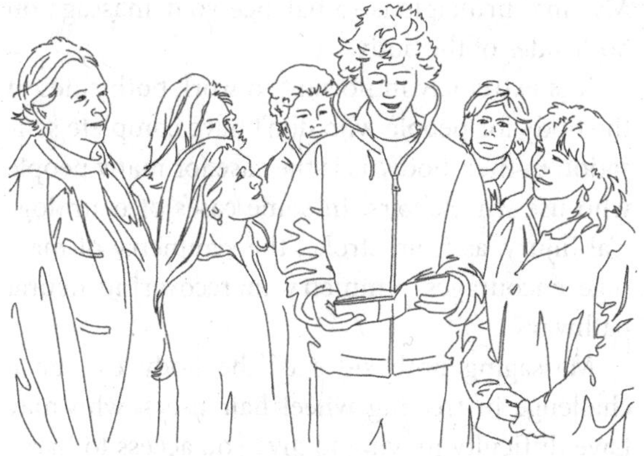

Mary Coletti's massage team reading from their logbook. Mary, who had ALS, had many people on her team. The logbook helped them coordinate their efforts, and kept them up to date on what worked best for Mary.

Principles of Massage

Over my years of teaching wheelchair massage, I have modified and changed some of the rules I originally learned that did not turn out to be true in real life. However, there are four basic principles that I always follow.

1. Uncork the Bottle

When massaging, always work the part of a limb (an arm or leg) that is hooked up with the trunk of the body first before moving down its length. I call this uncorking the bottle. Think of it like this: if you want to get the contents out of a bottle, you need to uncork it first. So, for example, when giving someone an arm massage, massage the shoulder first, and then the upper arm, and then the lower arm. It's the same with the legs: massage the hips first, then the thigh, and then the calf.

Loosen up the area at the top of the arm or leg first. This makes sense of having what is below that area be able to drain up and out of the extremity more easily. The principle of working shoulder to fingers and hips to toes is sound in terms of circulatory theory.

2. Apply Pressure Toward the Heart

I don't have many massage rules written in stone, but the direction of massage pressure is one. Although you start at the trunk and move out to the extremity, the pressure of each stroke must always go toward the heart. Don't push "downward" on the arms or legs with any stroke, whether it's your starting general strokes or the nitty-gritty of therapeutic pressure—each stroke of pressure should go in an "upward" direction, always toward the heart.

This principle is based on the way blood travels around the body. The heart is the pump of the

FIGURE 2.1. Veins of the Body

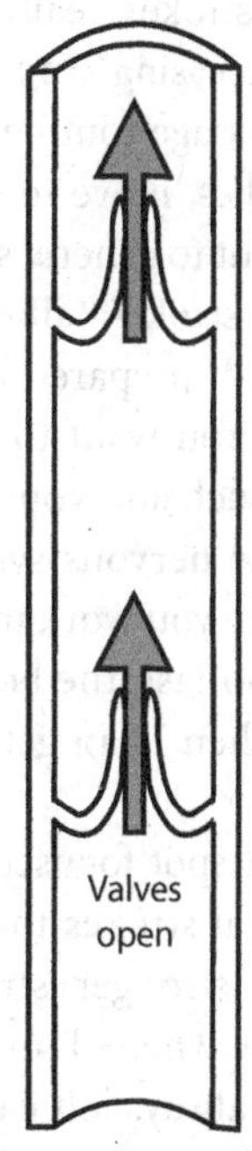

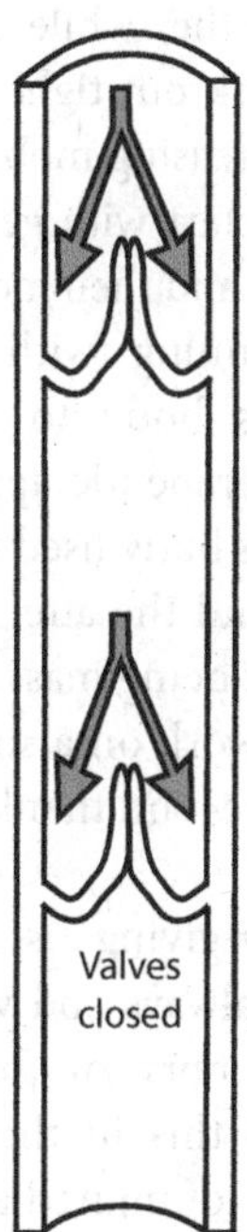

Veins have one-way valves that open as the heart beats, permitting blood to flow through, and then close between heartbeats, stopping the blood from moving backward. These valves keep blood moving toward the heart.

circulatory system. It gives the blood a big push from the center of the body out to the arms and legs, right to the tips of the fingers and toes. These extremities must then work against gravity to return blood to the heart, so our veins are designed with little one-way valves like gates to keep blood moving in the right direction. Directing your massage pressure up toward the heart helps promote the movement of blood back to the heart.

So, I repeat! Pressure toward the heart!

There is only one exception to this rule: when massaging the trunk of the body. The heart is near the middle of the body and the circulatory system is more deeply buried, so the venous return is not directly affected by your direction of pressure in the trunk of the body.

3. Move from General Strokes to Local Strokes to General Strokes

Massage strokes include some superficial, general, large strokes and other smaller, focused, and intense strokes. The superficial strokes tend to smooth out and soothe, while the local strokes really get in and work out tight spots, decreasing contractures and increasing mobility. A massage routine should always start with general strokes, move to specific strokes, and then move back out to general strokes.

Beginning with general strokes allows the patient's body to adjust and prepare for further therapeutic application. You want to get the patient's body used to your touch and you want to command the attention of the nervous system to the part being massaged before you work into it. If I start work on a sore spot too fast, the body will repel me—no thanks!—and then I can get locked out.

After giving a sore or tight spot focused attention, I always end with general strokes that erase the memory of the deeper, stronger strokes. I learned this in the barnyard where I massaged all sorts of injured animals. I always left each animal I worked on with a stroke memory that was positive, if not necessarily therapeutic. If the animal remembered me as the person making them uncomfortable, even if there was later therapeutic gain, then it was going to be a lot harder to repeat the treatment. The animal would take one look at me coming into the barn and head for the other side of the stall. So, I learned early to "trick" the tissues and leave a lasting impression of positive contact. I usually use whatever is my client's favorite stroke for my finale. You want to leave the tissues happy to see you again.

4. Work Both Sides of the Body

My final principle is to balance your massage on both sides of the body.

It is extremely important to work both sides of the body for people who don't have complete sensation in their body, as is the case for many people who use wheelchairs. In some cases of neurological injury, as from stroke, the symmetry of massage encourages symmetry in recovering neural pathways.

Massaging both sides of the body can be a challenge in treating wheelchair users, who may have difficulty moving to give you access to hard-to-access areas. There are techniques for gaining access, such as levering, taught in this book.

Wheelchair users have helped me to design new massage strokes that I never would have discovered without trying to meet their needs. My career has included wheelchair massage in all kinds of environments, from gymnasiums to office cubicles. Wheelchair massage has taught me even more about the importance of being adaptable to unique situations and individuals.

Basic Anatomy

Professionally trained massage therapists have extensive knowledge of anatomy, which is critical for their work. However, you can apply effective massage therapy at home with just a little knowledge of human anatomy. Figures 2.2 to 2.5 provide some of the basic anatomic knowledge and vocabulary you will find helpful as you work through the massages in this book. Understanding the human skeleton will help you understand the body's bony spots that are prone to bedsores.

Basic Massage Movements

The common movements used in massage include:

1. **Effleurage:** stroking movement.
2. **Petrissage:** alternating pressure with wringing, kneading, and scooping.
3. **Levering (modified petrissage):** pressing down with back of hand to provide leverage and strength in order to lift up; single-handed, bilateral, and reinforced fingertip kneading.
4. **Fisted:** levering the back of the leg, back of the thigh for supine patient, back of knee, as well as unlevered on the back between shoulder blades and spine.
5. **Frictioning:** adaptive for patients and traditional techniques for the caregiving team.
6. **Compression:** chest compression, chest pumping, and alternating digital compression.
7. **Stretching:** thumb stretching, fingertip stretching, and palmar stretching.
8. **Percussive tapotement:** cupping, adaptive single-handed pounding, beating, and hacking.
9. **Vibration:** fine, coarse, static, running.
10. **Light reflex stroking:** longitudinal, circular, backhanded.

We're going to go through each of these in detail.

Effleurage

Effleurage is a French term that means "to cover" or "to cloak." Fittingly, this stroke is most often used to cover or spread the body with oil. It is a warm-up stroke with a gentle, double-loop shape. This is the introductory stroke I use most often to get my hands accustomed to my patient and the patient accustomed to my touch. With my wheelchair patients, this stroke can start to alleviate uncomfortable skin tension from swelling. Effleurage also has its own stand-alone merits of promoting better circulation. The stroke encourages congested circulation to move more effectively, helping to reduce swollen limbs, as well as reducing stress and inducing relaxation.

Introductory effleurage strokes are done at least three times on whichever part of the body you are going to massage: back, arms, legs, or chest and abdomen. The first time spreads the oil, the second time allows you to get comfortable with the stroke, and the third time establishes pressure and gets the circulation moving.

To begin a back massage, for example, put some oil or lotion on your hands. It is important to get the right amount of oil, which may take some practice. You want enough oil to provide ease of movement, but not so much that you make the person's back slippery. You want your hands to have good contact and not just skate over the surface. Start with just a few drops (not a dollop) and then add more as needed. You don't need to put on the total amount of oil you will use throughout the massage at the beginning. You can add lotion as the massage progresses. If you get too much, towel some off.

Place one hand on each side of the spine, applying firm, even pressure. Use the whole palmar surface of your hands, including fingers. Don't be dainty! Effleurage is a flat-handed stroke: keep your fingers together but flat, and make good contact with your entire hand, from the base of your palm to your fingertips.

Move your hands together from the shoulders down to the lower back. At the base of the spine, loop your hands out to the outer back and sides and continue the pressure as you return along the length of the torso to the shoulders. Be firm, especially on the return stroke up the sides. At the shoulders, begin the stroke again.

When effleuraging the arms or legs, use a technique similar to the one described above, but always push up toward the heart and never down toward the extremities. On the back, it doesn't matter—you can apply pressure in both directions, as the direction of massage pressure does not directly affect venous return.

As this is the beginning of the massage routine, this stroke gives you lots of information about the part of the body you are getting to know. As you effleurage, you can sense the areas of tension underneath your hands.

HELPFUL TERMS

Posterior: back	Transverse: across	Supine: face-up	Inferior: below
Anterior: front	Ascending: upward	Lateral: side	
Proximal: close	Descending: downward	Medial: middle	
Distal: far	Prone: face-down	Superior: above	

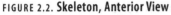

FIGURE 2.2. Skeleton, Anterior View

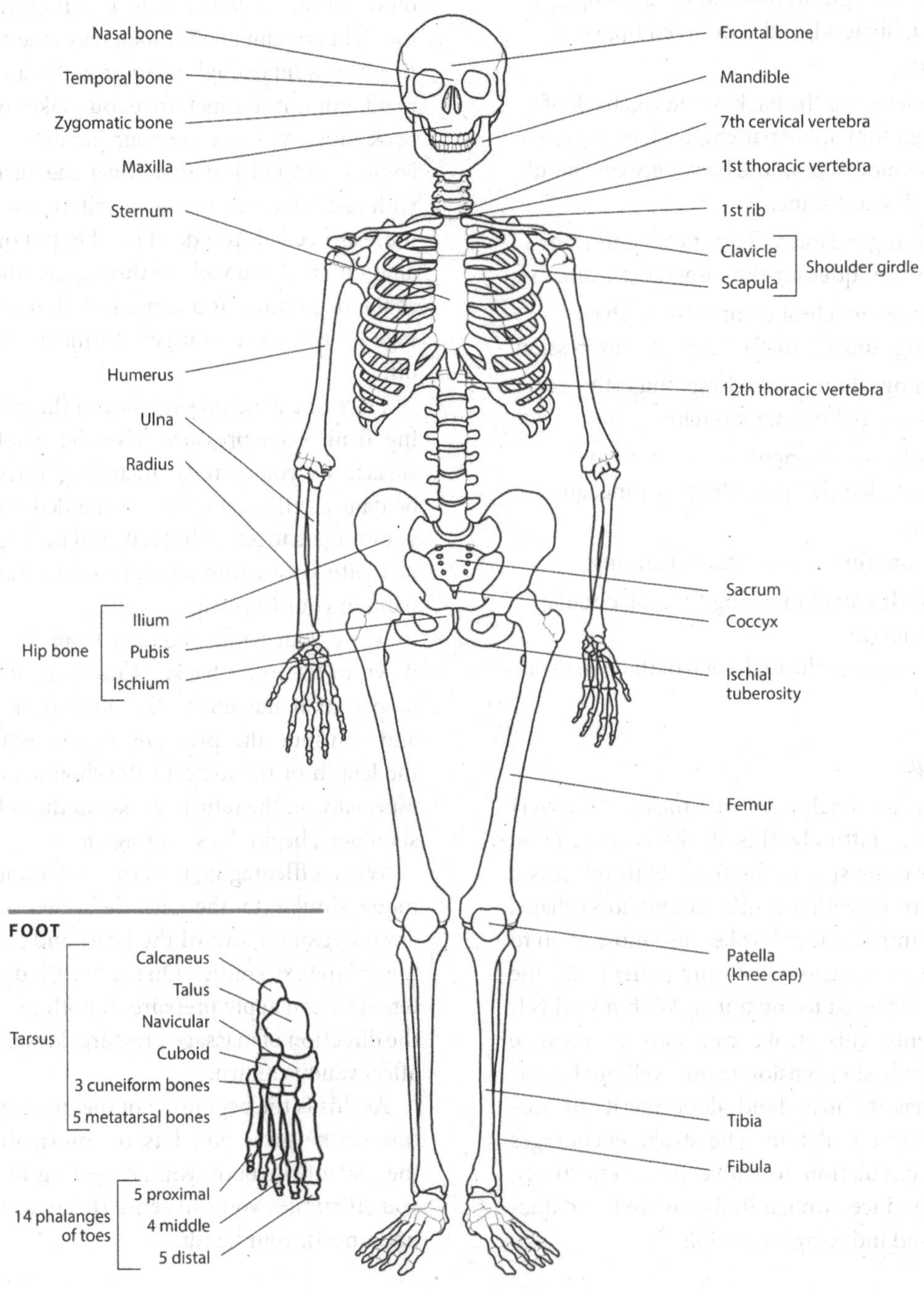

FIGURE 2.3. Skeleton, Posterior View

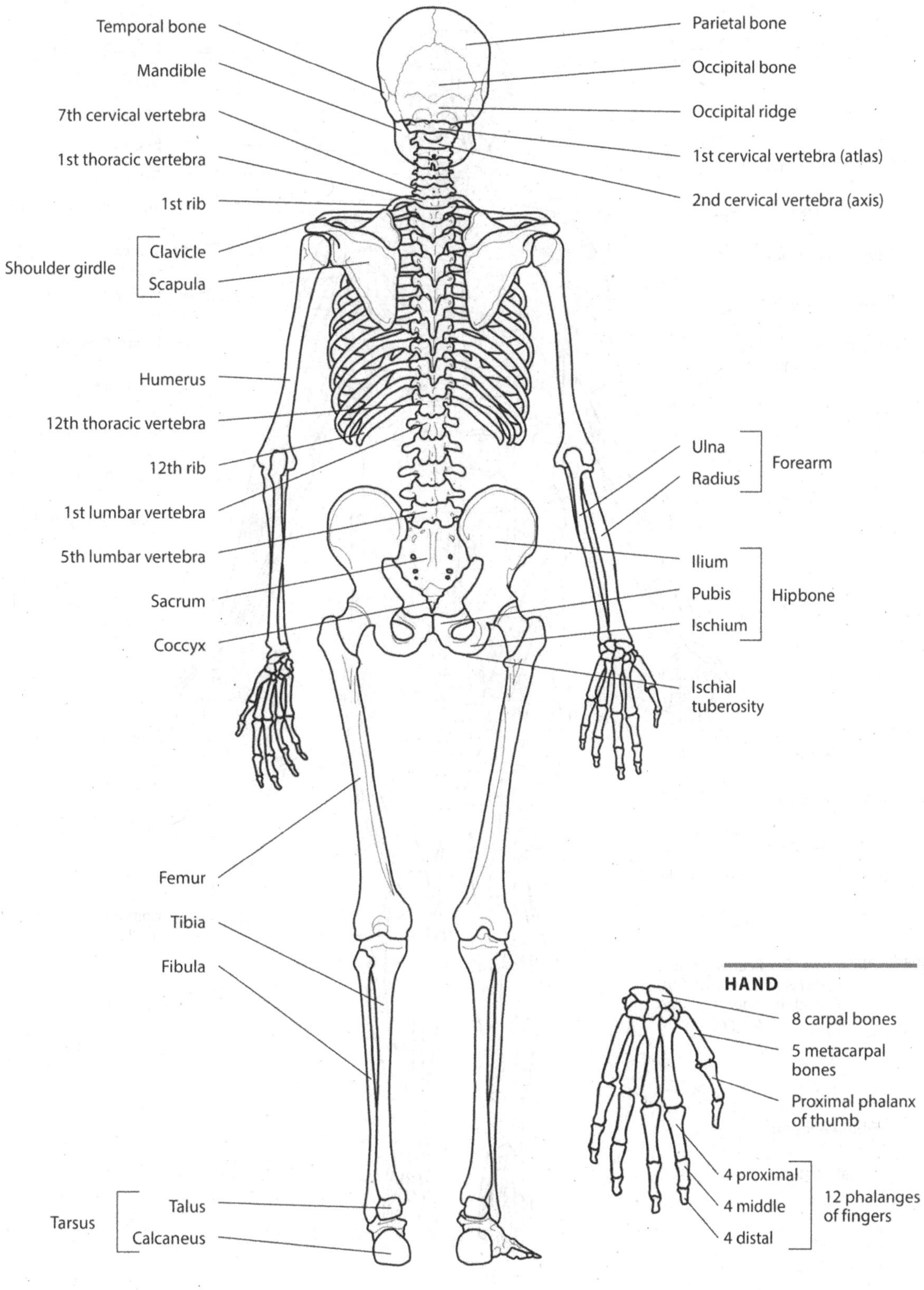

Temporal bone
Mandible
7th cervical vertebra
1st thoracic vertebra
1st rib
Shoulder girdle
Clavicle
Scapula
Humerus
12th thoracic vertebra
12th rib
1st lumbar vertebra
5th lumbar vertebra
Sacrum
Coccyx
Femur
Tibia
Fibula
Tarsus
Talus
Calcaneus
Parietal bone
Occipital bone
Occipital ridge
1st cervical vertebra (atlas)
2nd cervical vertebra (axis)
Ulna
Radius
Forearm
Ilium
Pubis
Ischium
Hipbone
Ischial tuberosity

HAND
8 carpal bones
5 metacarpal bones
Proximal phalanx of thumb
4 proximal
4 middle
4 distal
12 phalanges of fingers

FIGURE 2.4. **Major Muscles of the Body, Anterior View**

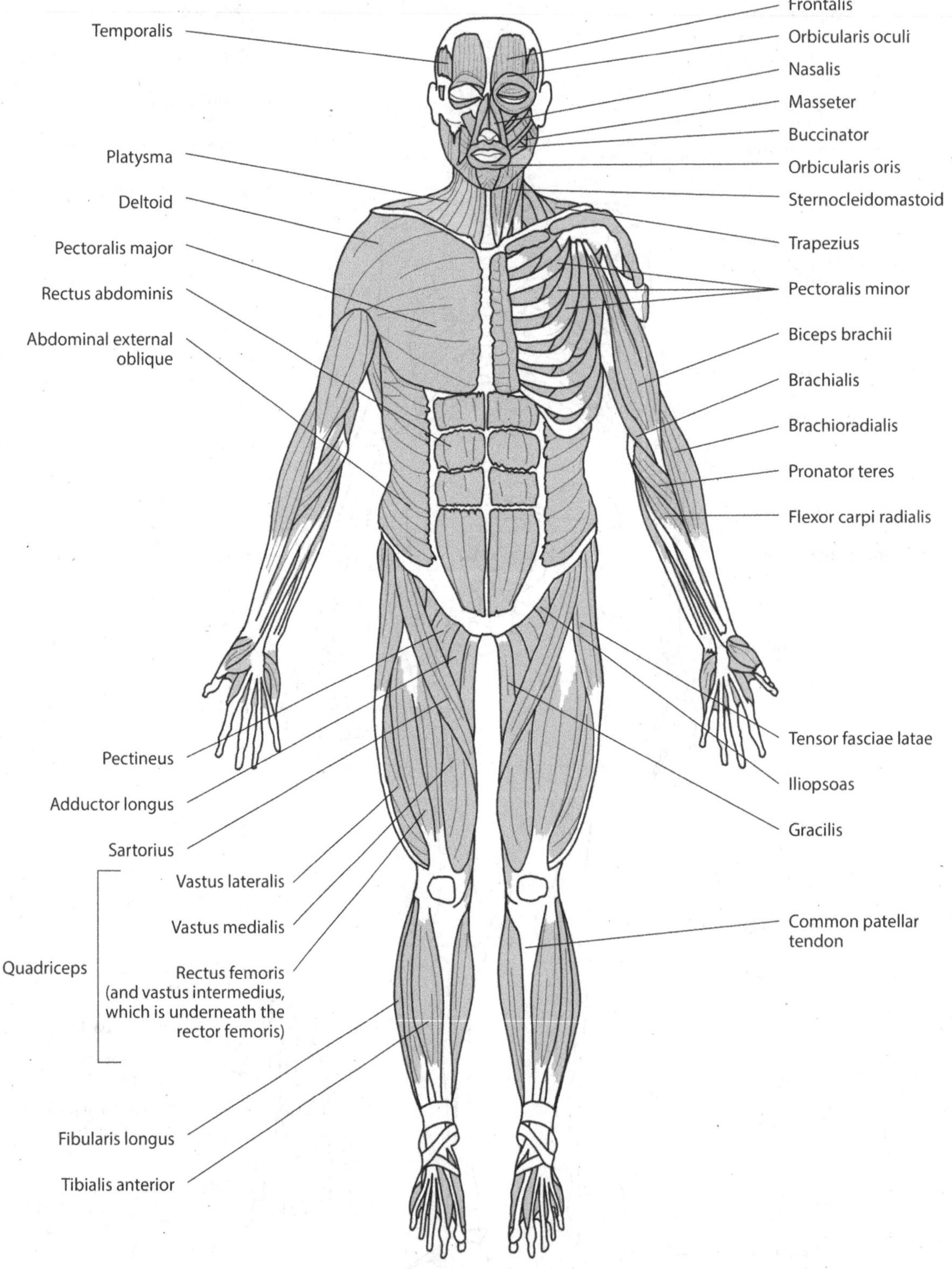
Temporalis
Platysma
Deltoid
Pectoralis major
Rectus abdominis
Abdominal external oblique
Pectineus
Adductor longus
Sartorius
Vastus lateralis
Vastus medialis
Quadriceps
Rectus femoris (and vastus intermedius, which is underneath the rector femoris)
Fibularis longus
Tibialis anterior
Frontalis
Orbicularis oculi
Nasalis
Masseter
Buccinator
Orbicularis oris
Sternocleidomastoid
Trapezius
Pectoralis minor
Biceps brachii
Brachialis
Brachioradialis
Pronator teres
Flexor carpi radialis
Tensor fasciae latae
Iliopsoas
Gracilis
Common patellar tendon

FIGURE 2.5. **Major Muscles of the Body, Posterior View**

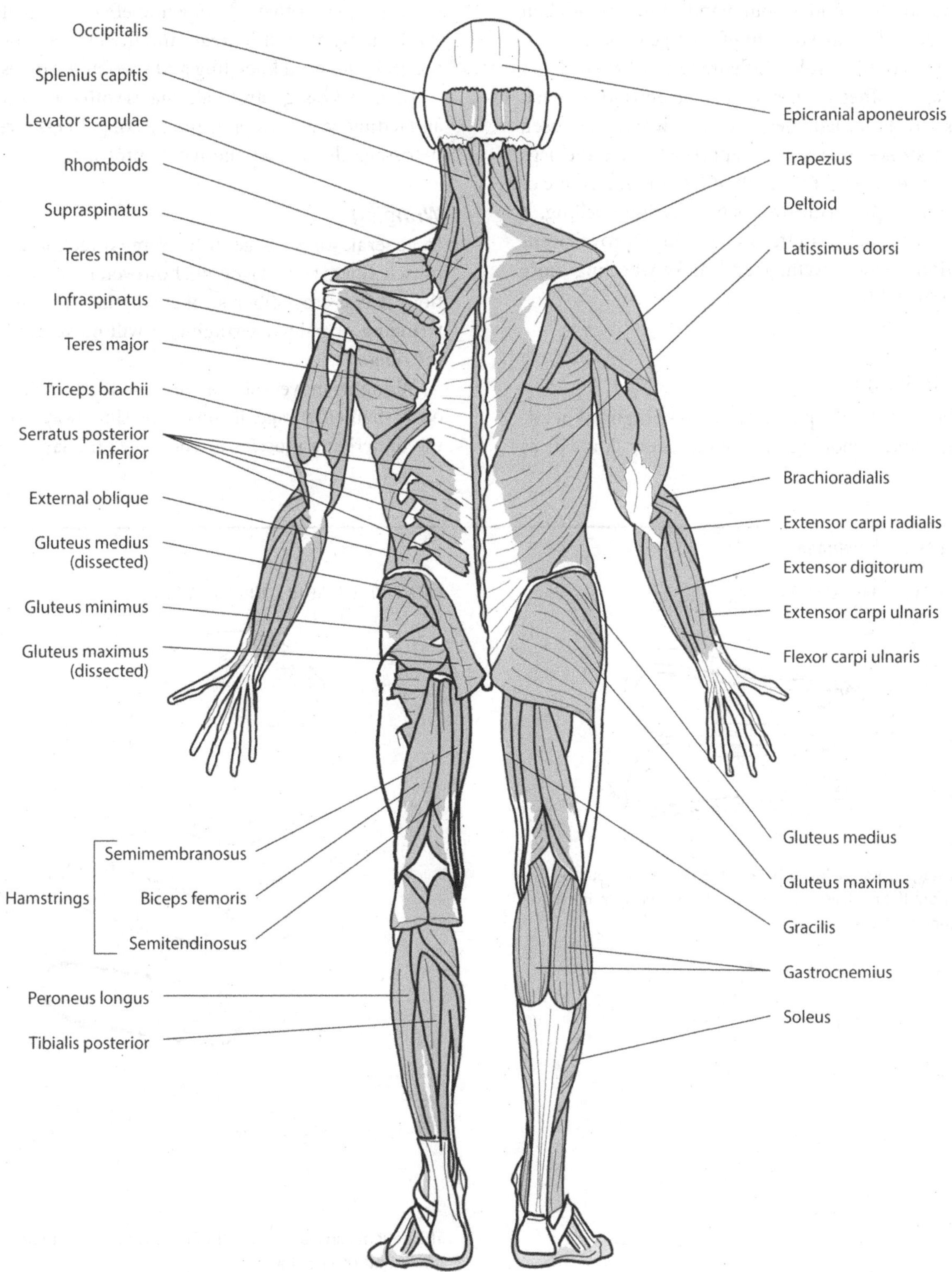
Occipitalis
Splenius capitis
Levator scapulae
Rhomboids
Supraspinatus
Teres minor
Infraspinatus
Teres major
Triceps brachii
Serratus posterior inferior
External oblique
Gluteus medius (dissected)
Gluteus minimus
Gluteus maximus (dissected)
Hamstrings
Semimembranosus
Biceps femoris
Semitendinosus
Peroneus longus
Tibialis posterior
Epicranial aponeurosis
Trapezius
Deltoid
Latissimus dorsi
Brachioradialis
Extensor carpi radialis
Extensor digitorum
Extensor carpi ulnaris
Flexor carpi ulnaris
Gluteus medius
Gluteus maximus
Gracilis
Gastrocnemius
Soleus

In some people, the skin bunches up as you push up or down the back. Go slow and allow the skin to slide under your hands and smooth out again in the wake of your effleurage stroke.

I love this stroke. Effleurage is what to do in between other strokes. When you don't know what else to do, effleurage! With any wheelchair user, this stroke is especially appreciated on the legs because of swelling and fluid retention. It is one of the most powerful strokes in reducing swelling. It offers a quick yet effective way to improve circulation, reduce swelling, and make wheeling more comfortable.

Petrissage

The next three types of strokes—wringing, kneading, and scooping—are collectively known as *petrissage*. If general effleurage helps surface tension dissipate, then specific petrissage strokes reach deeper in their therapeutic effect. I usually do wringing after effleurage, and then move on to the really focused kneading and scooping strokes.

Every petrissage stroke alternates with squeezing and letting go, or grasping and relaxing. In essence, petrissage always uses alternating pressure.

Wringing

In general, we massage in the same direction that muscle fibers run. Wringing, however, is an exception. It is a cross-fiber stroke: whether it's finger wringing or palmer wringing, it will move across the fibers.

Wringing moves the muscles around more vigorously than effleurage. It moves the skin away from the underlying muscles to encourage the layers of

FIGURE 2.6. Effleurage

SIDE-LYING BACK EFFLEURAGE

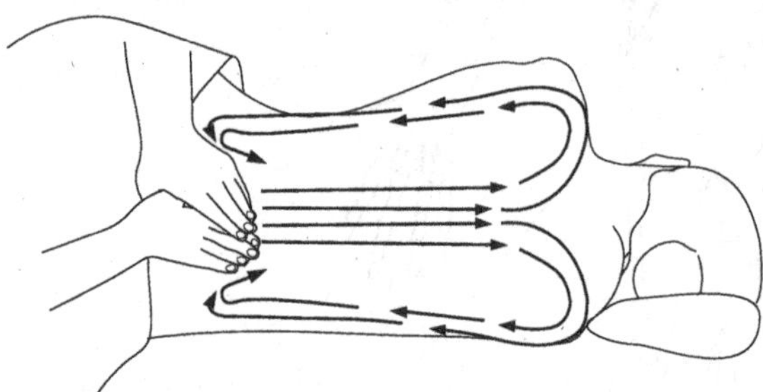

Massage from the lower back to the neck and shoulders or from the neck and shoulders to the lower back. Both directions work.

BACK EFFLEURAGE IN A WHEELCHAIR

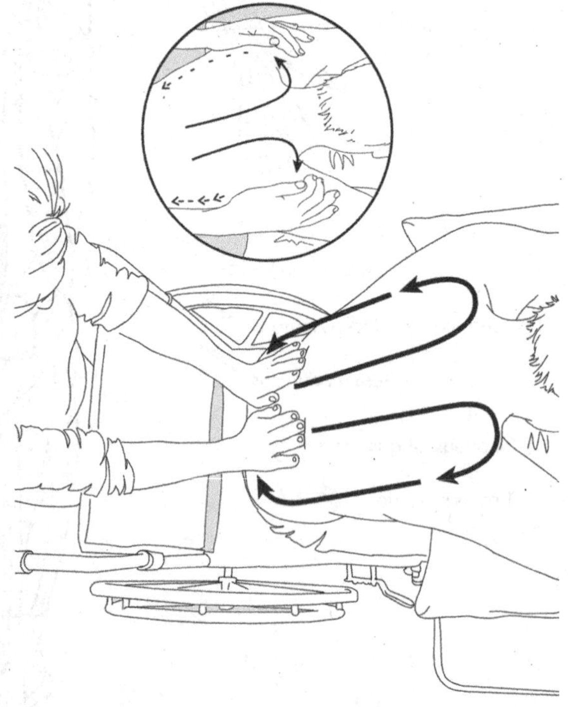

The patient can lean forward in their chair and rest their upper body on a pillow.

FIGURE 2.6. CONTINUED

SIDE-LYING LEG EFFLEURAGE

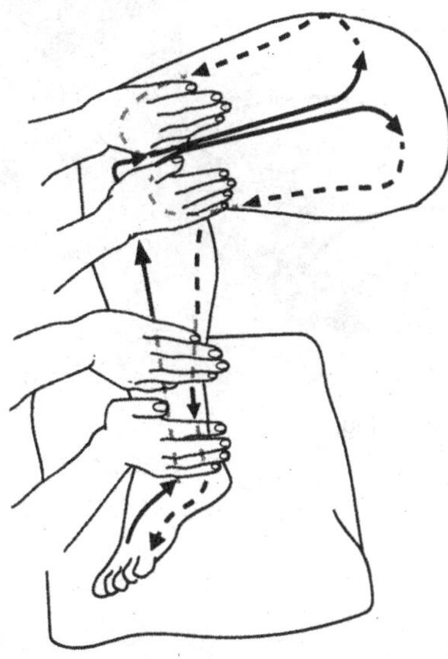

The solid line shows the direction of pressure, and the dotted line shows the return with a light touch.

tissue to not adhere so tightly to each other. Wringing is another general stroke that helps establish or restore tolerance for more focused strokes from the thumbs and fingertips. Wringing lengthens muscles by working transversely (across) the tissue.

This stroke can never be overused. It is like the effleurage stroke that I use between other strokes.

PALMAR WRINGING

For closed palmar wringing, keep all five fingers beside each other. When massaging the patient's back, work at right angles to the spine and move your hands in opposite directions: one hand pushes the skin and underlying flesh away from you around the curve of the ribs, while the other pulls the skin toward you, from the other side of the back. Be sure not to apply any pressure directly onto the spine as you cross over it.

Your hands should be beside each other—close enough to touch—as they move in opposite directions back and forth across the muscles. If you are wringing with the correct technique, you can see the skin and tissues underneath your hands torqueing. Work up and down the whole length of the back. You will find you can move the skin and muscles quite easily. Go slowly: if the patient has loose skin, it will not be a problem. All that skin torqueing might look awful, but it feels wonderful!

Use a similar technique when massaging other areas of the body.

This stroke is a favorite among my patients, both wheeling and non-wheeling. There is something about the cross-fiber direction of the stroke that works on the nervous system differently from other massage strokes. Even the sleepiest and most relaxed of patients often make the effort to make a positive comment (especially when I'm working at the knee, a favorite spot for wringing).

FIGURE 2.7. Palmar Wringing

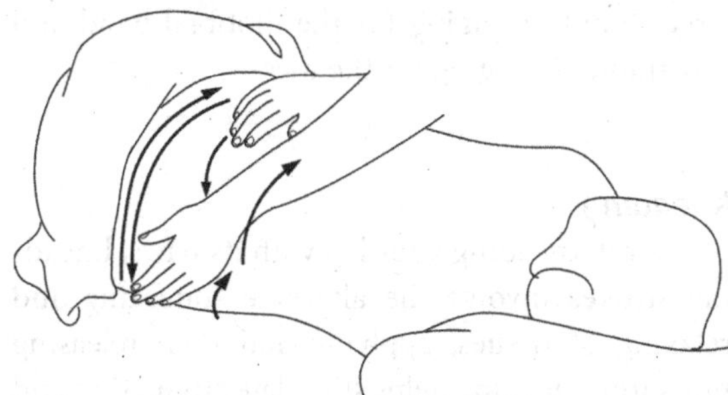

Side-lying bilateral wringing. Work across both sides of the body at the same time.

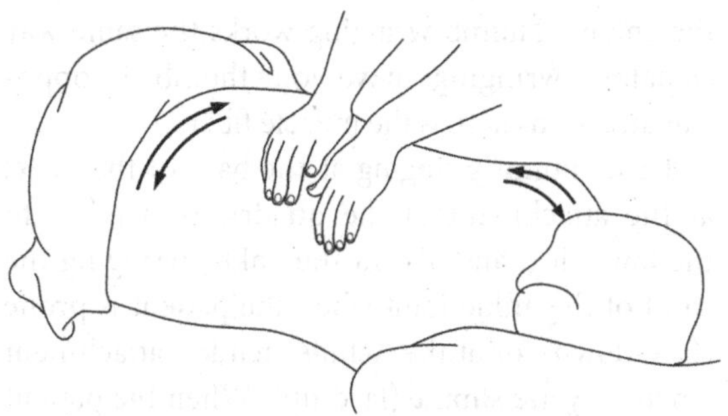

Side-lying unilateral wringing to back and shoulders. Work one side of the body at a time with hands side by side and close together.

FIGURE 2.7. CONTINUED

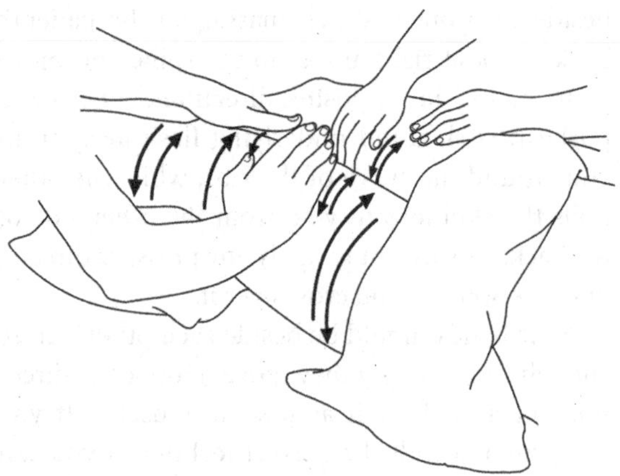

Upper leg wringing.

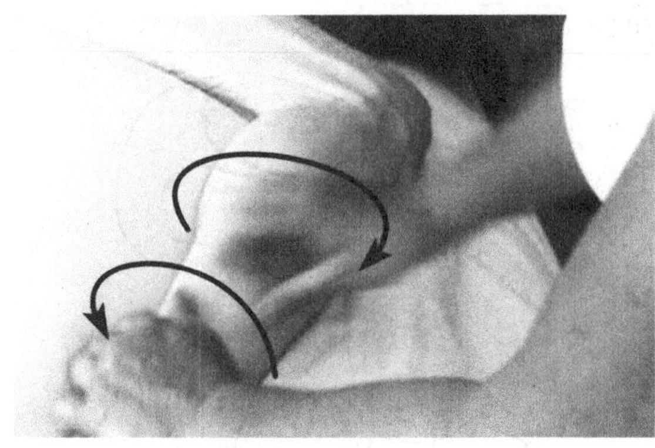

Lower leg wringing.

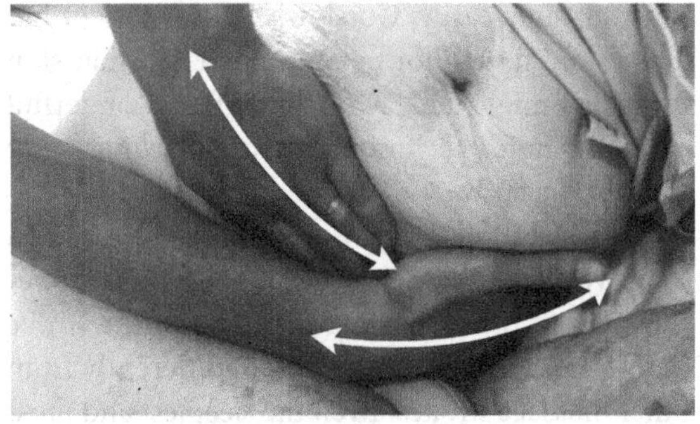

Wringing the abdomen with a side-lying patient.

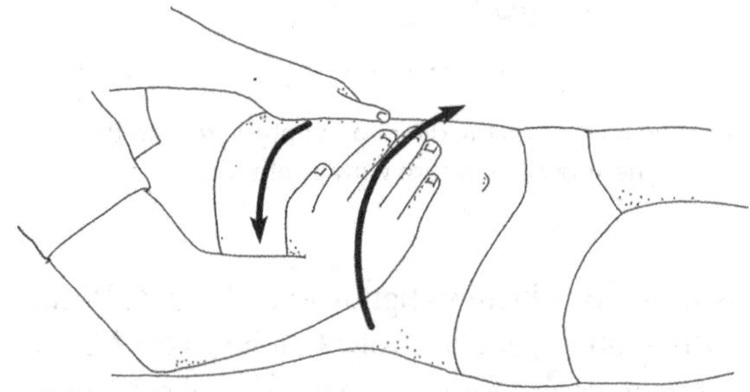

Wringing the abdomen with a supine patient.

THUMB WRINGING

Although you most often use your whole palmar surface for wringing, you can also use your thumbs for smaller areas, such as around the knees or on the ankles. Thumb wringing works the same way as palmar wringing: move your thumbs in opposite directions across the muscle fibers.

I use thumb wringing at the base of the knee, at the attachment of the quadriceps tendon to the lower leg, and also at the ankle, wringing the front of the ankle joint when the patient is prone (face-down), or at the Achilles tendon attachment when they are supine (face-up). When the patient is side-lying, I use thumb wringing at the head of the femur (hip joint) and the side of the thigh (iliotibial band).

A person using a wheelchair every day for the long term will need focused massage on the knees and ankles to help maintain mobility and reduce tendinous shortening at those joints. You can use large thumb wringing for the iliotibial band and tiny thumb wringing for the toes.

Kneading

Like a cat kneading your lap with its paws, kneading strokes involve the alternate squeezing and relaxing of tissues, applying and then releasing pressure. Kneading helps stimulate circulation and in turn promotes the natural healing of injuries, tears, and strains by bringing fresh blood to damaged tissue. Every kind of kneading is essential

FIGURE 2.8. **Thumb Wringing**

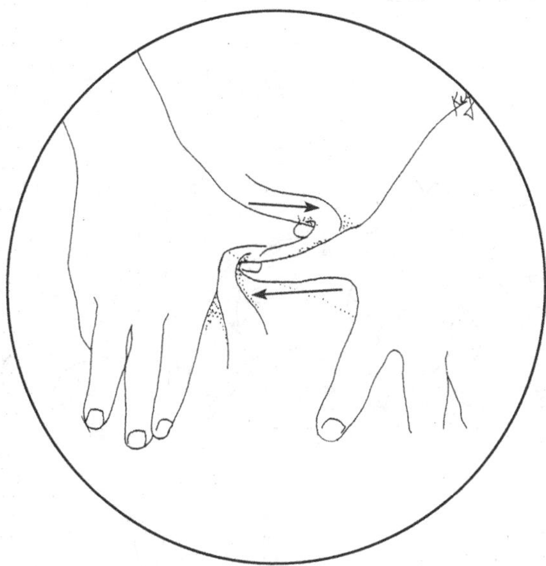

Use your thumbs to wring across the erector spinae muscles. Work up and down the back.

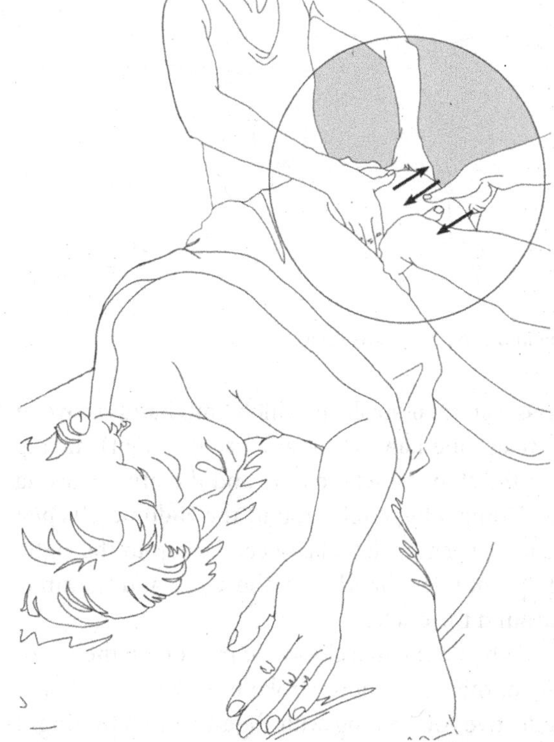

Thumb wringing at the hip joint and along the iliotibial band can soften tight spots and prepare them for more intensive work.

therapy for wheelchair pressure sore sites. Remember, this can be lifesaving.

There are many kneading strokes to use with wheelchair users. They range from big strokes using the entire palmar surface of your hand to nitpicky strokes using just the thumbs or fingertips. Sometimes you might put one hand beside the other and move them in the same direction, alternately pushing the muscle and then releasing it, usually in a semicircular pattern. Other times, you might use one hand to knead while the other hand rests on or supports the patient's body.

Some of my most common kneading strokes are discussed briefly in this section.

REINFORCED PALMAR KNEADING

Reinforced palmar kneading is when you put one hand on top of the other and make kneading circles. This helps you put the weight of your body into your strokes to really focus on achy spots in large muscles, such as the hip or shoulders. On the back, the direction of pressure should always be up and away from the spine. On the legs or other extremities, the pressure always goes up toward the heart.

In my classes, I often see how people take the name "palmar kneading" literally. They use only the palm of the hand, sometimes keeping their fingers off the skin and just polishing with the heel of their hand. Palmar kneading is intended, however, to be more of a cupping movement that uses the entire hand. Give as much skin-on-skin contact as possible with the whole palmar surface of the hand, right to the tips of the fingers.

OVERHANDED PALMAR KNEADING

Overhanded palmar kneading is another stroke I use often, especially on the abdomen or hips in seated, supine (lying down), or side-lying postures.

FIGURE 2.9. Palmar Kneading

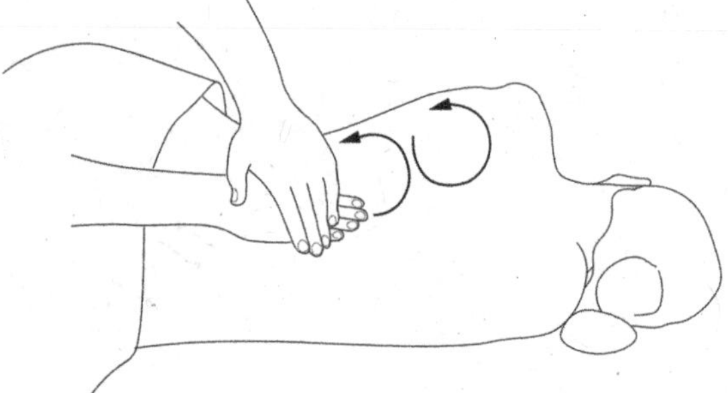

Reinforced palmar kneading.

It is a circular stroke in which both hands move in circles, one hand (I usually use the right) staying on the skin the whole time and the other chasing it. Doing a big circle around the abdomen. When your "chasing" (left) hand catches up to the right, hop your left hand over the right and continue around the circle.

When done in a clockwise motion on the abdomen, this continuous stroke is very thorough and effective for helping with digestive functioning. I also use overhanded palmar kneading at the head of the femur when I am massaging the hip in side-lying positions. I often change back and forth between reinforced palmar kneading and overhanded palmar kneading.

I use overhanded palmer kneading with shoulders, often at the end of the introductory effleurage. I find this large massage stroke over the shoulders is really effectively done by standing in front of the person and pushing out and around. It's as though you're pressing their shoulders back and stretching the chest muscles. If a person is stretched out—on a bed or the floor, for example—I use a lot of overhanded palmer kneading, positioning the person on their side with the knees bent up and focusing attention on the head of the femur. This can be a lifesaving technique for wheelchair users.

When teaching someone else to do overhanded palmar kneading, get right beside the learner and put their hands on your hands so they can feel the rhythm and pattern. Do the circle three times so the imprint will carry into their attempts to do it on their own.

FIGURE 2.10. Overhanded Palmar Kneading: Navigating Drains and Tubes

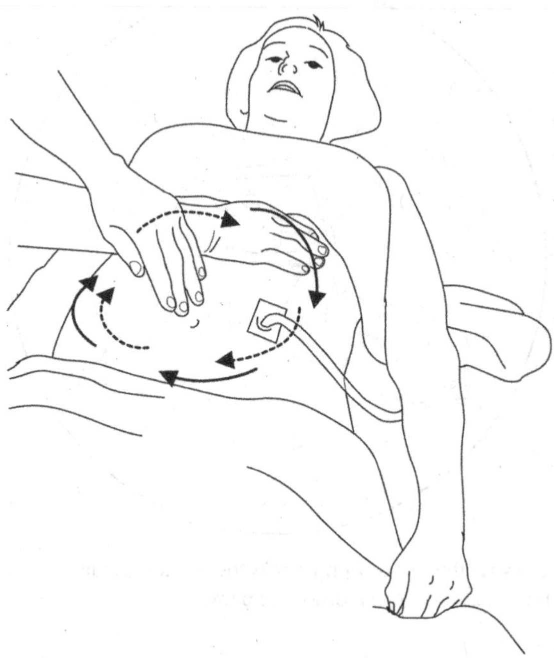

If your kneading passes by any drains, tubes, or stoma sites, just hop over and gently massage around them.

ALTERNATE THUMB KNEADING

The thumbs and fingers are also excellent instruments for kneading strokes, especially in areas of the body that require focused attention. In alternate thumb kneading, the whole hand (including fingertips) contacts the skin, but the thumbs do the work. First one thumb and then the other makes small, half- to three-quarter overlapping circles on the skin. If your thumbs get tired, give your hands a good shake to loosen up, refresh, and reset.

You want your thumbs balanced in their alternating rotations, pushing up and out along the direction of the muscle fibers. Always ensure that the pressure of each circle goes toward the heart. I encourage my students to talk out loud to get their thumbs into a rhythm, saying "up and out...up and out...up and out" or "right and left...right and left...right and left." I learned early on in my teaching that there is something about saying something three times that glues it into the brain the right way. I also often take my students for a "ride" on my thumbs so they can feel the momentum and balance of alternate thumb kneading.

This stroke is a staple of my massage routine. I find that the tiny focus of this stroke really works to ease tension in muscles. I use alternate thumb kneading everywhere; probably the only place I don't use it is on the face. It tends to be particularly appreciated in the arms and legs, at the inner elbow and inner forearm, and around the knees and ankles, which are ideal spots to do long, relaxing sessions of alternate thumb kneading. Use this stroke, too, on the attachments of muscles, in the bulk of muscles, and in any knots or tight spots. I use this stroke after general strokes to the iliotibial band, head of the femur, or any other structures at the top of the leg.

This stroke is wonderfully designed to treat wheelchair aches and pains. Simply going over an area that is sore repeatedly with your alternating thumbs will slowly and steadily relax the tissues. With massage for wheelchair users, alternate thumb kneading is extremely important over every pressure site and potential pressure sore location.

But don't wear out your welcome with too much alternate thumb kneading! Move back and forth between alternate thumb kneading and the more general strokes of palmar kneading or wringing. Use general strokes to smooth things out, effectively erasing the discomfort; then you can go back to do another set of thumb kneading. I knead with a circular movement of my thumb on the muscle and then I switch hands and do the same with the other hand.

Wheelchair users who propel themselves, in particular, need a lot of single-handed thumb kneading on the upper arm, elbow, forearm, hand, and fingers. I use my other, non-massaging hand to hold the person's arm at either the elbow or the wrist, and then I always switch hands and do extensive single-handed thumb kneading to the inner aspect if I've just finished the outer aspect of the arm itself. Any individuals with arm mobility, excluding or including the hand, will benefit one hundred percent from your single-handed thumb kneading, especially the inner elbow.

The other location of extreme importance is the outside of the upper thigh (iliotibial band). This band of fascia shortens because it is made of inelastic connective tissue. Therefore, single-handed thumb kneading has endless possibilities, running up and down the outside aspects of the thigh. Any shortened muscles from prolonged sitting should be massaged with a single hand, because you can often get more focus using one thumb.

UNILATERAL THUMB KNEADING

With single-handed thumb kneading, you need to secure the person with one hand while your

FIGURE 2.11. Alternate Thumb Kneading

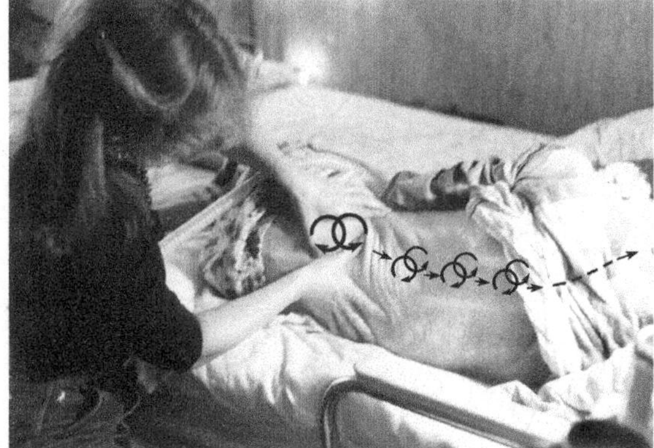

Alternate thumb kneading to the lower back. Massage one side at a time, up and down the erector spinae muscles. Negotiate around any folding or bunching of skin.

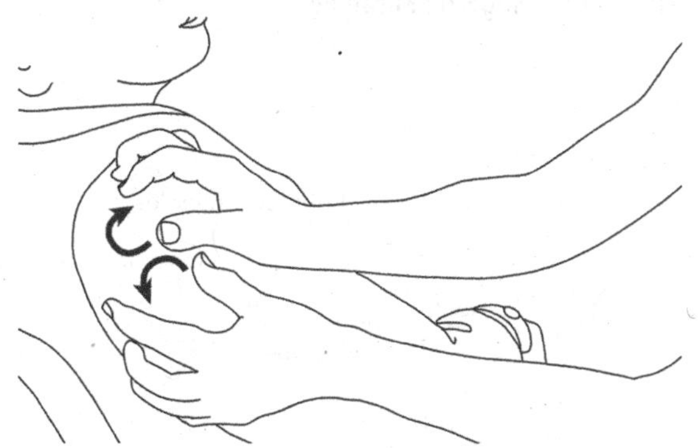

Alternate thumb kneading for the shoulder.

FIGURE 2.11. CONTINUED

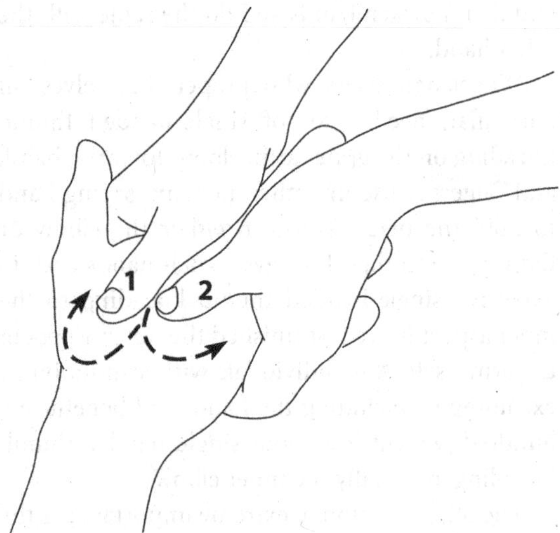

Palmar alternate thumb kneading.

other hand is massaging. I use one hand to hold on to the side of the person's shoulders and use the other hand to massage the rhomboids between the shoulder blades and the spine, and right through the rhomboids to the levator scapula. Single-handed thumb kneading is extremely important. It is very common to use bilateral single-handed thumb kneading at the soreness in hip muscles.

BILATERAL THUMB KNEADING

Bilateral thumb kneading is a classic shoulder massage. For wheelchair users, use it to focus on those hard-working or immobilized shoulders. Whether these wheelchair shoulders are highly functioning or immobilized, they are in high need of this bilateral stroke. You can spend hours just doing this stroke in the posterior aspect of the shoulders and get tons of relief for the entire shoulder girdle. However, so many times the posterior aspect is not easily available, especially if the person is in a tilted chair. Face-to-face bilateral thumb kneading is called for. You can work out lots of tension, especially in wheelchair athletes, by doing this bilateral thumb kneading along the pectoral muscles, along the sternum, and right up to the armpits.

I use thumb kneading (alternate, single, bilateral) probably as thirty percent of my total full body massage stroke allocation. It is very popular in adapting to parts of the person that are easy to get to in a wheelchair. Although this is my most popular stroke for easily accessible areas, I have found it impractical for levering applications.

FINGERTIP KNEADING

Fingers can also be used to knead, usually with reinforced fingertips: stack your hands on top of each other and keep your fingers straight and stiff. Then knead with a pivoting action of your wrist so your fingertips are like a soft drill. As with thumbs,

FIGURE 2.12. **Fingertip Kneading**

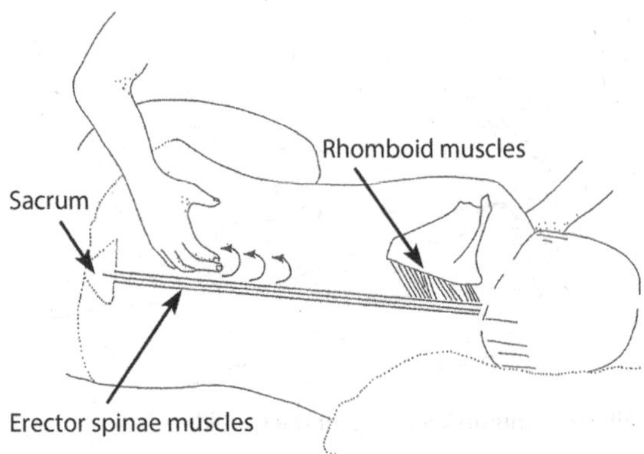

Fingertip kneading to the rhomboids and erector spinae muscles.

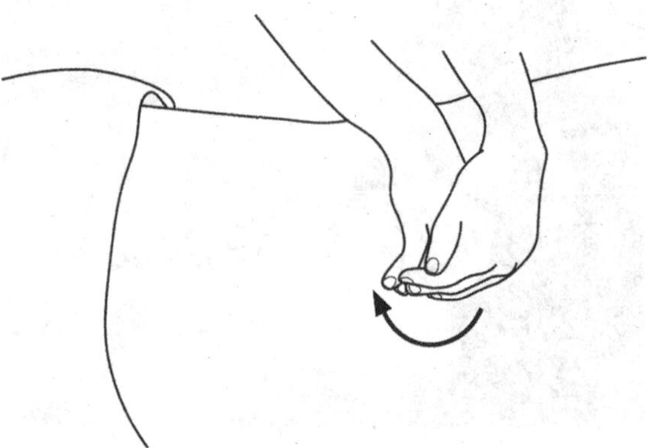

Reinforced fingertip kneading (both hands, fingers stacked).

FIGURE 2.12. CONTINUED

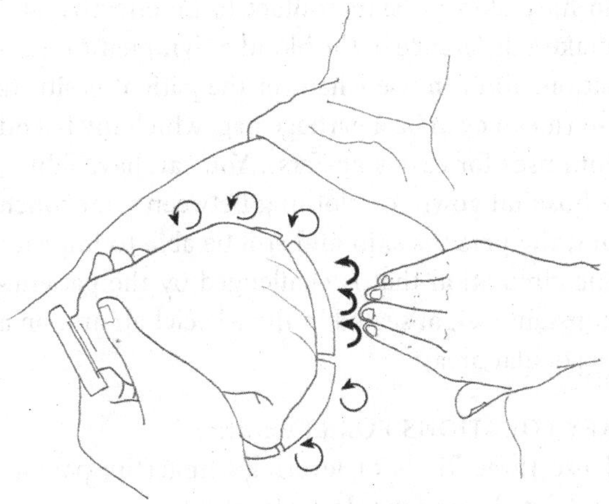

Single-handed fingertip kneading around a stoma site.

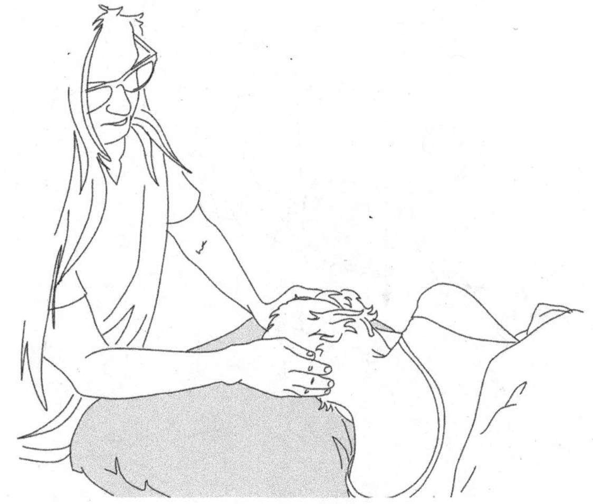

Side-lying, single-handed fingertip kneading to the occipital ridge with the head supported by the upper hand.

FIGURE 2.13. Therapist Postures to Provide Leverage, Supine Patient

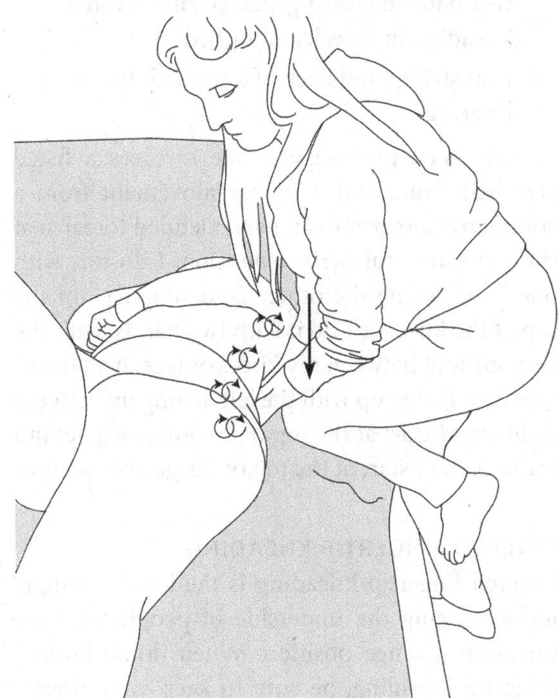

One knee up.

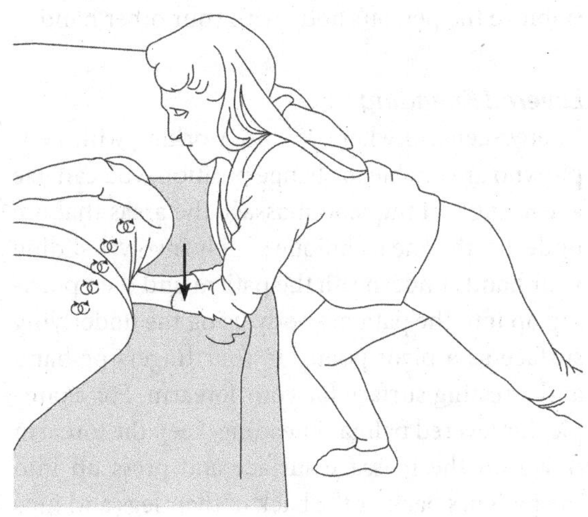

Stride.

FIGURE 2.13. CONTINUED

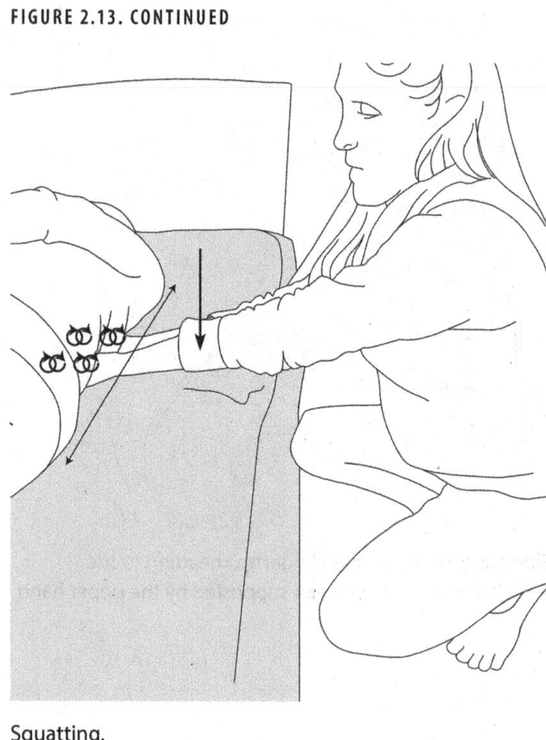

Squatting.

you can also knead with one hand if you need to stabilize the person's body with your other hand.

Levered Kneading

In any scenario where you are working with people who are unable to change position, you can use a levering technique to massage the areas that are underneath. The technique simply involves sliding your hands underneath the patient and then pushing up into the patient's body using the underlying surface as a pivot point for your fingers or hand and a resting surface for your forearm. For example, for levered palmar kneading, keep the forearm down on the massage surface and press up into the patient's back or the back of their legs and hips with your hand.

For this underside massage technique, slide your hand beneath the person, with your palm up; then press down with the back of your hand, lift all of your fingers in a straight line (keep your fingers together), and start your massage. Although traditional skin-on-skin contact is always advantageous, it isn't helpful when working from underneath a person. You don't need to have skin-on-skin contact to be effective and make a difference in the blood or lymphatic circulation. You can use whatever the patient is sitting on (it can even be a garbage bag, which my friend Joni uses for easy transfers). You can have fabric, a hospital gown, or clothing between your touch and the person's skin and still be able to improve the circulation that is challenged by the patient's constant weight seated in the wheelchair and on a particular area.

KEY LOCATIONS FOR LEVERING

I use three kinds of levering—fingertip, palmar, and fisted—on four classic locations:

1. Hips with bent knee and stabilizing hand supporting the knee as you lever up into the hip muscles, gluteal muscles, and ischial tuberosity whether in a wheelchair or supine in bed.
2. Shoulder (back of the shoulder in the rhomboids) in wheelchair or bed.
3. Along the erector spinae muscles, with single-handed fingertip kneading, alternating two-handed levering, and palmar levered kneading in wheelchair or bed.
4. Hamstrings and back of knee with fisted levering.

The fisted petrissage stroke involves a fisted clenched hand, and a rolling movement from a contracted forearm to an overextended forearm at the wrist, to a full wrist extension. I do this with one hand, while the other hand supports on the top of the knee, or I do it with two hands, with the person's foot between my knees or legs. And then I alternate fisting up with the left, fisting up with the right, etc. I start at the top of the lower leg behind the knee, so I start at the top of the gastrocnemius.

LEVERED FINGERTIP KNEADING

Levered fingertip kneading is the best technique for massaging the underside of people who are unable to change position. When doing levered fingertip kneading, be sure to keep your fingers straight and stiff so they act as one unit.

FIGURE 2.14. Levered Fingertip Kneading, Supine Patient

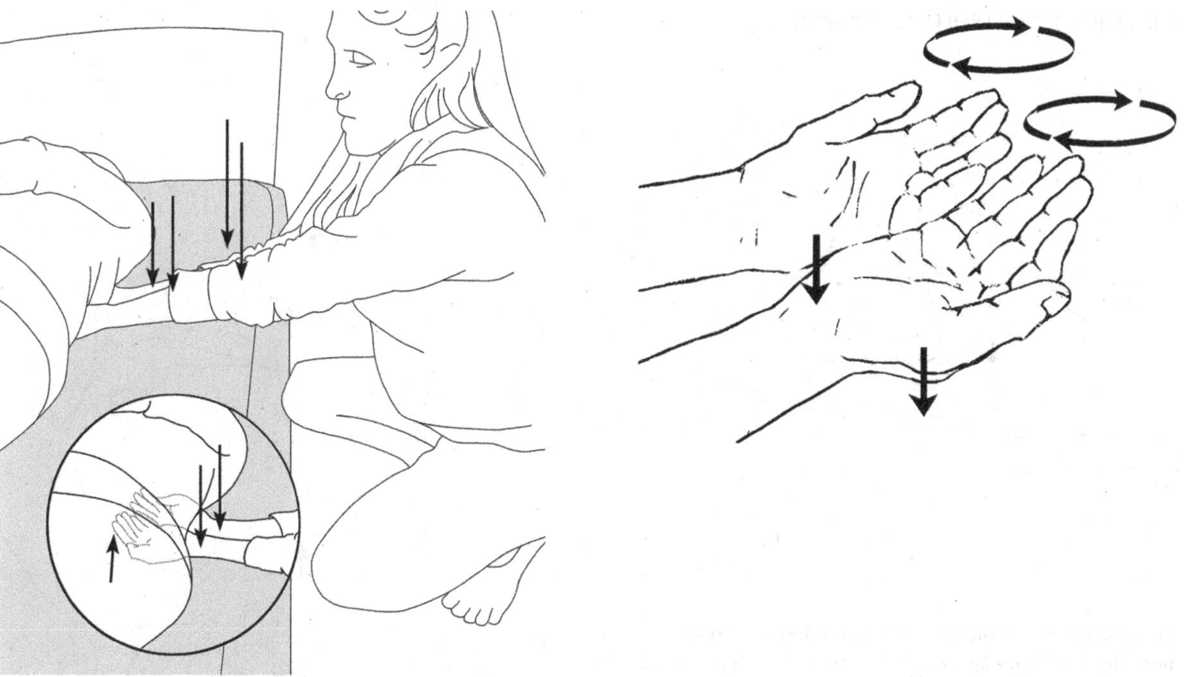

Levered fingertip kneading is the stroke I use most often under supine patients.

Single-Handed Levered Fingertip Kneading

For supine patients who cannot change position, I usually put one hand on top of their knee so that I can move their leg and easily access their lower back and hip. I can then gently rock their leg back and forth as I massage under their hips and back with my other hand. I find that the rocking motion makes it easier for me reach underneath and helps amplify the effects of my kneading into the gluteal muscles.

To reach the back of the shoulder girdle with a supine patient, I use the same technique with one hand on the elbow to allow me to slip my other hand onto the rhomboids between the scapula and the spine. I use a rocking motion with my hand on the patient's bent elbow as I knead the rhomboids with the fingertips of my other hand.

Levered Fingertip Kneading, Side-Lying Adaptations

This is an adaptable posture for confined spaces where there might not be room to stretch out the legs. In a side-lying, bent-leg position, you can lever your hands up, single-handed or double-handed, especially focusing on the hips or shoulders. The person can roll to the other side to make it a perfect balance. This can all be done in a stretched-out wheelchair!

Levering for a side-lying patient works basically the same as for a supine patient, but you might need to use one hand to massage and the other to stabilize. For example, when massaging underneath the hip that a person is resting on, you can slide your massage hand under them to begin levering and use your non-massaging hand to stabilize their upper hip. Use the top hand to gently rock the patient as you lever up into the underside of their bottom hip and lower back.

Scooping

Scooping is done with a closed-fingered, C-shaped hand like you would use to scoop a handful of water. In wheelchair massage, I use scooping primarily with breast and abdominal massage, but it can be used at the knees or on other large muscle groups. For example, I also use this stroke on the

FIGURE 2.15. Levered Fingertip Kneading

SINGLE-HANDED LEVERED FINGERTIP KNEADING

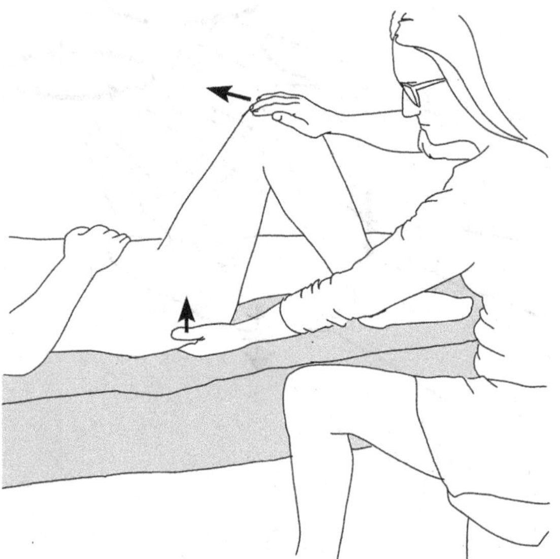

Working a patient's glutes with levered single-handed fingertip kneading. You want to be sure to massage around the ischial tuberosities to prevent pressure sores.

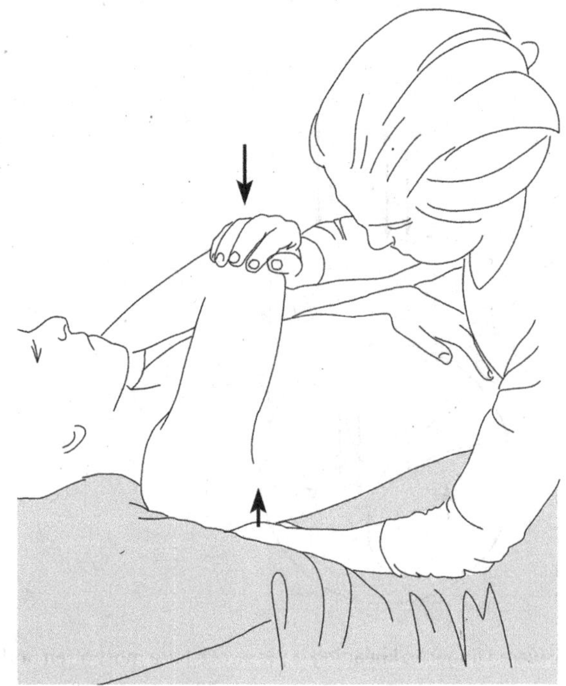

Levered single-handed fingertip kneading to the shoulder with elbow support.

TWO-HANDED LEVERED FINGERTIP OR PALMAR KNEADING

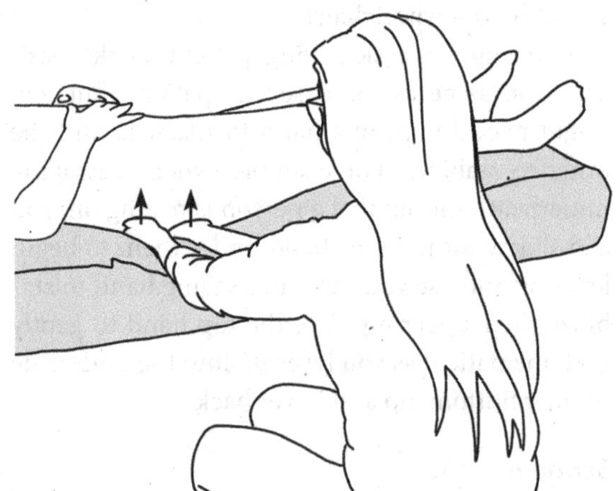

FIGURE 2.15. CONTINUED

LEVERED FINGERTIP KNEADING, SIDE-LYING PATIENT

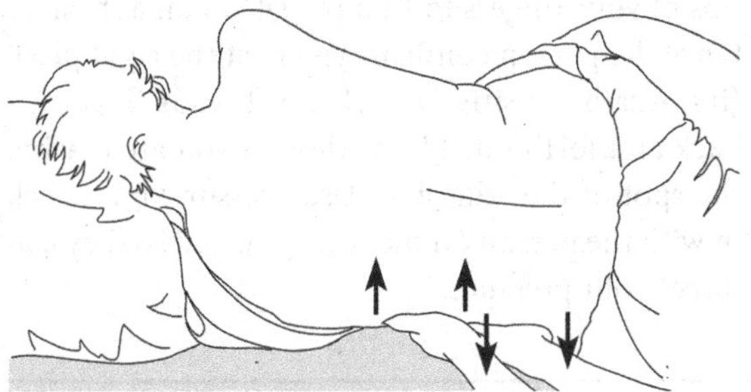

Side-lying levered fingertip underside massage.

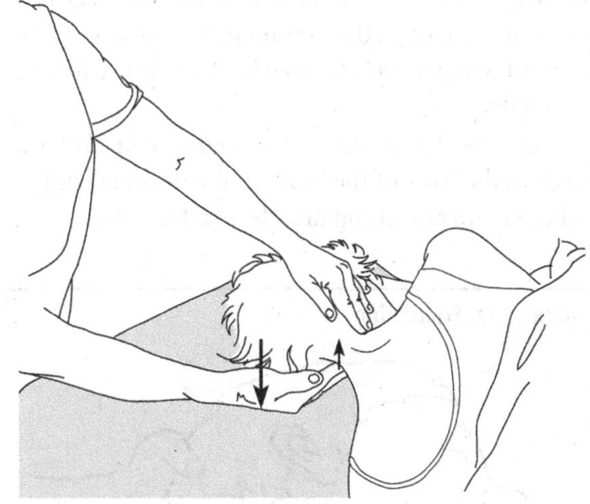

Side-lying bilateral fingertip kneading to the neck with levering from the lower hand.

neck, scooping up toward the head, or on the back with my patient lying supine, scooping from the bottom of the shoulder blades up the neck with alternating hands.

Scooping to the abdomen is very helpful for digestion, especially since people in wheelchairs are not moving their hips in a natural walking gait that would mobilize peristaltic action. This scooping to the abdomen can be effective even if the person has pouches, drains, a colostomy bag, or other obstacles: you can work around the obstacles with a modified scooping stroke, using one hand instead of two hands to fit the special-needs location. Tilting back the chair allows the tummy to be more exposed and less cramped for your massage!

This scooping stroke to the abdomen can be started with massages in ICU, if the wheelchair person suffered a traumatic injury or spinal cord break.

FIGURE 2.16. Scooping

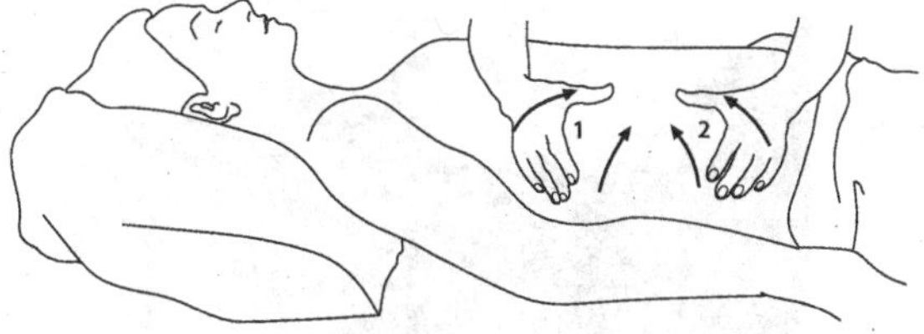

Scooping with a wide-open, C-shaped hand. Alternate between your hands as you scoop.

Frictioning

Traditional frictioning is a highly therapeutic, cross-fiber stroke used to wear down adhesions, which are areas of tissue that build up in response to injuries, infection, or postsurgical conditions. Tears or other injuries in the belly of muscles or their attachments to ligaments and other structures are healed by fibrin, a glue-like substance. Fibrin adhesions are inelastic, which can limit normal function, movement, and flexibility. If it is done properly, frictioning can break down adhesions and improve elasticity in muscles and ligaments, leading to decreased pain and increased function.

I use frictioning frequently with my wheelchair patients because those who have old injuries from childhood or adolescence that limit their hip mobility for walking can benefit from work done on their adhesions. Sometimes a person can tell you where they've had an injury or where they have tight spots. You can feel the adhesion area as a thickening in the muscle. Your patient will give you feedback when you've found the right place.

For wheelchair users, frictioning can also be used at the back of the head on the occipital ridge, where there are strong muscle attachments.

To start the cross-fiber stroke, put your fingertips together. I usually use my pointer and middle fingers, but sometimes I use my thumb. Use the tips of your fingers to find the site of an adhesion. Once the person confirms you're at the right place (it's usually sensitive), start to rub your fingertips back and forth quickly, as though you are erasing the spot of the adhesion. Use pressure, but check in with the person on the receiving end so they can direct your pressure.

FIGURE 2.17. Frictioning

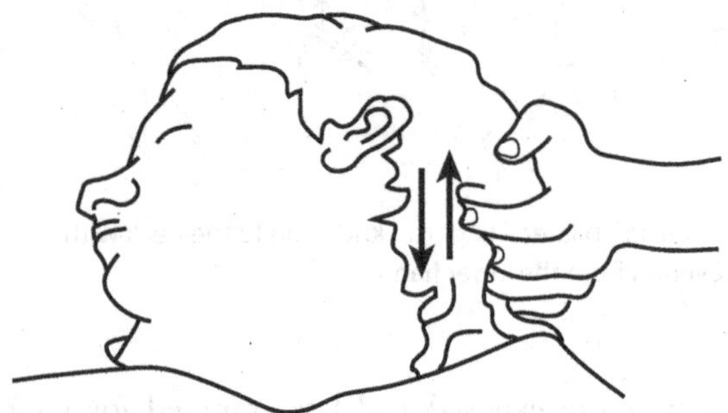

Use gentle, single-handed frictions to the occipital ridge. Use one hand to hold the head with the patient's face rotated to the opposite shoulder.

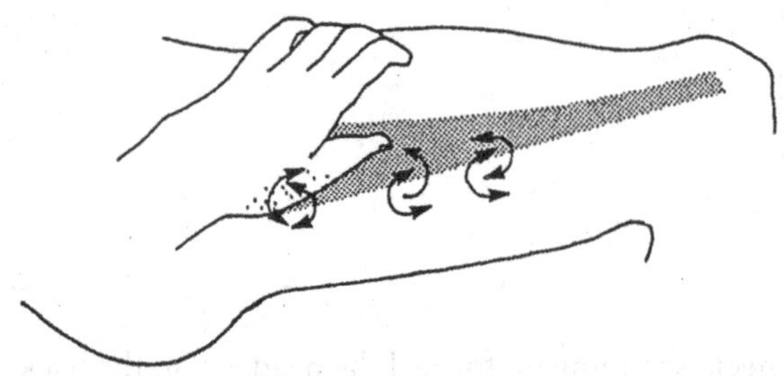

I use palmar frictions along the iliotibial band to loosen up stiffness.

FIGURE 2.18. Ice Frictioning

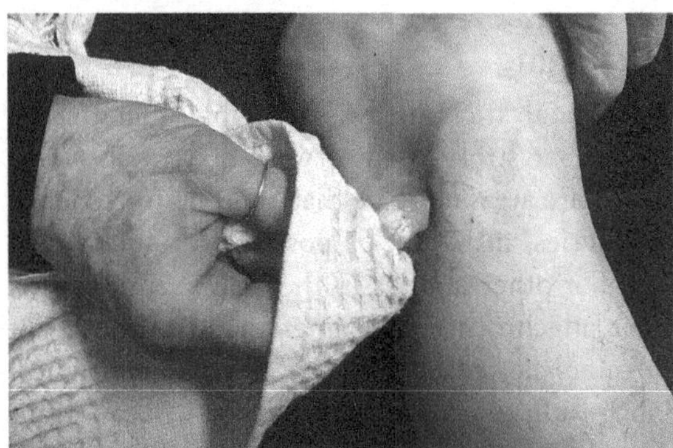

Ice frictioning around the ankle.

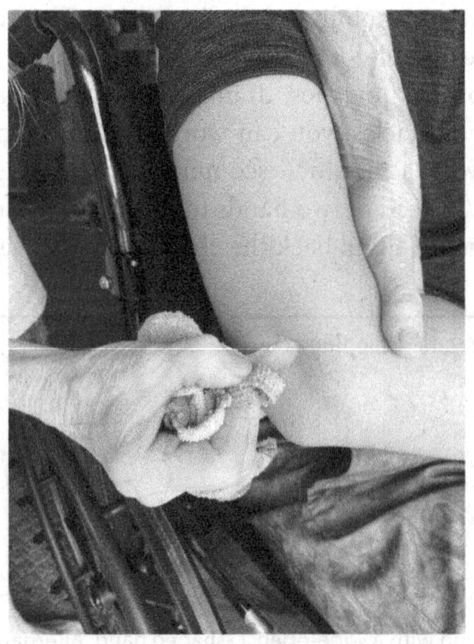

Ice frictioning around the elbow.

You are basically working to soften and stretch the tough adhesion under your fingers. You will have to use pressure to get this result but, as always, ask the person whether your pressure is too much, not enough, or just right. Usually, if you have the right location—the place where the tension centers—the patient will find the stroke uncomfortable, but tolerable. Use this stroke in the middle of your treatment, not the beginning. Other, more general strokes will have "primed" the adhesion area for this focused treatment.

Ice Frictioning

I love the combination of ice and frictioning! The cold has an anesthetizing effect, while my fingers soften and break down hard muscle fibers. In a recent massage of a wheelchair user, the patient, Di, insisted we keep frictioning and kneading her sore spots to lessen her muscle spasms. She specifically asked for ice frictioning because it gave her needed relief. Wheelchair sports massage is a classic ice frictioning opportunity. Any place that has an overabundance of tension can benefit from ice frictioning.

Compression

I always use alternating digital thumb compression in massaging the head, neck, and shoulders of wheelchair users. I usually start right away with this alternating digital thumb work in the upper back areas of the trapezius, rhomboids, or the full length of the erector spinae muscles. I spend quite a bit of time working the full length of the erector spinae muscles. I work from the occipital ridge at the top down into the rhomboids with the thumbs on either side of the spine. When my recipient indicates one side favored compared to the other, or a particular spot on one side where they would like extra attention, I take both thumbs to that one side and work along the top of the trapezius.

To get my body weight rolling onto the tips of my thumbs, I am careful to use a locked-arm stride position rolling my body weight forward on to my front leg and down my arms to my thumbs. This digital compression is a static noncircular pressure alternating from one thumb to the other. As I alternate, I move, I never stay in the same spot (not wanting to wear out my welcome). Alternating

FIGURE 2.19. **Compression**

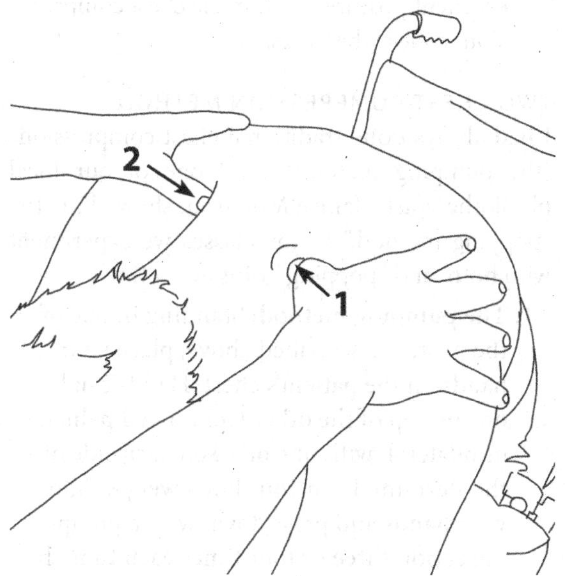

Alternating thumb compression to the upper trapezius.

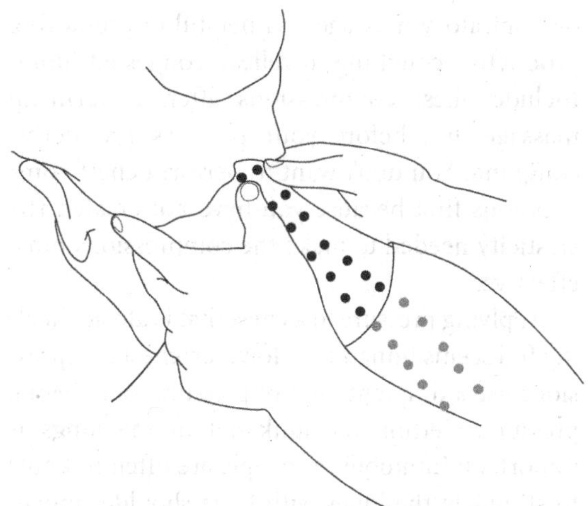

Alternating thumb compression on the back of the neck.

digital thumb, fisted, or palmer compression is not moving across any muscular surface but rather staying in one place exerting the pressure and then lifting off and moving to a new spot. That alternating lifting off is the differentiating feature of compression compared to the steady contact of most petrissage circular strokes. I also use this favorite stroke (alternating digital thumb compression) when I am working on the hips.

These compression strokes ease a significant amount of tension at the same time as encouraging a deeper relaxation response. You can use firm compression pressure, deep pressure, or very light pressure, and get a wide variety of positive, therapeutic responses.

If I'm running out of time in a full body massage, I will often use compression up and down the legs (whichever part hasn't been massaged yet, including the abdomen). When I'm on the extremities, I will compress with one hand under the extremity, one hand over, squeezing the hands together and compressing the extremity between my two hands. This squeezing technique is often a favorite. Bilateral, two-handed compression is good for all extremities, especially wheelers.

Chest Compressions

Chest compressions are an important component of respiratory massage and helpful in promoting productive coughing to relieve congested lungs. Include chest compressions after a warm-up massage and before your patient's productive coughing. You don't want to perform chest compressions first because you have not created the elasticity needed to make the compressions most effective.

Applying pressure to a chest that is already feeling full seems unnatural. However, chest compressions use a different kind of pressure—a relieving pressure. Getting the junk out of the lungs is important; immobilized people are often not able to stimulate the lungs with large shoulder movements, so getting the congestion out manually is important. With chest compressions, we can dislodge sticky stuff from the side of the lungs so it can be spit out during productive coughing.

THREE CHEST COMPRESSION POSTURES WITH A SUPINE PATIENT

1. **Reinforced palmar compressions:** With your patient lying supine, stand at their head (either beside or behind them at the head of the bed) and place both hands, one palm on top of the other, on the sternum or breastbone. Lean forward with your body weight transferred onto your hands to compress the chest three or four times as the patient breathes out.
2. **Bilateral palmar compressions:** Standing at the head of the person, place both hands on the upper chest, one on either side of the sternum, hands about six inches apart.
3. **Thoracic compressions:** Stand at the patient's side in a stride position. Have the patient breathe slowly and deeply. Do compressions, leaning onto your hands, along the side of the patient's body at the regions of the mid- and lower lobes. In each location, pump three times and compress on the out breath. If your patient has a bony rib cage, place a soft towel between their body and your hands so that you do not bruise or damage their ribs during the pumping. If your patient is able to lie prone (hips up, so that they're nose down, looking like they're diving), this is also an excellent posture for thoracic chest compression to clear the lungs.

TWO CHEST COMPRESSION METHODS

I had always done traditional chest compressions (the pumping method) until one of our local physiotherapists, Janice Morrison, showed me the "popping method." In my classes we experiment with both, and "popping" wins every time!

1. **The pumping method:** Standing in one of the postures described above, place your hands on the patient's chest. Hands can be one on top of the other (reinforced palmar) or bilateral, with one hand on each side of the sternum. Lean your body weight onto your hands and press down with a pumping action three or four times each time the patient exhales.

FIGURE 2.20. Chest Compressions

REINFORCED PALMAR COMPRESSIONS, SUPINE PATIENT

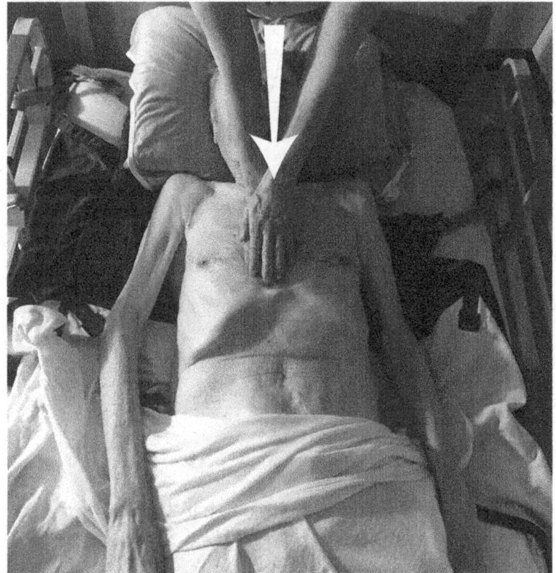

Reinforced palmer pumping on the sternum (standing at the head of the patient).

BILATERAL PALMAR COMPRESSIONS, SUPINE PATIENT

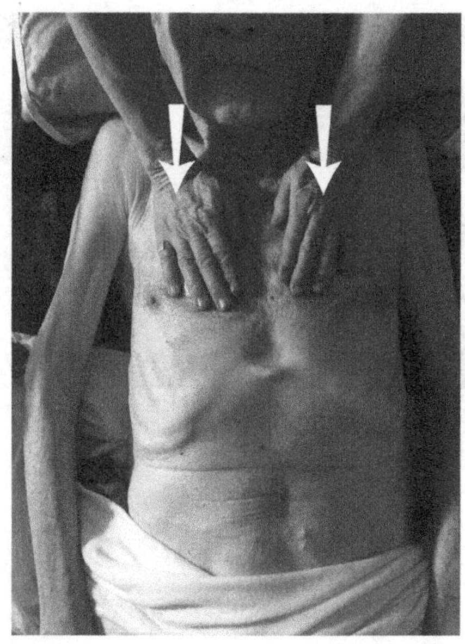

Bilateral palmer pumping (standing at the patient's head). Pump the chest three times.

THORACIC COMPRESSIONS, SUPINE PATIENT

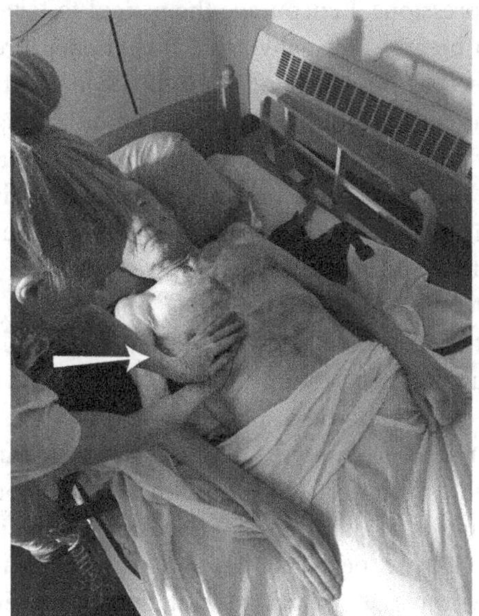

Reinforced midlobe compression.

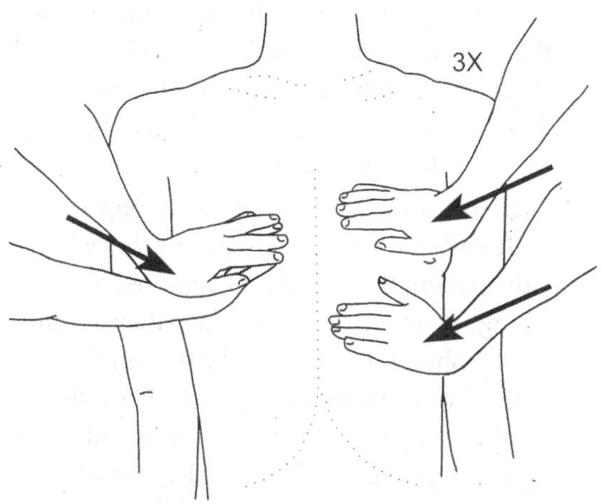

Reinforced and bilateral midlobe compression.

FIGURE 2.20. CONTINUED

THORACIC COMPRESSIONS, SUPINE PATIENT

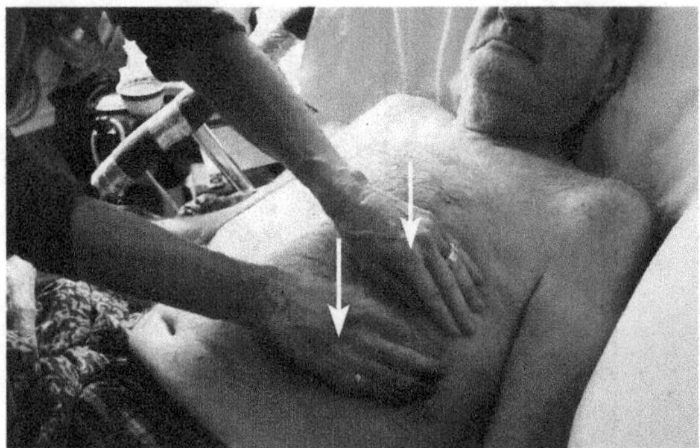

Thoracic compressions from the far side.

THORACIC COMPRESSIONS, PRONE PATIENT

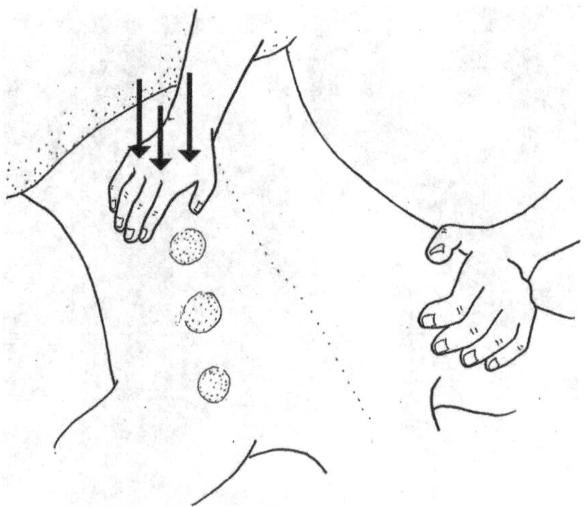

Support the patient's body with one hand while the other moves down the back, pumping three times in each position. Then do the other side.

2. **The popping method:** Stand in one of the postures described above and place your hands as described in the pumping method. Press down, leaning your body weight into your hands, on the breath out. At the end of the breath, as your patient starts to breathe in, continue to hold the downward pressure. Then let go suddenly, about a fifth of the way through the breath in.
   - Holding down the compression longer at the end of the out breath means that when the patient tries to take a deep breath, their lungs meet resistance. As the patient begins to fill their lungs against the pressure, you "pop" your hands off the chest. The effect of this popping technique is profound—the patient automatically gets a deep surge of new air. It reminds me of a toilet plunger, keeping the suction going and pulling the stuck material up and out of the lungs. It also reminds me of how we strengthen a muscle. When you are training against resistance, the work feels hard—but when the resistance is removed, you get a stronger reaction than you did before.

CHEST COMPRESSIONS ROUTINE

Massage your patient before doing the chest compressions to loosen things up. Massaging after compressions helps the body recover. During compressions, I encourage the patient to take big, deep breaths. I usually say, "Take a deep breath, as deep as possible, and then focus on breathing out as empty as possible before breathing in again. Slow your breathing down, making each breath a little bigger than the breath before." Although the routine here uses the pumping method, you can substitute the popping method.

During chest compressions, the patient may want to clear their lungs by spitting and coughing. I pause for bouts of productive coughing and then start again with the compressions.

Another technique, thoracic shaking, can be added as you perform the compression. Thoracic shaking is a rolling motion, rocking the patient's body as you perform the compression. You can apply thoracic shaking throughout your entire respiratory massage—beginning, middle, and end.

The motions of chest compression are controlled and performed while the patient's body is still. The patient's breathing is connected to the compression. Compressions can be a short pumping action during the out breath. On the inward breath, we can start again with fresh compression.

FIGURE 2.21. Chest Compressions and Thoracic Shaking for Productive Coughing

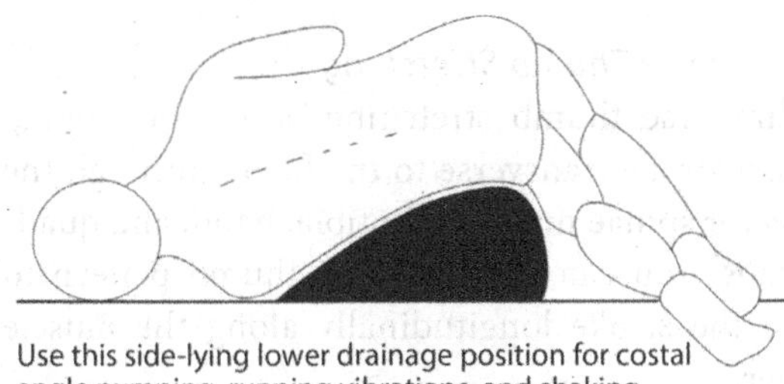

Use this side-lying lower drainage position for costal angle pumping, running vibrations, and shaking.

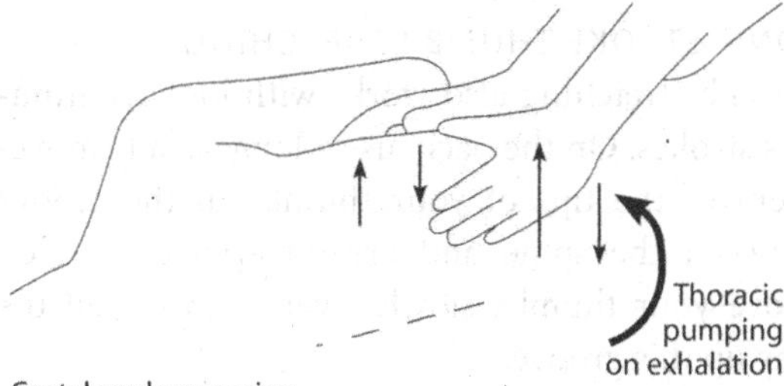

Costal angle pumping.

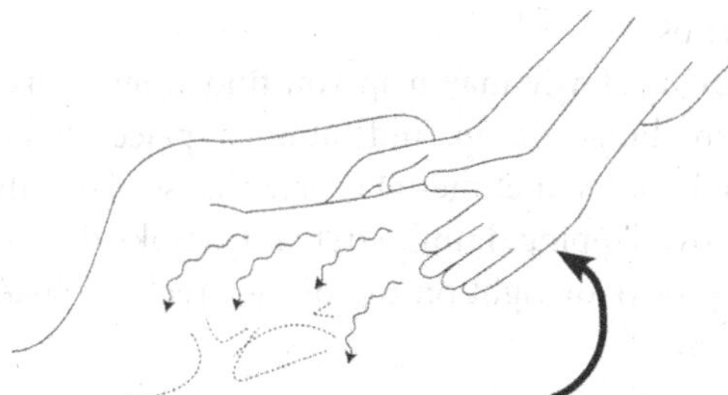

Running coarse vibrations towards the bronchia.

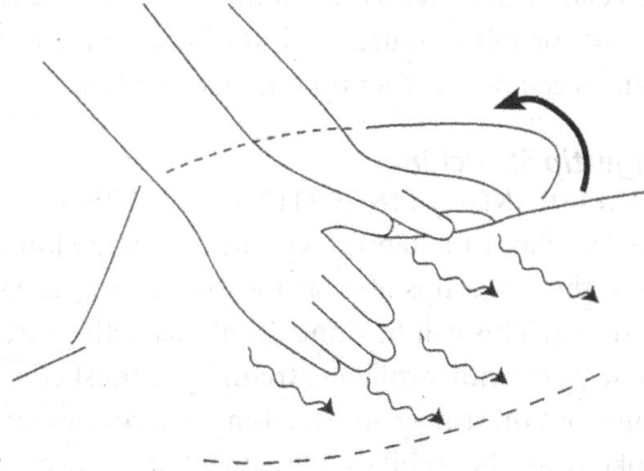

Thoracic shaking.

In massage, compression is steady pressure with no circular action. For wheelchair users, it is primarily used in the thoracic area to aid in expectoration after respiratory massage. The pumping action of the compression helps to move the congestion up and out of the lungs.

Chest Compression Menu

1. **Reinforced palmar pumping to the sternum:** Standing at the head of the bed or table, do some reinforced palmar pumping to the sternum.
2. **Bilateral palmar pumping to the sternum:** Move to bilateral palmar pumping to the upper chest and clavicular area.
3. **Thoracic pumping:** Move to the side of the table or bed and stand in a stride position. Do some bilateral thoracic pumping around the breast.
4. **Reinforced palmar pumping on the side of the chest:** Perform reinforced palmar pumping all over the side of the chest closest to you.
5. **Pumping on the opposite side:** Repeat steps 1 through 4 on the opposite side.
6. **Running vibrations:** Use running vibrations from the bottom up—the direction that the lungs would like to clear. Adding vibrations to chest compressions increases the mobilization of the lungs. I move in different angles over the chest with running, shaking vibrations that combine compression with movement. Turn to page 42 for how to do vibrations.
7. **Rib raking:** Try rib raking combined with a shaking, vibrating compression. Turn to page 38 for how to do rib raking.
8. **Costal angle pumping:** Try some single-sided or tandem costal angle pumping.

Stretching

Stretching is a continuous pressure stroke from beginning to end. The steady pressure increases the elasticity of the muscles because it stretches the muscle fibers. Wheelchair patients, because their joints and muscles are often constricted and increasingly fixed, are perfect candidates for stretching connective tissue and muscle contractors. These slow, stretching strokes can give patients better mobility and help ease the discomfort and pain of their constricting muscles.

Stretching strokes can be done with the thumbs (pads, tips, and sides), fingertips, and palms (reinforced and overhanded). Ideally, stretching strokes are done very slowly, with the pressure adapted to the patient's tolerance and mobilization restrictions.

Thumb Stretching

Thumb stretching can be done double-handed or single-handed. Do what works best in the situation!

SHORT-STROKE THUMB STRETCHING

Thumb stretching with short strokes is a little like alternate thumb kneading, but instead of the thumbs moving in overlapping circles, the thumb tips or sides move in short, overlapping, straight strokes of steady pressure to stretch out the tissue underneath. Push your thumbs alternately ahead and away from you. Start with the thumb pads and move to the thumb tips for greater focus, pokiness, depth, and precision. This can also be a transverse stroke that can be performed using the side of the thumbs—not the tips—across the erector spinae muscles as the patient is leaning forward. Especially when people are spending long periods of time in their wheelchair, I use this stroke down the iliotibial band, from the hip to just below the knee.

FIGURE 2.22. **Transverse Thumb Stretching**

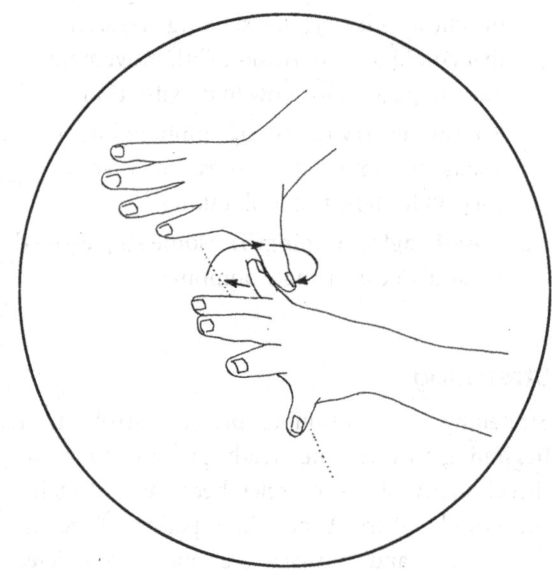

Transverse Thumb Stretching

Transverse thumb stretching is an overlapping short stroke transverse to the fibers, through the erector spinae muscles, iliotibial band, and quadriceps. You can use the same thumb pattern to run the stroke longitudinally along the muscle fiber.

LONG-STROKE THUMB STRETCHING

Thumb stretching also works with long, continuous strokes. On the back, use a long, steady movement of the tips of your thumbs in the groove between the spine and erector spinae muscles. Move your thumbs slowly—very slowly—all the way up this groove.

I use long-stroke stretching also with the fingertips.

Moving slowly may help you find where muscles are bunched up, indicating a place to be worked on. I sometimes alternate this stroke with short, overlapping thumb-stretching strokes in the same groove or right on top of the erector spinae muscles.

DOUBLE-HANDED THUMB STRETCHING

This can be done with one thumb on either side of the erector spinae muscles for the back, or the two thumbs can be together on one side at a time.

Fingertip Stretching

SINGLE-HANDED FINGERTIP STRETCHING

Use one hand to stabilize the nearest large joint, while the fingertips stretch the connecting muscle slowly. This can be done deeply, as with sports massage, or with swollen extremities. I most commonly use this fingertip stretching in a continuous stroke from the Achilles attachment at the heel of the foot to the back of the knee.

FIGURE 2.23. Palmar Stretching

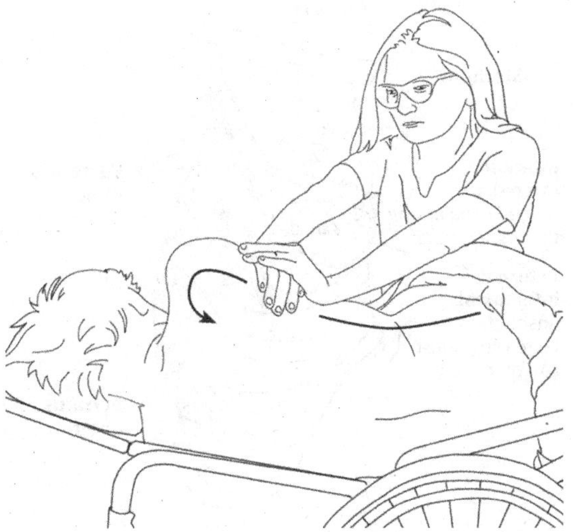

Side-lying reinforced palmar stretching.

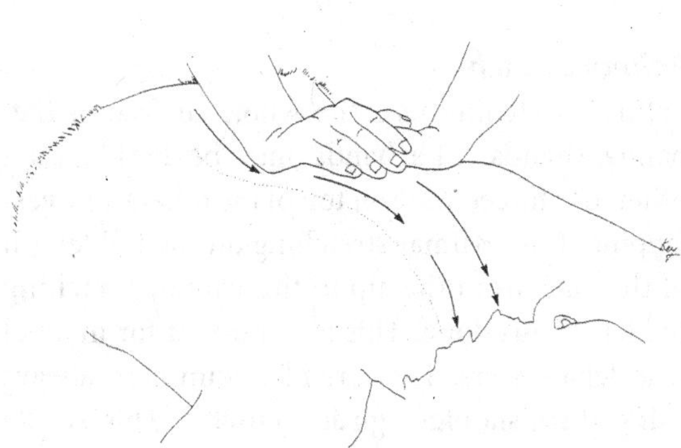

Prone reinforced palmar stretching.

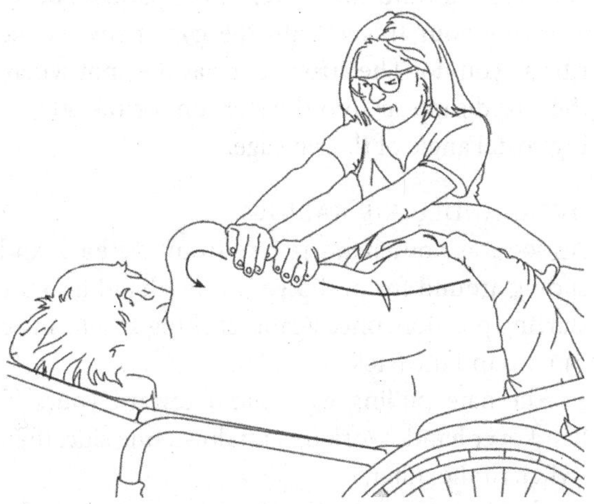

Side-lying side-by-side palmar stretching to the latissimus dorsi.

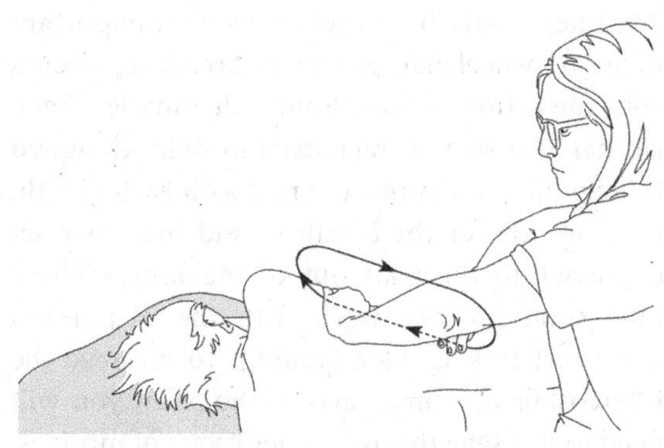

Side-lying overhanded palmar stretching.

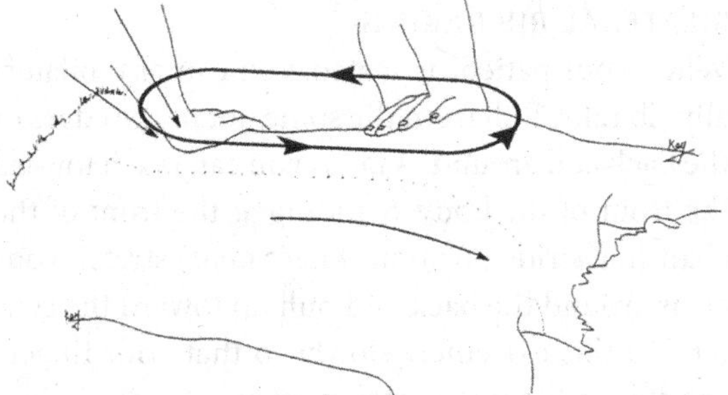

Prone overhanded palmar stretching.

FINGERTIP STRETCHING WITH BOTH HANDS

I use my fingertips together from both hands as one unit so that the backs of the fingers of each hand are touching each other. I use this stroke most commonly to split the gastrocnemius muscle, pulling up from the Achilles tendon at the heel, again to the back of the knee.

Palmar Stretching

Palmar stretching uses the whole surface of flat, palmar hands. The hands may be beside each other, reinforced (one on top of the other), or overlapping. I use palmar stretching on the full length of the back from the hip to the armpit, stretching the latissimus dorsi. This is important for manual wheelchair users. They are like swimmers, always using their shoulder girdle muscles. This stroke can be done in a continuous, overlapping manner or with one hand starting as the other hand finishes. It can be done in either direction, up or down the back.

Rib Raking

The intercostal rib muscles are another important focus of wheelchair massage: breathing occurs with the action of these tight little muscles. Each rib has two sets of intercostal muscles designed to help lift and depress the ribs with each breath. One set lifts for the breath in and the other set depresses to push air out of the lungs. These intercostal muscles work with the diaphragm and heart to keep us breathing. To massage the intercostals on some parts of the body, you will need to massage through other layers of muscles, such as the pectoralis minor and serratus anterior muscles.

Rib raking is the most effective respiratory massage stroke. Your fingers groove in between the ribs to stretch the tiny, tough intercostal muscles, making them more elastic and helping them to simply allow the person to breathe more easily. Rib raking can ease a patient's breathing in a minute (or less)! Standing at the side of your patient, reach across to the far side of the patient at the midlobe to lower-lobe level. Try to reach as far as you can, if possible to the patient's spine where the ribs attach.

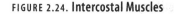

FIGURE 2.24. **Intercostal Muscles**

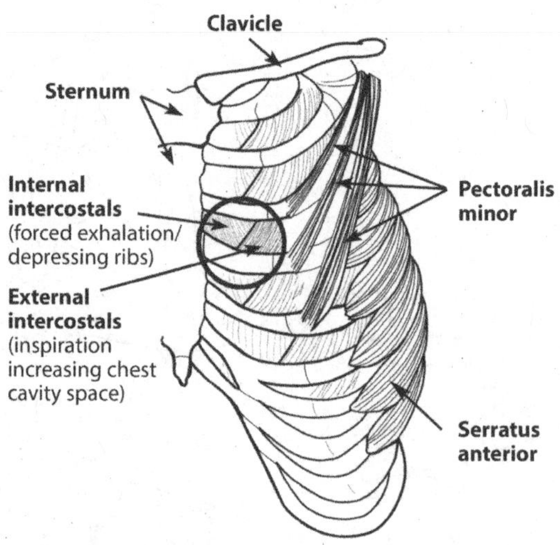

With fingertips in a clawlike position, pull your hand toward the center of the patient's body, grooving your fingers into the gaps between the ribs as you do. The stroke ends at the spot where the ribs disappear into the sternum or the attaching costal angle of the rib cage.

OVERHANDED RIB RAKING

As soon as your hand is free from the back and sliding around front, slip your other hand into the starting position, once again reaching as far as you can around the back.

Alternate pulling each hand toward yourself, hand over hand. Work up and down one side, then switch to the other.

If the patient is female, move around the breasts, lifting the breast out of the way of rib-raking strokes if necessary

BILATERAL RIB RAKING

When your patient is seated, you can also bilaterally rib rake. Pull from the spine out to the edges of the back and around as far as you can reach toward the front of the body. Standing at the front of the chair in a stride position (knees bent) stretch your arms around the back and pull up toward the center. Do this extremely slowly so that your fingers can stay in the intercostal grooves.

FIGURE 2.25. Rib Raking

HAND POSITION IN ALL STYLES

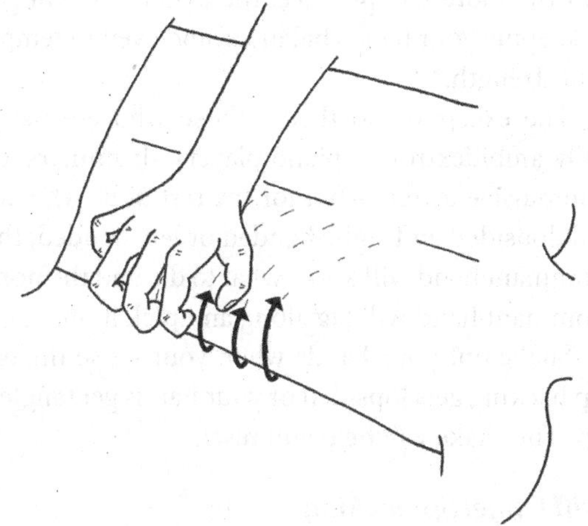

For all styles of rib raking, use a clawlike hand, fit your fingers between the ribs, and pull to help stretch the intercostal muscles.

SINGLE-HANDED RIB RAKING

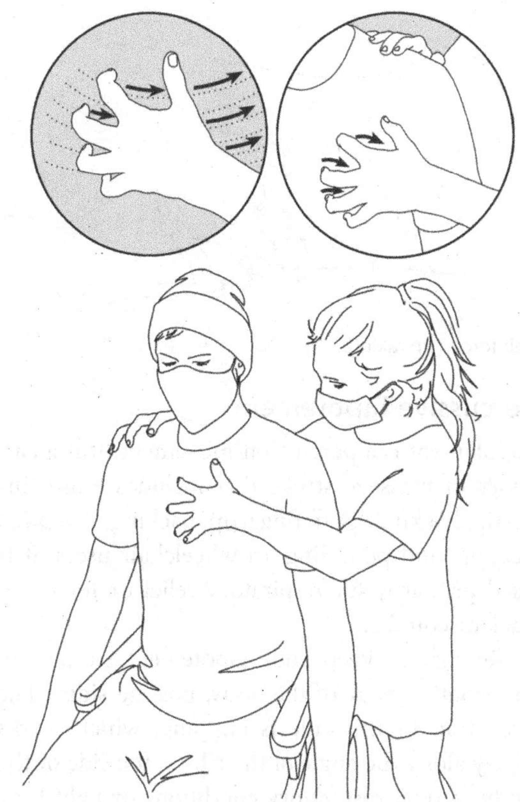

Single-handed rib raking on the upper chest.

BILATERAL RIB RAKING

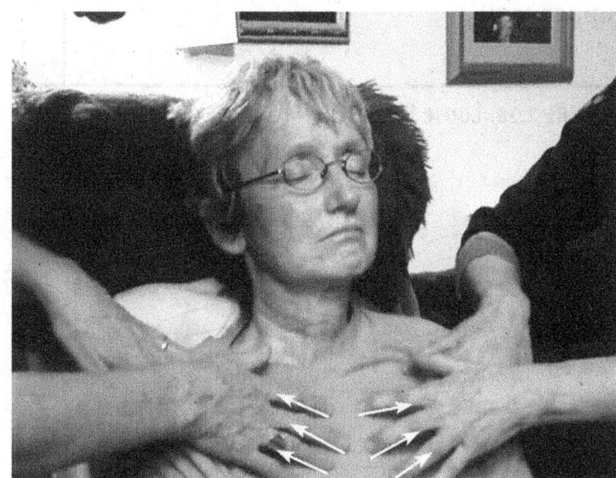

Press down at the start with your fingertips and move out firmly across the upper chest, grooving your fingers between the upper ribs.

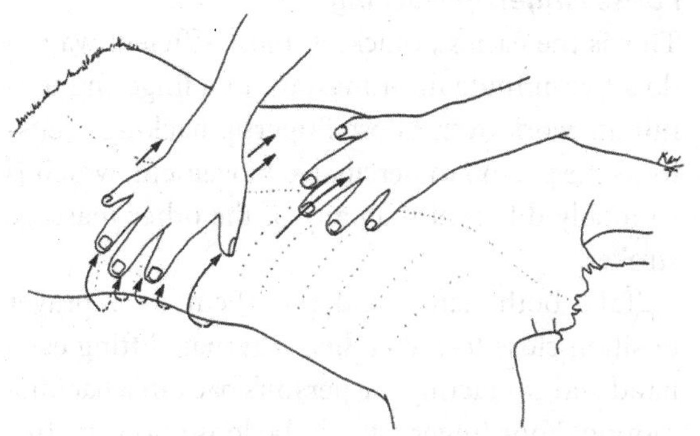

Overhanded rib raking: one hand follows the other repeatedly.

FIGURE 2.25. CONTINUED

BILATERAL RIB RAKING

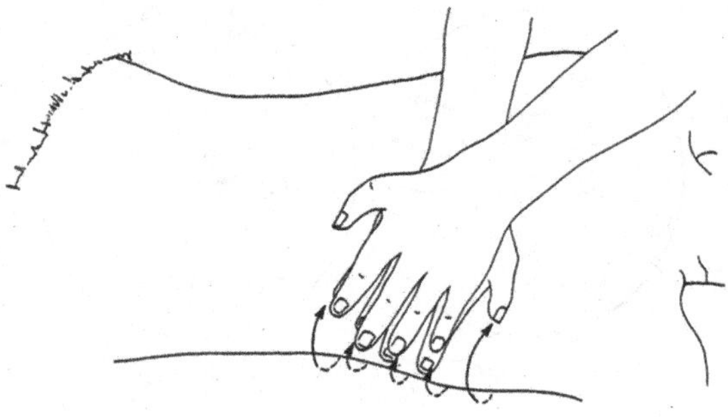

Reinforced rib raking.

Percussive Tapotement

Tapotement is a percussion movement. It is a category of massage stroke that includes loose fingertip hacking, stiff fingertip hacking, cupping, beating, and pounding. In wheelchair users, it is used primarily for respiratory relief or for lower back discomfort.

Be sure to keep your tapotement strokes on the front or back of the body, not the sides. The exception to this rule is cupping, which works nicely along the angle of the ribs at the side of the body to treat respiratory conditions or light lung congestion.

The following strokes are listed in order of how they would normally function in a massage.

Loose Fingertip Hacking

This is the easiest, quickest, most efficient way to do a two-minute mini-massage or a lingering ten-minute work over. Loose fingertip hacking accustoms the person to percussive movement, which is so totally different than any of the other massage strokes.

Take both hands and put them in a prayer position close to each other. Alternate lifting each hand and contacting the person's back in a hacking motion. Your fingers should be loose, so your fingertips will flick against each other. Only the little finger side of the hand will contact the person on the receiving end of this invigorating stroke.

Once you get a rhythm, speed it up so your hands are a blur of activity. The trick is to keep your hands from tangling up with each other. Most people find that one hand will keep a steady rhythm, while the other will be all over the place. But the more you practice, the better you will get at keeping your hands balanced and even in tempo and strength.

The exception to this is those who are naturally ambidextrous—piano players, drummers, or compulsive texters—but for the rest of us who are still lopsided and right-handed or left-handed, the dominant hand will know what to do, and the non-dominant hand will tag along and pick it up.

Shake out your hands when your loose fingertip hacking gets lopsided or your hands get tangled up. The shake will help you reset.

Stiff Fingertip Hacking

This stroke is similar to loose fingertip hacking, but instead of keeping your fingertips loose, you keep them tight together. The action of the hand lifting up and down is also more controlled in this stroke. The fingers do not flick against each other, but hold tight to each other as the hand moves in a chopping motion.

Both loose fingertip hacking and stiff fingertip hacking strokes are used on the upper shoulders and the entire back. A face-down position gives you access to the entire length of the erector spinae muscles into the lumbar lower back, including the sacrum and upper hips. You can also work the stroke from the top of the arm (deltoid) down the upper arm.

FIGURE 2.26. **Loose Fingertip Hacking**

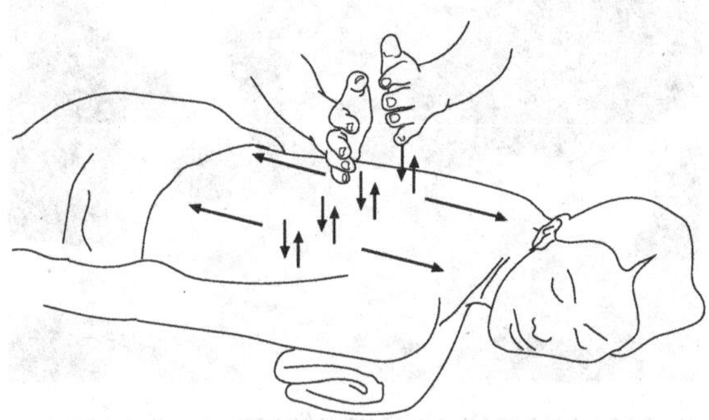

Loose fingertip hacking can be performed on a person lying prone or sitting up.

Cupping

Cupping is a traditional treatment for respiratory conditions, such as chest colds, shortness of breath, congestion, coughs, or end-stage lung saturation. People in wheelchairs are more susceptible to respiratory illnesses, sometimes due to limited mobilization and activity in the thorax, especially for high-level spinal cord injury people. The stroke helps dislodge congestion in the lungs and aids in expectoration.

Cupping is usually done on the back and the ribs. Remember that the thorax goes all the way up to the collarbone, occupying the entire trunk of the body from the waistline up in the back.

Cupping is my favorite tapotement stroke, and for conditions with congestion in the chest, this stroke is a godsend. Before modern medications for drying up mucus in the lungs, traditional cupping tapotement was the most effective way to aid expectoration. It was even part of nurses' training! Helping to get junk out of the lungs helps people breathe better, taking pressure off the heart.

Cup your hands and bring them down in a fairly fast drumbeat, which should create a hollow sound. The most common mistake students make is keeping their fingers straight; be sure to keep the curve of your palm extending all the way out to your fingertips. The sound of cupping done properly is distinctive: the hollow sound differs audibly from the slapping sound made when the hand starts to flatten out. If the sound is not hollow or if your patient says the stroke stings, cup your hands more. Your hand should be cupped as though you're scooping water.

When you soften the stroke by cupping your hands properly, you will hear the difference immediately. I use a towel to insulate the stroke and check in with the patient about the strength of my impact.

When you apply this stroke fast, it becomes very superficial in effect. When it is slowed it down, it has a chance to reverberate throughout the thorax and loosen material from the lung wall to be coughed up and out.

Beating

Beating sounds terrible but feels wonderful. Tuck your thumbs into your hands to make fists. Then

FIGURE 2.27. **Cupping**

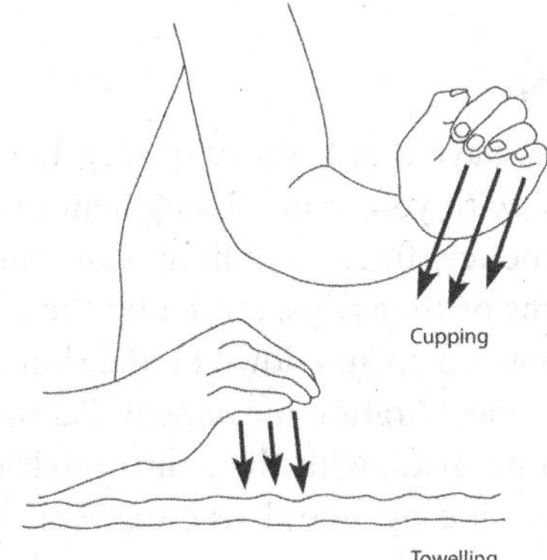

Extend the curve of your palm all the way to your fingertips.

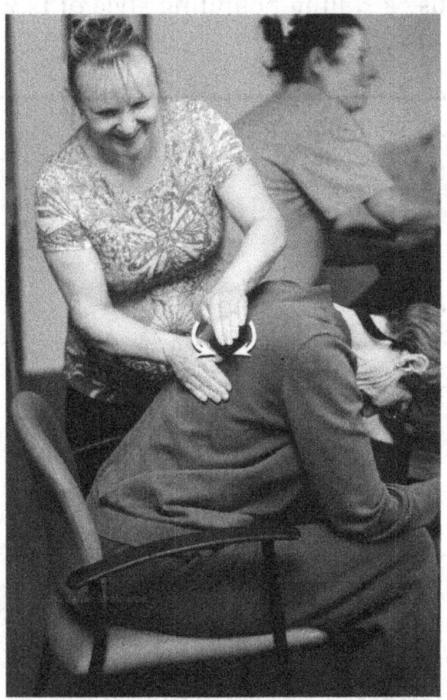

Cupping on the back in a chair, with clothing insulating the stroke.

FIGURE 2.27. CONTINUED

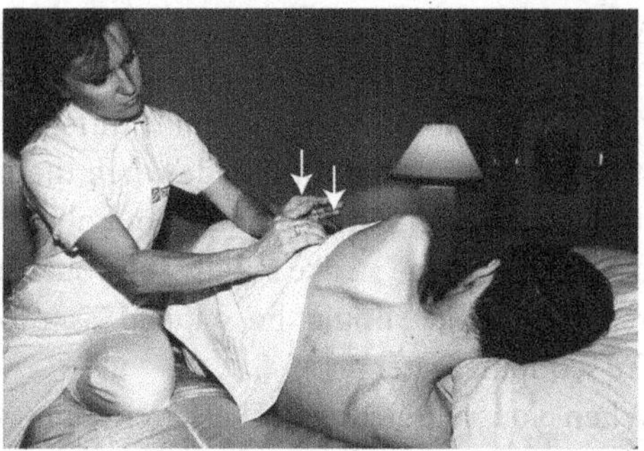

Cupping to a side-lying patient.

flatten out the fists into "monkey paws." Make contact with the person's skin using the knuckled surface of the hand in a palms-down posture. Beating is a movement of the hands up and down from the wrists, not the whole arms. The hands alternate up and down with loose wrists. Your whole flattened fist, not just the fisted fingers, will make contact with the person.

Pounding

For the patient, the pounding stroke is like a local anesthetic: it numbs areas that feel the discomfort of prolonged sitting or lying, usually the lower back. I use a rolling pounding style of tapotement on the sacrum for this purpose. This rolling tapotement is the same stroke I use when mountain climbing to relieve lower back tension from backpacks or prolonged hiking. About one minute of rolling tapotement on the lower back will erase the achiness of the hike and freshen the lower back for another few hours of hard work.

Make tight fists, thumbs tucked in. This makes a cushion on the ulnar border (little finger side) of the hand that makes contact. A tight fist has a softer impact than if the hand is loose, which can feel bony. You don't want the stroke rebounding off the back; instead, use a rolling application where the fists make a circular movement between impacts. The result is a sort of pounding caress.

I use two types of pounding, single-handed and double-handed (both hands side by side). With double-handed, keep your hands close together so they're just about brushing each other, and make this a continuous stroke close to the surface of the skin up to about six inches away from the skin. You can vary the distance.

For single-handed, rest one hand on the patient, and pound on top of your own hand with the fisted hand. I use this adaptive style of pounding, using one hand to cushion the pounding stroke of the other, usually in the thorax.

FIGURE 2.28. **Beating**

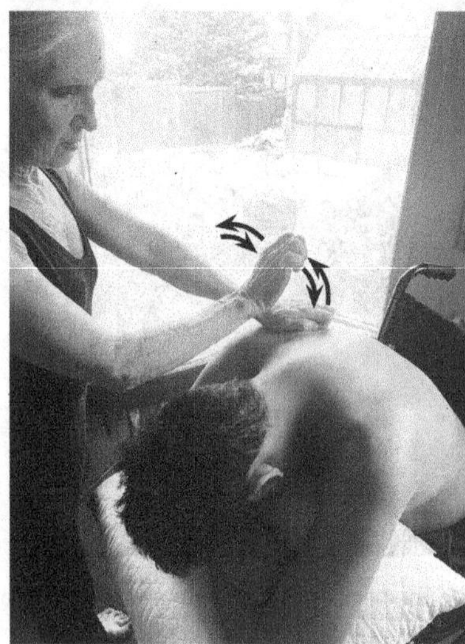

Vibration

Vibrations have a fast, shaky quality, like getting "nervous" with your hand. Using bent or straight arms, produce fine, trembling vibrations with your palms or fingertips. Stiffen up the arms and quickly bounce up and down on the skin or make a side-to-side vibration movement. Palmar vibrations can be made with the palms stacked (reinforced) or side by side. I use a several types of vibrations:

- **Fine:** Move your hands as if you have a light tremor.
- **Coarse:** Move your hands side to side and up and down actively. The movements are larger and more obvious than with fine vibrations. I use these after an application of fine vibrations.

FIGURE 2.29. **Single-Handed Pounding**

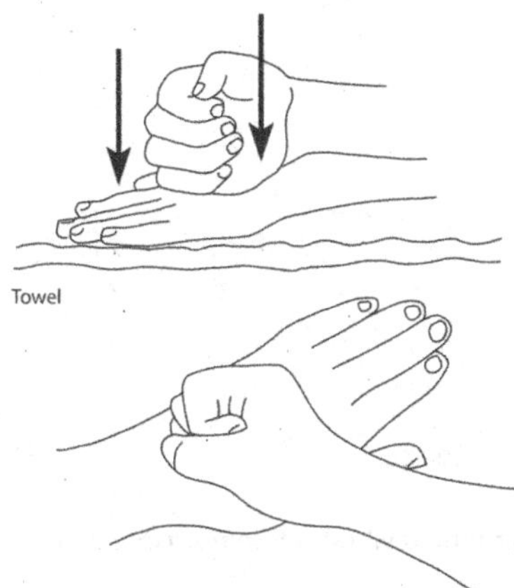

Cushion the stroke by pounding on top of your own hand.

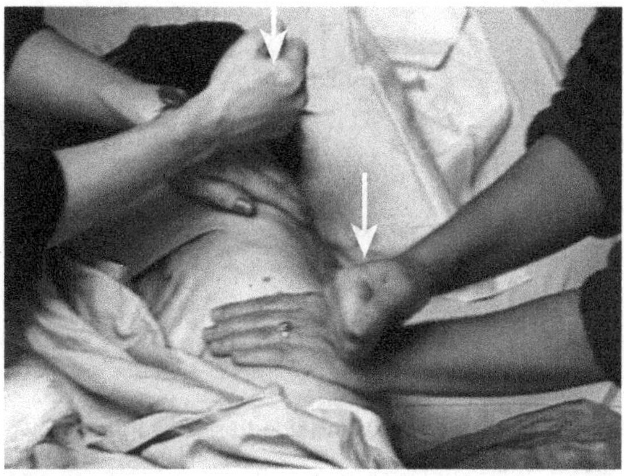

Tandem pounding to a side-lying patient.

- **Static:** Picture your hands as a jackhammer, with the hands angled down on a specific spot and moving up and down without changing location on the body. Drill in one spot, then move to the next location and repeat. Both fine and coarse vibrations can be done in a static way.
- **Running:** Either coarse or fine, these vibrations move. They can go in any direction, although an excellent spot to use them is down the descending colon as a fix for constipation.

Vibrations are useful for respiratory and digestive blockages, and very light, fluttering types of vibrations can work along nerve routes for neurological soothing. Most North American massage therapists use electronic vibrations, but European massage therapists commonly use a bent elbow or stiff, straight arm to apply this traditional massage stroke. These strokes were the most difficult for me to master. Most people have one hand that vibrates more easily, while the other is less skilled. I like to use reinforced hands (i.e., one hand on top of the other) to accomplish these fine movements, where the hand that vibrates better helps its partner.

In my early instruction, I was taught not to apply pressure with this stroke, but today I use firm pressure, copying my experience on the receiving end of vigorous vibrations in Germany. My massage therapist there, a Roman Catholic nun wearing a full habit, drilled away with running and static vibrations with a huge tremor quality. I had a deep relaxation response, sleeping two rejuvenating hours immediately after that massage session.

With wheelchair patients, vibrations can be delivered even over areas that might be bandaged or tumorous. Because it can be applied in just one spot, it is easy for the person receiving the vibrations to get used to them and sink into them.

For the person delivering the massage, this stroke requires some endurance. After years of practice, I can out vibrate anyone, but years ago, I would be good for short bursts only. Practice this stroke for two minutes and you will see that it is easy for the first thirty seconds, and then it gets more difficult to maintain. If you shake out your hands and start fresh again, you can develop more stamina.

When receiving this stroke, organize an experiment in which someone will tell you when one minute is up and then two and then three and four and five. Experiencing the effect at two minutes is nothing like the effect at five minutes, when there is often a numbing reaction and a diminishment of local pain, as in abdominal cramping.

FIGURE 2.30. **Vibrations**

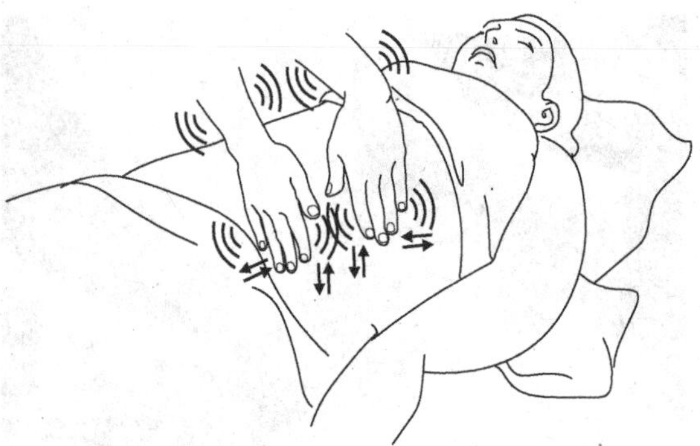

Vibrations can be done with a side-to-side or up-and-down movement.

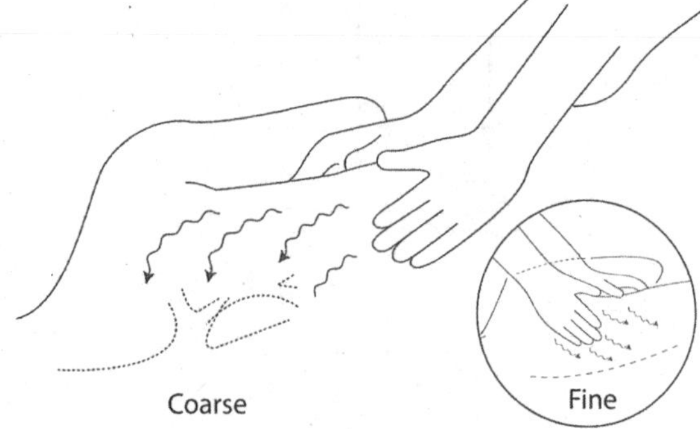

Side-lying running vibrations in both directions.

Just as it can take minutes for the stomach to tell the brain it is full, the body takes time to register the strokes throughout the nervous system. It takes time for the skin to register the pressure of the stimulation and get the message to the brain to turn off the pain. The vibrations work by overstimulating the skin, which eventually overtakes any painful sensations—there just isn't room for both.

Light Reflex Stroking

A good stroke with which to finish to the therapeutic section of any massage routine is light reflex stroking: moving your hands with a light touch over the body. Reflex stroking is a modified form of wringing. This variation uses the back of your fingers for the stroke away and then palmar side of your fingers as you move toward yourself. When stroking away, start with the knuckles closest to your palms, then gradually move to the middle knuckles, and then the fingertips.

On the back, simultaneously glide your fingers along each side of the spine from the neck down to the lower back. Then, switch to overhanded stroking with your hands moving like a conveyor belt of continuous movement: one hand lifts off at

FIGURE 2.31. **Light Reflex Strokes**

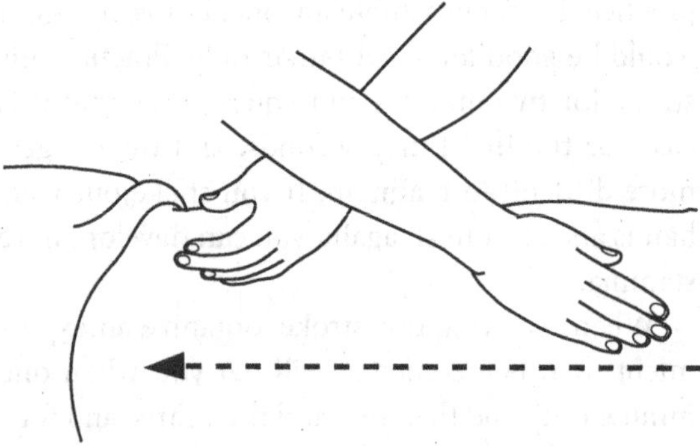

Continuous overlapping light reflex stroking from the neck to the sacrum/lower back. Light reflex stroking is a nice finish. For butterfly stroking, add a flicker of movement to your fingers like playing a piano!

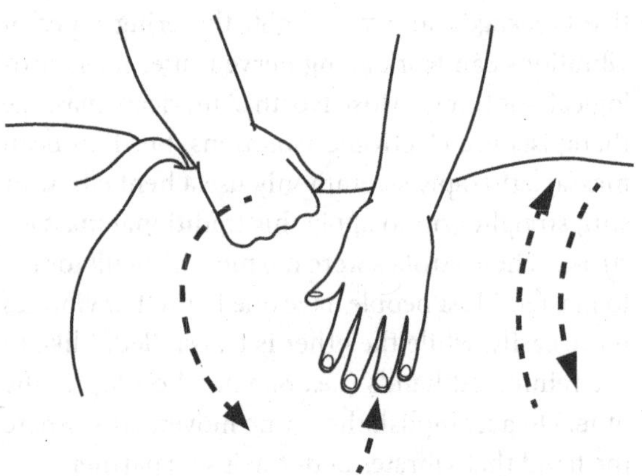

Back-of-the-hand variation of light reflex stroking.

the lower back and the other hand makes contact at the neck. After this, switch back to both hands at once. Whatever combination you use, keep the flow going for at least five or six strokes (at least one minute). Make each stroke lighter or slower than the last so you finish with your hands hovering over the person's skin.

The light reflex stroke, applied continuously over minutes at a time, creates an anesthetizing effect, a numbing accompanied by relief. It is a genuine "neurological eraser." When I am teaching this stroke, I demonstrate this by asking my audience to find a sore spot on their forearm and press on it with their thumb going back and forth for 10 to 30 seconds while I am explaining the phenomena of this neurological eraser. Then I ask them stop pressing and see how they can still feel the sore spot when they are no longer touching it. With a focus on the discomfort, I ask them to then lightly stroke the area with their fingertips and with the back of their hand, making it as light as a caress. When they finish and they are hands-off, there is no sensation of that uncomfortable thumbprint.

Always end any massage treatment with soft strokes.

It is a useful stroke to help people (and animals) get to sleep. Some people cannot sleep no matter how medicated they are, but they get easily hypnotized by this stroke. The length of time that you can deliver the stroke is usually in direct proportion to the depth of sleep or relaxation achieved.

I use light reflex stroking when I finish each part of the full body massage, doing the stroke five or six times each time as I go along. At the end of the full body massage, I use light reflex stroking from the top of the head, all the way down the arms, continuing down the legs, to the very bottom tip of the toes. I lift off at the end of the stroke (instead of stroking back up) and then I start again at the top of the head, so my light reflex stroking is continuously on a downward direction. You can also vary the pressure, making each time a little lighter than the time before.

The Finale

For all massage routines, try to back out of the massage the same way you went in. The three strokes of effleurage, wringing, and reinforced palmar kneading are used as the final bookends when I am finished with the more focused massage strokes that make up the middle of any massage sequence. I start with these three strokes and usually end with the same three strokes.

All you need to do is remember to always finish by smoothing out with wringing, then reinforced palmar kneading, and finally effleurage. Light reflex stroking is a nice finish if you're ending the massage or moving to a new body part.

In tandem massage, we often finish with "the wave." We start at the head of the patient with two team members, in perfect unison, lightly stroking down the patient's whole body with their fingertips, restarting again and again and again, lighter and lighter each time until they are barely touching the patient's skin. When it is a team of four to six people, the wave is longer and bigger but it is still deeply relaxing, soothing, and fun at the same time. The person in the wheelchair should be floating off the chair by the time we're finished.

Post-Massage Treatments

All your massage work will generate warmth in the patient's body by increasing their circulation. Take advantage of this warmth by covering them up and allowing them to just lie peacefully still. They could be lying forward in their wheelchair onto an eating tray or stack of pillows to rest. This is an excellent time for meditation, prayer, or visualization. The patient can use the massage as a vehicle for a deeper experience of letting go. An Epsom salt bath can deepen the relaxation effects of the massage and help the patient get more mileage out of your treatment.

You might also use hot water bottles, Tiger Balm for the hands or feet, cold cloths, or an alcohol rub to finish.

VIDEO LIBRARY

Visit brusheducation.ca/wheeling-in-good-hands to watch these videos:

- **The importance of communication:** Feedback, feedback, feedback with Sylvia
- **Principles of massage with Molly and Fernanda**
- **Effleurage with Molly and Fernanda**
- **Adaptive arm effleurage:** In the classroom with Christina and Val
- **Petrissage:** Wringing the legs – in the classroom
- **Petrissage:** Alternate thumb kneading and adaptive therapist postures
- **Petrissage:** Alternate thumb kneading to the knee
- **Petrissage:** Alternate, single, and bilateral thumb kneading and fingertip kneading to the arm
- **Petrissage:** Bilateral thumb kneading and bilateral fingertip kneading to the ankle
- **Petrissage:** Fingertip kneading and alternate palmar kneading to the calf
- **Levering:** Key locations – back (erector spinae) – in chair
- **Levering:** Key locations – back – supine
- **Levering:** Key locations – hamstrings – levered fingertip kneading
- **Levering:** Key locations – levered fingertip kneading to the back – in chair
- **Scooping:** Fingertip kneading and scooping to the occipital ridge
- **Chest compressions with supine patient in ICU**
- **Rib raking:** Overhanded rib raking – in chair
- **Percussive tapotement and light reflex stroking with Barbara**
- **Light reflex stroking with Molly and Fernanda**

Barbara

Barbara Turnbull was a tireless activist who devoted her career to reporting on and advocating for people with disabilities. I met Barbara in 1986 when she helped me teach wheelchair massage by being my wheelchair massage movie person. She had suffered a high-level spinal cord injury at cervical level 4 after being shot in a holdup at her job at a convenience store when she was only seventeen. After she graduated from Arizona State University in journalism and was working for the *Toronto Star*, we met in Toronto. She was my inspiration for massaging people in wheelchairs, as massage was a mainstay of her health and well-being beginning when she was young and until she died at the age of fifty in 2015.

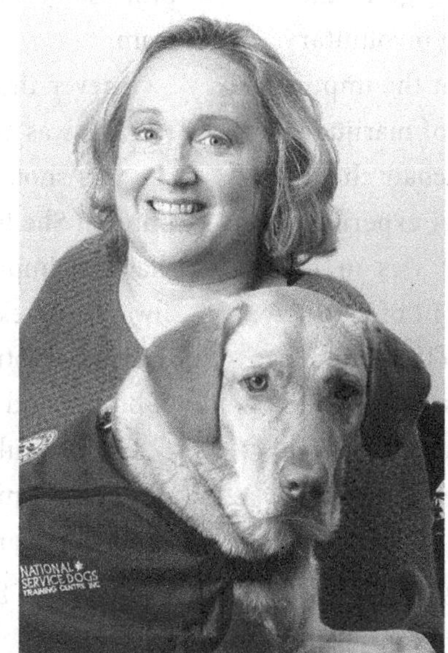

Barbara Turnbull.

I and so many others have benefited from her willingness to help me teach the significance of massage for a working woman in a wheelchair.

For Barbara Turnbull, who had no use of her arms and limited use of her shoulders, her head was her only means of movement. Massaging her head and face was magic to her.

From Barbara, I learned how people in chairs were able to control their chair with a head pad using very slight movements of the head to turn, back up, and park with exactness. This was perfect for the head, neck, and shoulder massages that I taught her friends and helpers. Although Barbara died a few years ago, you can still see our first wheelchair massage film on my YouTube channel.

Barbara was a famous Canadian even when I met her in her early twenties. She had a presence, a sense of confidence and conviction, that is still felt all these years later. I have used the film we shot in 1988 all over the world. In this high tech and social media way, she has traveled to Haiti, Guatemala, South Africa, and the Yukon, teaching people about high-level spinal cord paralysis wheelchair massage.

In the film *Strength and Courage of Barbara Turnbull*, Barbara says: "We have to take things one day at a time. Things don't work any other way. Everybody has to carry on. Everyone has to have determination in this day and age to carry on."

I think that the most dramatic part of our wheelchair massage film is when she experiences involuntary tremors and shaking as I pick up her arm to massage her. This is the most powerful image. When Barbara's arm is in spasm, it looks like I should stop massaging, but I don't. We are able to show that it is important to continue until the spasms subside. This is counterintuitive. It is more natural to stop massaging, but you would never complete a full body massage if you were constantly waiting. Barb taught me to keep massaging!

Recently, I watched a talk that Barbara gave several years ago to a large audience in Toronto at Ideacity. Her talk was about the significance of cannabis for people experiencing involuntary tremors. I had already known about the importance of the antispasmodic effects of marijuana through my work with other wheelchair clients. I had also rediscovered my original experience with "contact highs" from when I was in my early twenties! I had the unusual trait of getting high simply being in the presence of those under the influence. I learned from a researcher who was doing brain wave studies, of which I was a willing subject, that this was an asset, not a scary liability.

This susceptibility to contact highs means I have to be careful around others using drugs. In the seventies and eighties, this was like tiptoeing through a minefield.

So, listening to Barbara speak at Ideacity about her experience with the medical restrictions for therapeutic use of marijuana, I was taken back forty years. Watching and listening to her way of handling the subject and working the crowd, she was the mature and experienced Barbara that I had gotten to know so many years ago.

After I moved home to British Columbia, I massaged Barbara every time I traveled to Toronto. She had a variety of teams, all of which massaged her continuously. Over the years she contacted me for recommendations on massage therapists in Toronto and I arranged new people to massage her from a distance. I loved visiting her and massaging her over the years. I found it difficult to learn of her death in 2015.

Barbara helped so many people simply by being in that first wheelchair massage film. She was well massaged throughout her career as a journalist and simply as a person who needed a care team. Her experience of massage was positive and practical. She was massaged as often as possible, not just by professionals like me but people on her daily care team.

I never thought that I would outlive Barbara. Her life was a miracle. That she did not die when she was shot during the holdup at her job was a miracle. She lived to teach the world about issues that were important. Her newspaper reporting was always interesting, but as I watched her talk for Ideacity, I noticed she had developed a keen sense of humor and a keen ability with large groups.

Coming full circle, I was struck by the influence she had on me, from my first encounter filming her at her apartment in Toronto in her twenties, to watching her give an address to a huge audience in her forties.

I remember taking her to my fancy women's club, the McGill Club in Toronto. I wanted to thank her for helping me and she was enthusiastic about coming to the club. The club had a new disability elevator at the front entrance and Barbara totally approved of it! The way she treated everyone exhibited her upbringing as she was both gracious and generous, funny and friendly.

I still miss visiting Barbara. I will forever be grateful to her family for allowing the use of her story in this book and of our film in the video library that supports this book. Barbara left the world better educated about issues that were controversial. Listening to her and watching her is a comfort and a blessing. She will stay with me forever as I continue to teach. Most importantly, through the gift of film, I will always be able to feel her at my fingertips.

Thanks, Barbara.

VIDEO LIBRARY

Visit brusheducation.ca/wheeling-in-good-hands to watch these videos:

Story of Barbara: Using her wheelchair

Story of Barbara: Using her computer and a massage with Sue

3

Massaging in the Wheelchair

Massage for wheelchair users can happen in or out of the chair, but a lot of the time, massaging in the chair is the most practical. If the wheelchair allows you to tilt the patient back, or even make them prone, take full advantage of these possibilities to adjust the position of the patient. Often, however, your patient will be in a wheelchair that keeps them in an upright, seated position. Adapting massage to this situation is the focus of this chapter.

Sometimes massaging in the chair is more than just practical—it's necessary. My friend from high school, Dixie Allard, taught me this. For years before she died of MS, Dixie could not be moved an inch from her ideal position when in bed, so I was well trained by her to massage the underside of her body with levered fingertip kneading. Every day Dixie was carefully transferred to a high-back wheelchair so that she could have her daily cigarette out on the balcony of her chronic care facility. That was our best five minutes of levered fingertip kneading—before and after she was transferred to the chair from her bed.

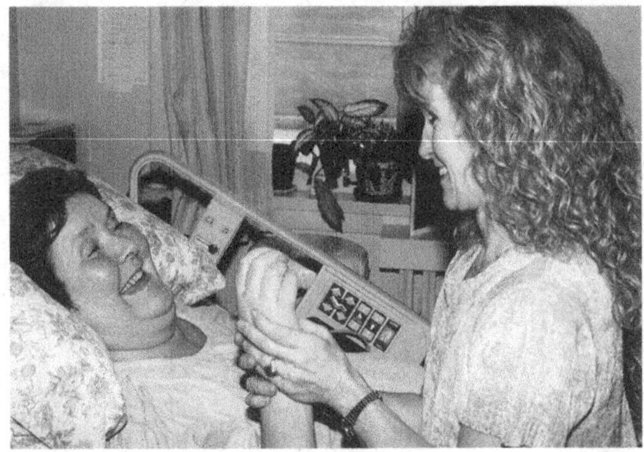

Dixie Allard and me.

First Steps Checklist

Before you begin to massage someone in a wheelchair, make sure you take these steps:

1. Put the brakes on.
2. Make sure the person has their seatbelt on.
3. Consider removing the armrests.
4. Check the position of the leg rests.

Negotiating Clothing

Most wheelchair massage is done with the patient fully clothed.

Clothes can get bunched and wrung in interesting ways during a wheelchair massage! I will give you the benefit of my extensive experience tangling up in people's clothing so you don't have to make the mistakes I made—for example, wringing the legs and undoing somebody's hidden leg catheter at the same time!

Adaptive Postures for Massaging in the Wheelchair

To massage someone seated in a wheelchair, you need to adapt your stances, and their positions, so that you can work with and around the chair. See Figures 3.2 and 3.3.

Wheelchair Massage for the Digestive, Circulatory, and Respiratory Systems

Lack of mobility is the source of most problems in the three major systems of the body: digestive, respiratory, and circulatory.

FIGURE 3.1. First Steps in Wheelchair Massage

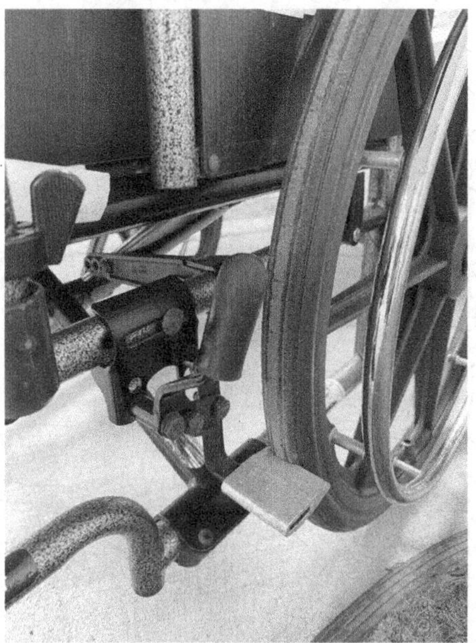

Every wheelchair is a little different as far as brakes go, but there is always a brake for each of the large wheels. Look for a lever on either side of the chair. When engaged, the brakes press a bar or wedge against the wheel of the chair to prevent it from moving.

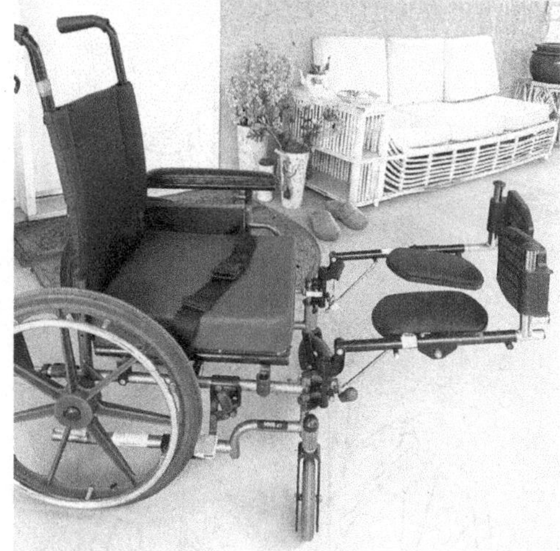

Make sure the seatbelt is on before you begin the massage, and especially before removing the arm rests. You could remove the armrests before you begin the massage, but you might also consider leaving them in place for support and safety until you need to remove them for access. Consider how you can manipulate the leg rests of the wheelchair (for example, up or down) to allow the best access for massage, while maintaining the patient's comfort. You might consider removing the leg rests altogether.

FIGURE 3.2. Therapist Stances

CLASSIC STRIDE

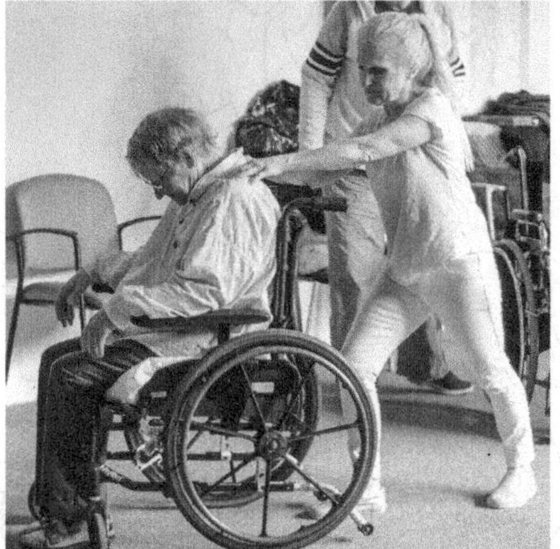

Keep the arms locked at the elbows and lean onto the front leg, which is bent at the knee. The back leg is always straight in order to lean onto the thumbs (rock and roll) with your full weight on the tips of your thumbs.

continued next page

FIGURE 3.2. CONTINUED

STRADDLING THE WHEEL

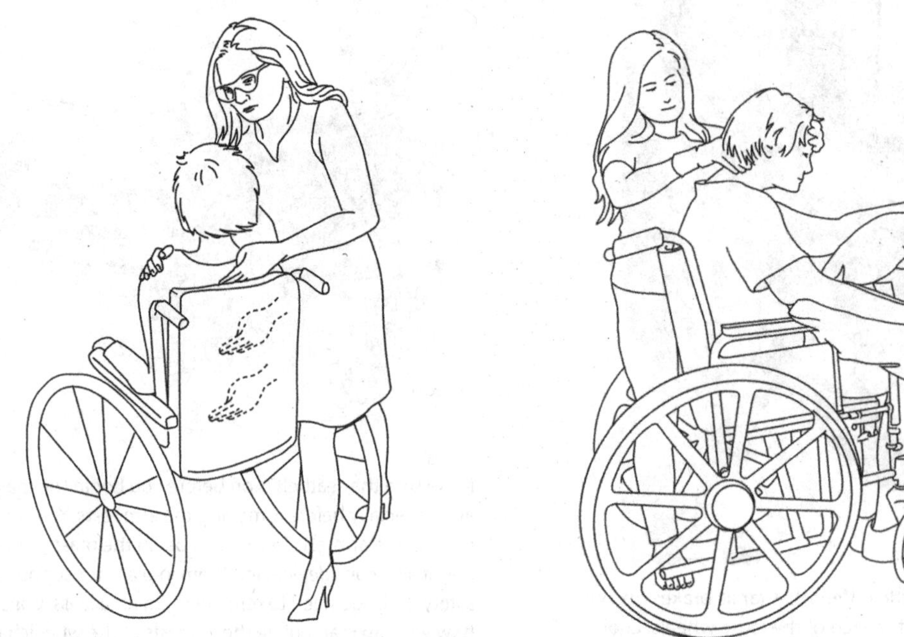

In the classic stride position, put the wheel nearest you under your front leg.

STANDING ON A STOOL

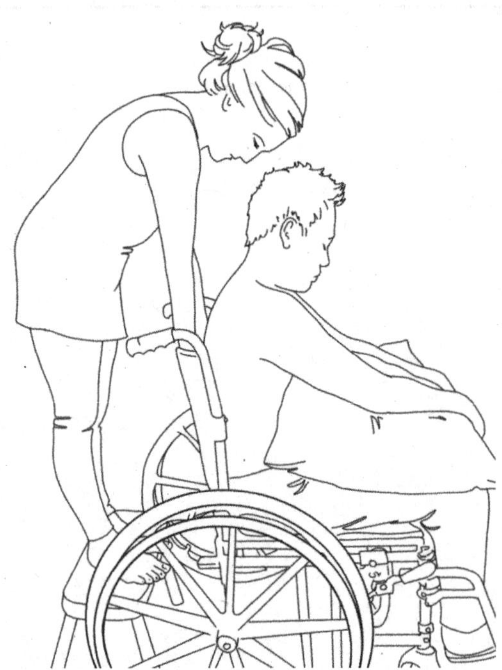

Stools give you a higher position relative to the chair.

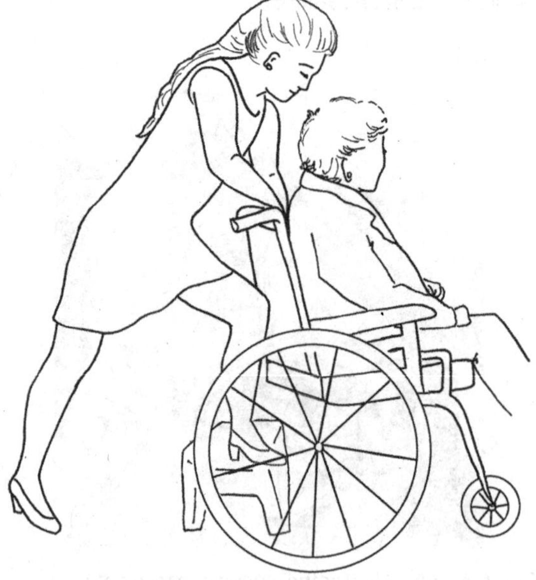

You can also half-stand on a stool.

FIGURE 3.2. CONTINUED

STRIDING BETWEEN THE LEGS

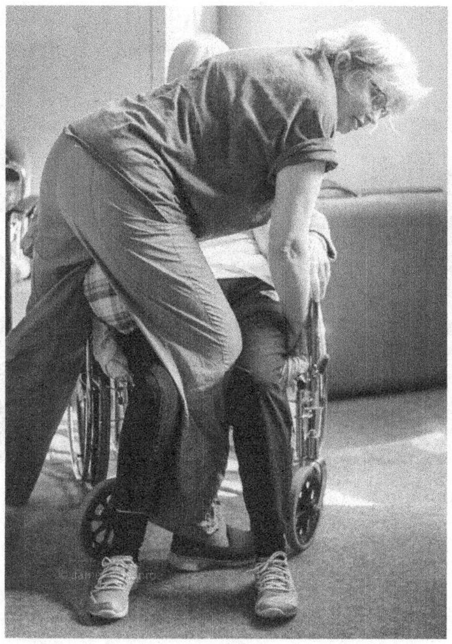

This is a classic stride, with your front leg (knee bent) positioned between the legs of the seated patient.

FACE TO FACE

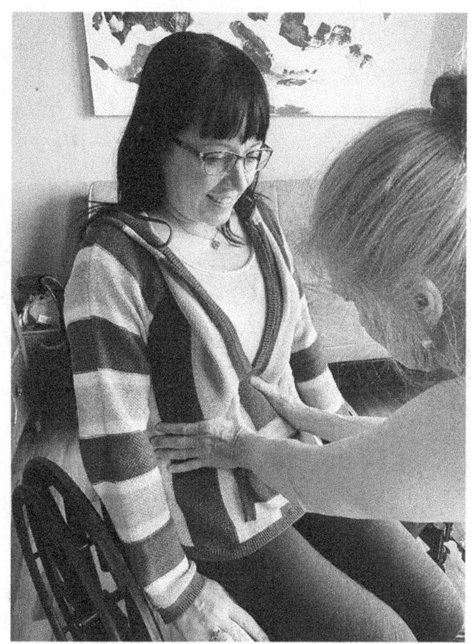

You can directly face a patient seated in a wheelchair.

HALF KNEELING

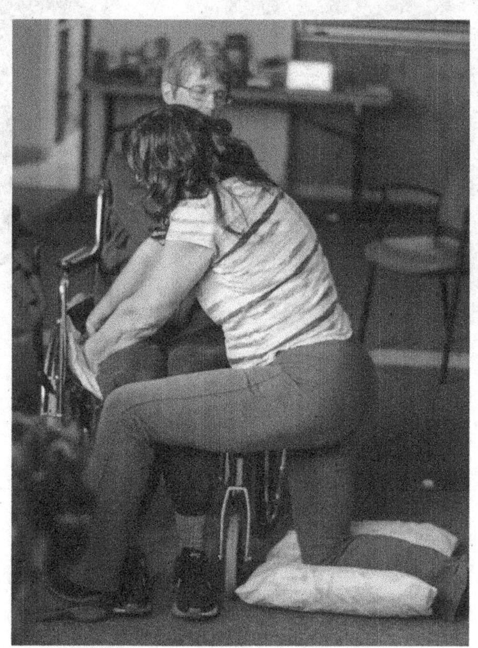

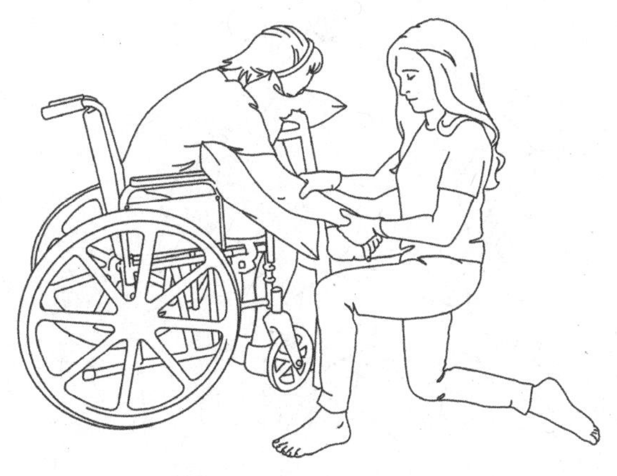

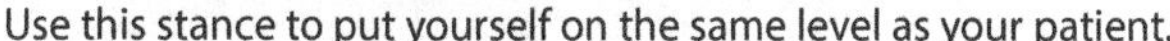

Use this stance to put yourself on the same level as your patient.

FIGURE 3.2. CONTINUED

FULL KNEELING

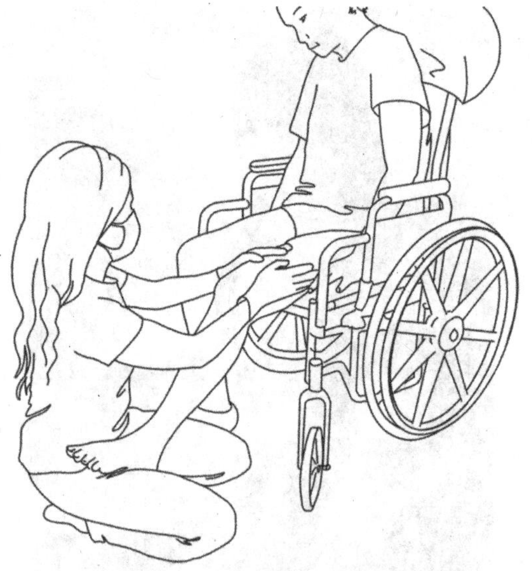

This stance is useful to work the lower parts of the body.

USING THE BACK OF THE CHAIR FOR SUPPORT

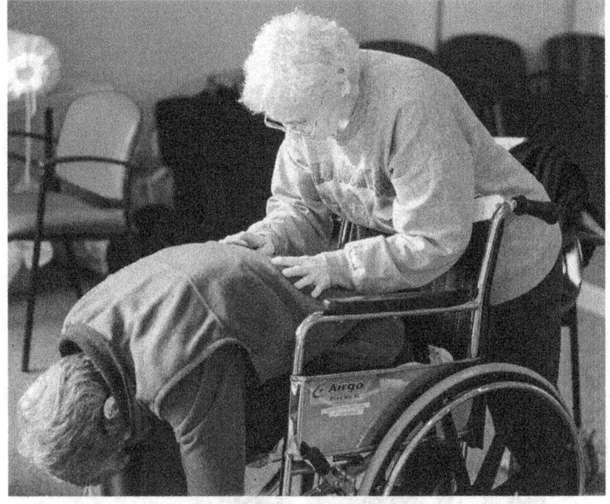

Put your tummy on the back of the chair.

FIGURE 3.3. Patient Positions

LEANING FORWARD WITH SUPPORT

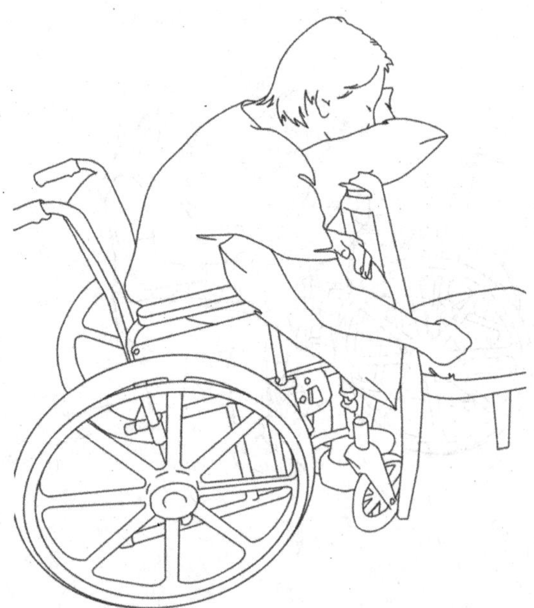

Position the back of a standard chair in front of the patient. Lean the patient forward, against the back of the chair. Use pillows to support the patient; help them position their hands (if possible) for comfort and stability.

ONE KNEE UP, FOOT ON SHOULDER

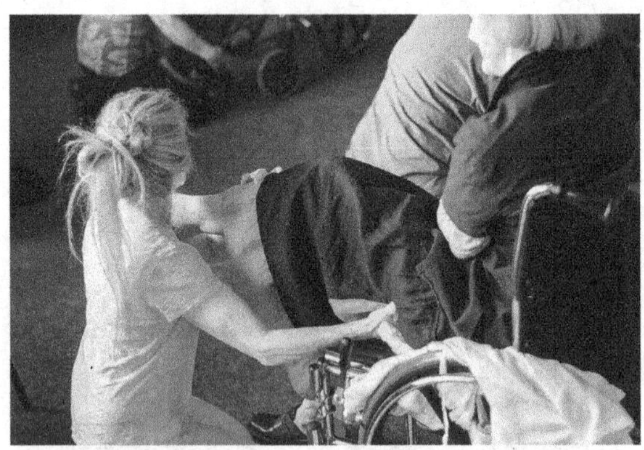

This position can give you access under the leg.

FIGURE 3.3. CONTINUED

SHOULDER SUPPORT WITH SIDE STRIDE

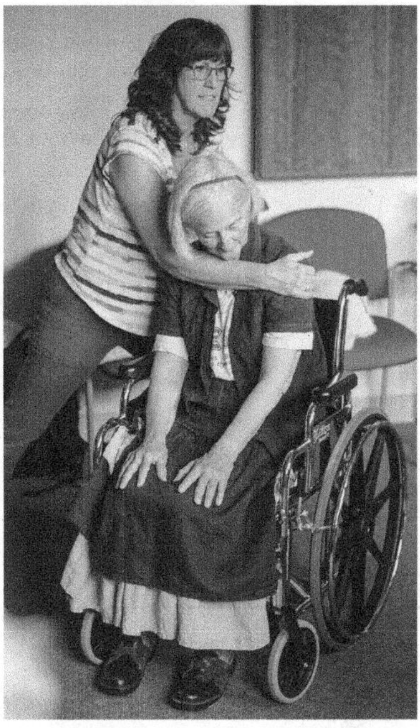

Reach across the patient and grasp their shoulder to provide support.

Wheelchair Massage for the Digestive System

When someone is not moving, their digestive system tends to slow down, and problems of constipation or indigestion of various kinds can appear. Mobilization of the hips will stimulate the peristaltic action of the colon, and, usually right away, there are productive results!

Massaging local to the abdomen is the same for the wheelchair massage as when the person is lying down in face-up position. But in the cramped confines of a wheelchair these same strokes must be adapted.

I use a "sandwich" stroke on the back and front of the abdomen at the same time. This is much easier to perform on a person in a wheelchair than when a person is lying down.

Upper digestive massage is easy to do in a wheelchair, because it involves the head and neck, and usually you have good access to these areas.

The lower digestive system is less easy to reach for a person seated in a wheelchair. Figures 3.5 and 3.6 show crucial anatomy and areas for massage in the upper and lower digestive system.

MASSAGING THE DIAPHRAGM

The abdominal massage includes the work between the digestive and the respiratory systems, on the diaphragm muscle. The diaphragm helps both systems, although it is usually only associated with breathing.

LEG PUMPING

Leg pumping is useful to the digestive health of all wheelchair users, from maternity wheelers to people with spinal cord injuries. Leg and hip activation keep the digestive system happy.

I use three kinds of leg pumping. In each case, the chair is pushed up against a wall, as this is a tippy chair adventure!

1. **Alternating:** This can be done in tandem or with just one person.
    - Bend the knee into the chest while sliding your hand supporting the knee from the lifting position at the beginning of the movement to the top of the knee at the end of the bend to press the knee firmly into the chest.

FIGURE 3.4. Sandwich Stroke

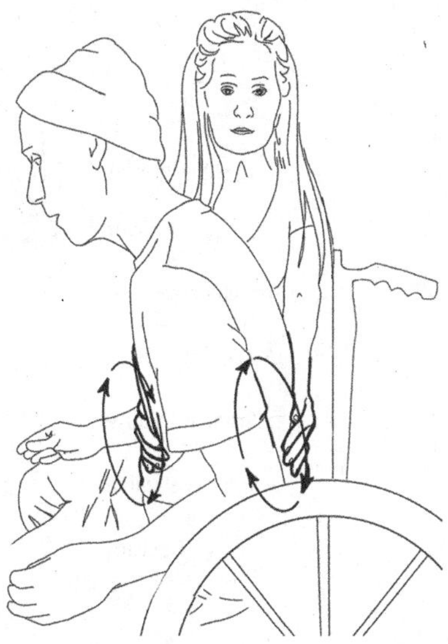

Sandwich the body between your hands, doing a sandwich vibration as you move your palms in alternating circles.

FIGURE 3.5. **Four Strokes for the Upper Digestive System**

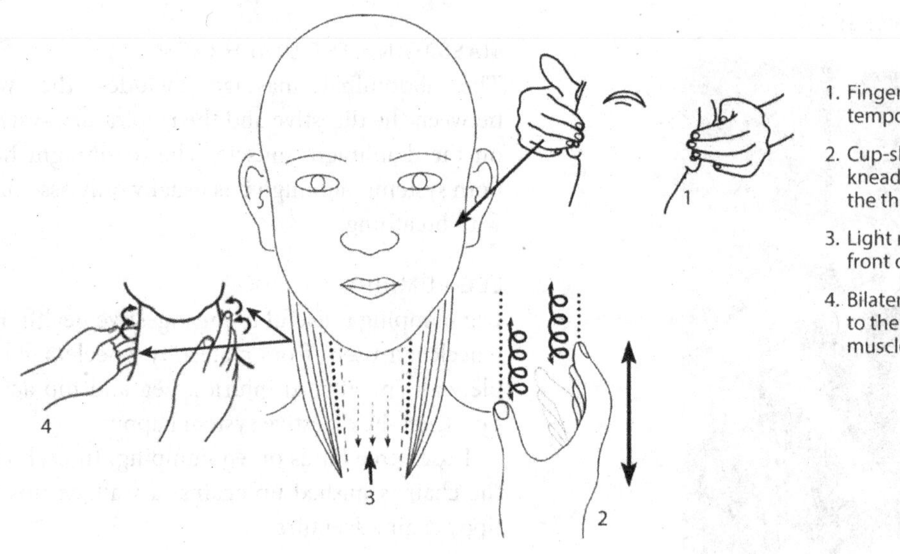

FIGURE 3.6. **Digestive Tract Anatomy and Key Massage Strokes**

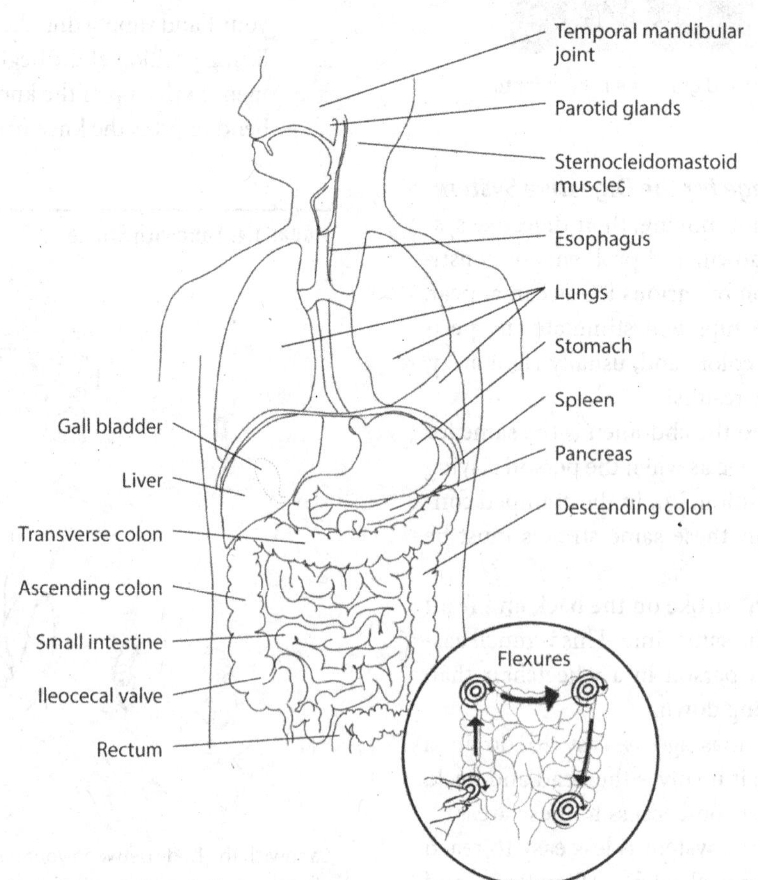

FIGURE 3.7. Diaphragm Strokes

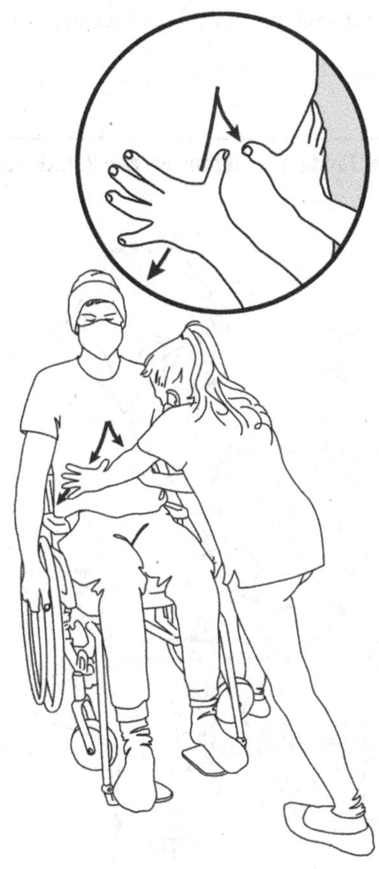

Bilateral diaphragmatic thumb stretching.

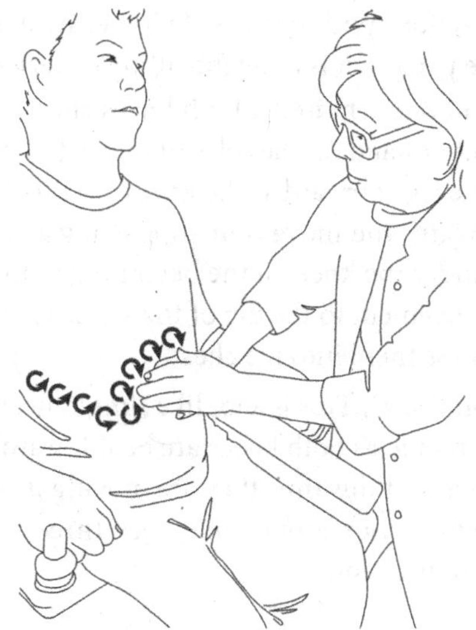

Reinforced fingertip kneading to the costal angle of diaphragmatic attachments.

FIGURE 3.8. Tandem Alternating Leg Pumping

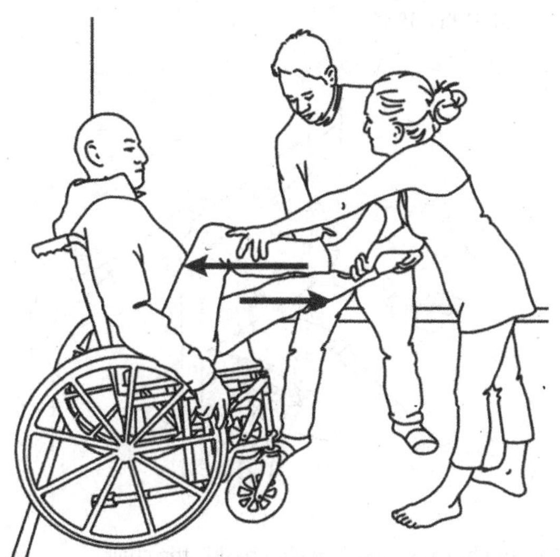

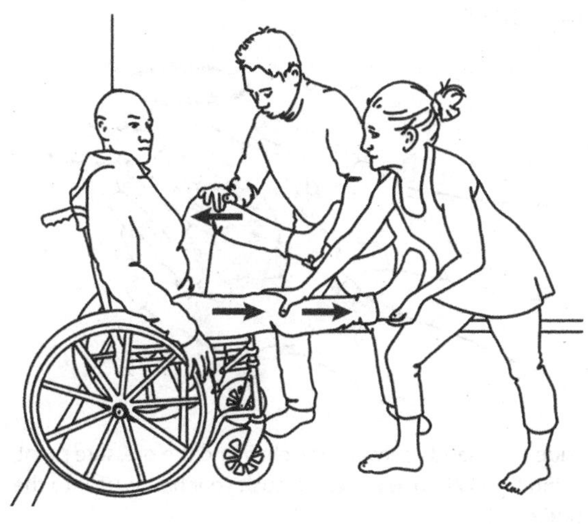

2. **Simultaneous:** This movement has both knees bending at the same time in the same direction. With two people it is easy. With one person, it is a weight-lifting experience.
   - Put one arm under both knees and your other hand on the soles of the feet to push the legs forward as the knees are lifted. Again, you move your supporting arm from under the knees at the beginning of the movement to the top of the knees to firmly press them into the chest.
3. **Rotational:** This is a lot like simultaneous leg pumping, as both knees are bent toward the chest. But this time they are moving in a bent-leg formation around in circles: three times in each direction.

Wheelchair Massage for the Circulatory System

COMMON SITES OF PRESSURE ULCERS

Key areas to focus on when you are massaging someone in a wheelchair are those places most vulnerable to pressure sores. The concentration here is on the lower extremities. Your objective is to stimulate blood flow, to maintain skin integrity, and to keep the limbs from forming ulcerations and permanent contractures.

Pressure sores come from contact between the body and the chair. With the person sitting in the chair, these points of contact are difficult to access.

FIGURE 3.9. **Tandem Simultaneous and Rotational Leg Pumping**

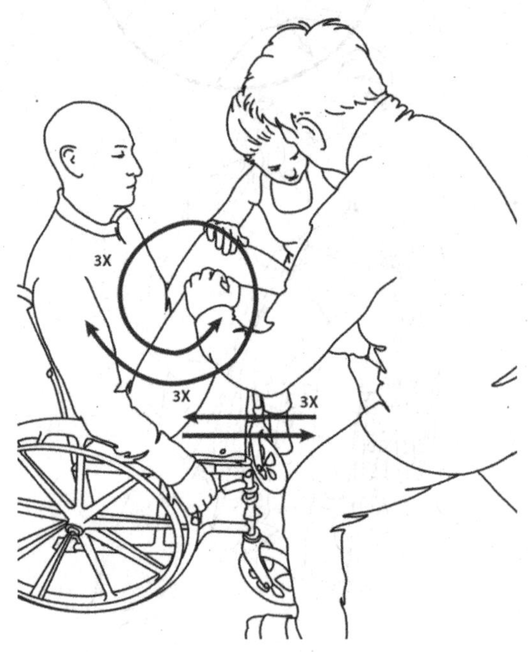

FIGURE 3.10. **Levered Massage for Pressure Ulcers**

BASIC STROKE

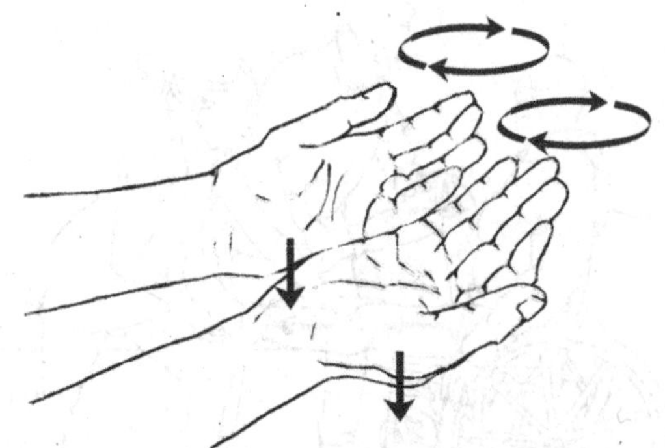

Slide your hands between the chair and the pressure point, using the chair to as a pivot to push your hands up into the body.

ISCHIAL TUBEROSITY

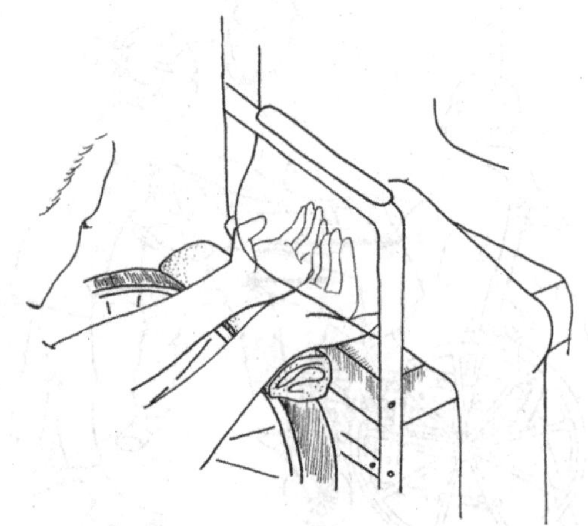

Levered hip massage, kneeling beside the chair.

FIGURE 3.10. CONTINUED

ISCHIAL TUBEROSITY

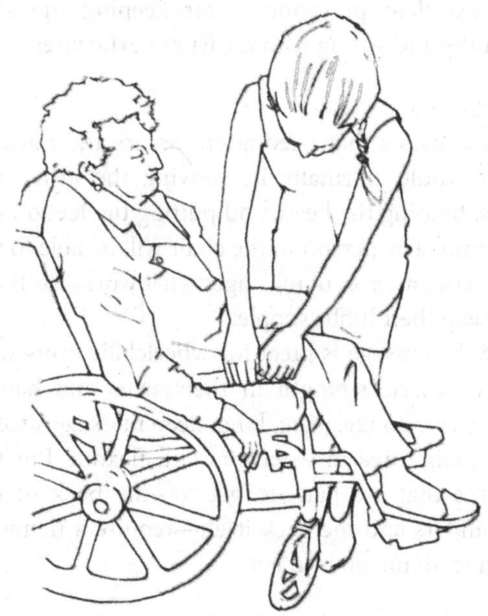

Levered hip massage, striding between a patient's legs.

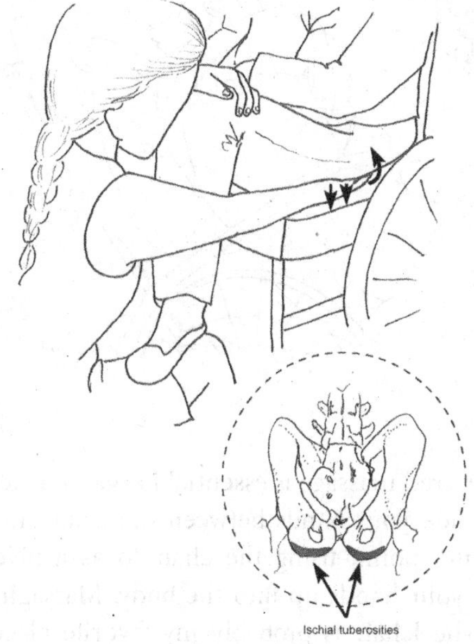

Levered hip massage, kneeling and face to face with the patient's foot raised to rest in your lap.

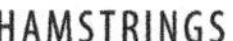

HAMSTRINGS

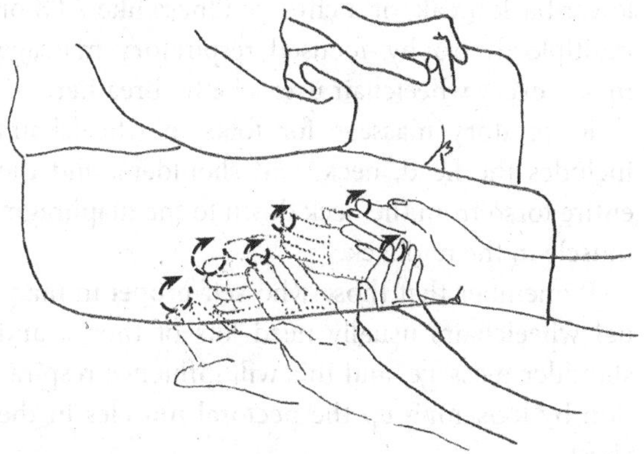

Levered massage along the length of the hamstring.

FIGURE 3.11. Foot Massage

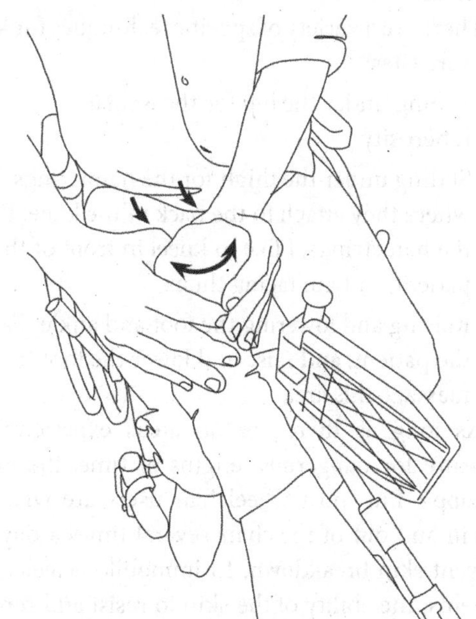

This figure shows a person in a wheelchair providing a foot massage. People in wheelchairs can give massages, as well as receive them, and reciprocity is important!

FIGURE 3.12. **Heliotherapy for Skin Health**

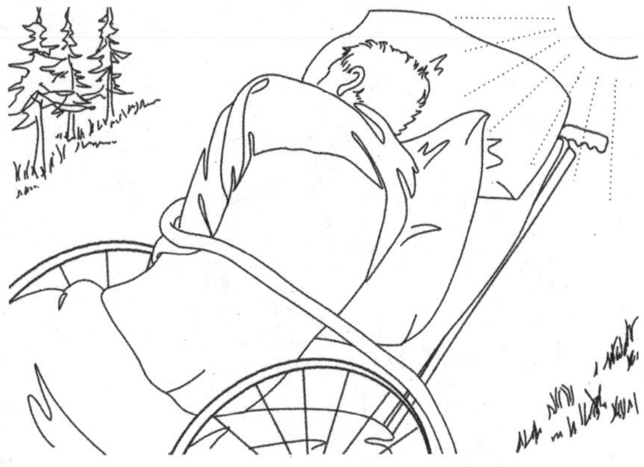

Levered massage is essential for gaining access: you slide your hands between the chair and the pressure point, using the chair to as a pivot to push your hands up into the body. Massaging in the wheelchair is probably my favorite place for levered fingertip kneading. This stroke allows wheelchair users to stay comfortable for long periods of time, because it can get to all those places that are hard to access when a person is seated in the chair.

There are a variety of specific techniques for key pressure sites:

1. Sliding under the hip for the ischial tuberosity.
2. Sliding under the thigh for the hamstrings where they attach to the back of the knee. For the hamstrings, I like to kneel in front of the patient, so I am facing them.
3. Raising and lowering the foot and ankle. Face the patient, and raise and lower the foot to massage this area.

As long as there are no areas experiencing pressure for dangerous lengths of time, the skin is happy. But most wheelchair users are wise to slip in and out of the chair several times a day to prevent skin breakdown. In immobile wheelchair patients, the ability of the skin to resist and repair is directly related to dry brushing, and applications of hot and cold temperatures, to get the skin reacting in a healthy and stimulating way.

Heliotherapy is a way of exposing the skin to ultraviolet rays that will disinfect and promote healing around the edges of ulcerations. It is also an excellent preventative for keeping the skin healthy and strong with measured exposures.

MUSCLES

The muscles that need attention are the muscles that would normally be moving the arms and legs, holding the head, and putting the feet on the ground. The person in the chair will be able to tell you after a series of massages what works for them to keep their limbs supple.

Self-massage is great for wheelchair users who have muscle strength in their arms and hands. They can do releasing, long, deep massage strokes for their forearm extensors and flexors. But the places that are hard to get to—the back of the shoulders and the back itself—require a therapist or a team member to help.

Wheelchair Massage for the Respiratory System

Everyone in a wheelchair benefits from massage for the upper and lower respiratory systems. Whether the person has a high-level spinal cord injury or a lower back break, or a chronic illness like ALS or multiple dystrophy, focused respiratory massage makes every wheelchair user a better breather!

Respiratory massage for folks in wheelchairs includes the head, neck, and shoulders, and the entire torso from the neck down to the diaphragm muscle in the midback.

Remember that those who self-propel in manual wheelchairs usually need lots of thorax and shoulder massage, and this will influence respiration by loosening up the pectoral muscles in the chest.

Prompting better breathing and lung health is extremely important for people in wheelchairs, especially those who have no use of their arms. These people are more susceptible to stiffening and developing contractures, which restricts movement in the truck and thorax. Even highly mobile wheelchair users are susceptible to lung congestion if they are not moving their arms over their head. For wheelchair people who can use their arms,

I always recommend the backstroke for swimming to mobilize the upper back with the shoulder muscles being stretched and strengthened.

The upper respiratory system is the place to start your wheelchair respiratory massage. The face and throat are often overlooked, and I like to emphasize the importance of this facial massage. Opening the sinuses is particularly beneficial for patients who have limited use of their shoulders and hands. For Barbara Turnbull, a high-level spinal cord injury patient with no use of her arms and limited use of her shoulders, her head was her only means of movement. Her lovely facial features were a delight to massage, and her upper respiratory breathing was always enhanced.

The same facial massage strokes outlined in our full body massage routines will open the sinuses and let the ears hear better. The work that I do around the ears has the effect of helping to open and stimulate the drainage of the eustachian tubes. I attribute my focus on temporal drainage around the ears to my first wheelchair facial massages with Barbara Turnbull. It is another case of the patient teaching the therapist!

For the diaphragm and thorax respiratory strokes, your patient's clothing can be lifted away from the skin so the respiratory strokes can be done more easily—for rib raking especially. Usually, I lift the person's shirt and, where possible, slip my hands underneath the clothing for these strokes.

Teaching productive coughing in the chair is also an important aspect of this respiratory treatment. I use all five percussive strokes: loose fingertip hacking, stiff fingertip hacking, cupping, beating, and pounding.

When using pounding with a person in a wheelchair, pull them forward so their lower back is about two or three inches away from the back

FIGURE 3.13. **Diaphragm and Thorax Respiratory Strokes in the Wheelchair**

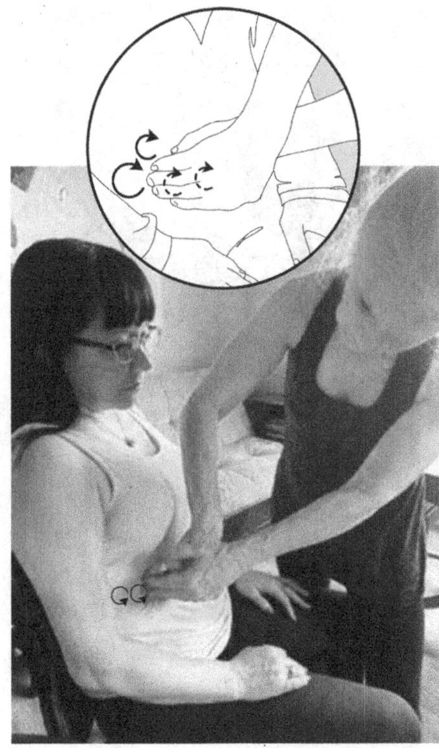

Reinforced fingertip kneading to diaphragmatic attachments.

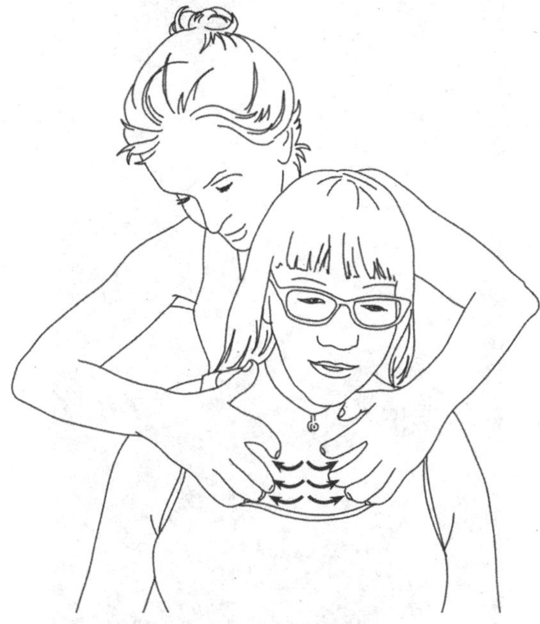

Skin-to-skin bilateral intercostal rib raking.

of the chair, so both your fists have room to roll (remember: it's an upward, rolling tapotement on the sacrum).

I use two postures for my wheelchair patients when doing percussive tapotement:

- I ask them to put their elbows on their knees and lean forward with their head down.
- I get them to lean forward onto the back of a chair or onto an eating tray, supported with pillows. For many wheelchair users, the tapotement treatment is easier to take with plenty of pillow support. I also often use a towel to cushion tapotement strokes for wheelchair patients.

Cupping is the most effective of all the percussive strokes for aiding in loosening material in the lungs and getting it up and out. The tempo can be fast for a superficial effect, or slow and plodding for a reverberating effect felt throughout the thorax.

In the wheelchair, single-handed cupping can be done to the upper respiratory system, using the other hand to hold the chair so it doesn't tip over. When the person is out of the chair, in bed at night or before they get up in the morning, this is the perfect time to put them in a side-lying position and apply cupping to the upper aspect of the ribs, which is often more accessible in this position than in the wheelchair.

I use compression when the patient is in the wheelchair, pressing on their upper chest and making sure the wheelchair is up against the wall so I don't tip their chair over. I do a lot of single-handed compression to the entire thorax by supporting the chair and patient with one hand while compressing with the other hand. I can use this

FIGURE 3.14. Percussive Strokes in the Wheelchair

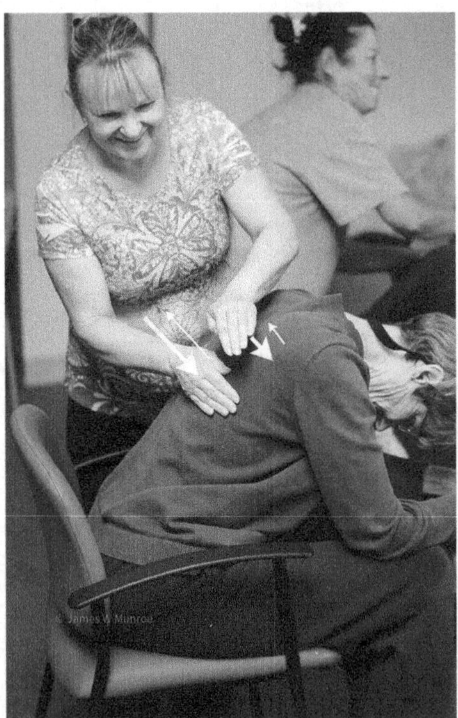

Percussive tapotement with the patient leaning forward on their elbows over their knees. Note the therapist's flat hands.

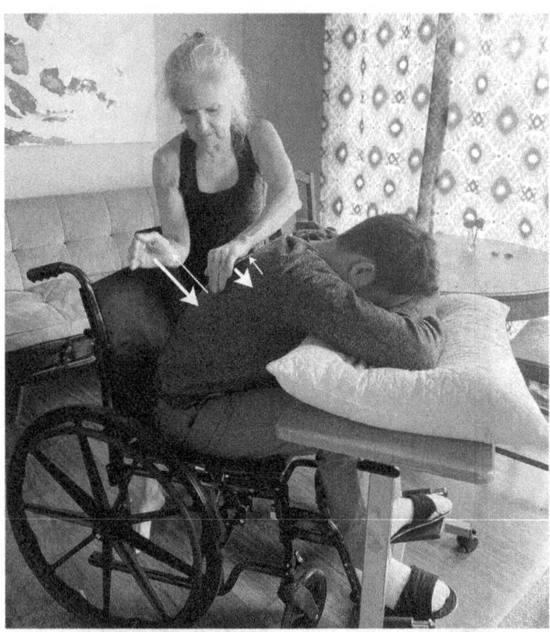

Cupping, with the patient leaning forward on a pillow. Note the therapist's C-shaped hands.

supported, single-handed compression along the front of the thorax or down on top of the shoulders or leaning the person forward in the chair. I can use single-handed compression throughout the posterior aspect of the thorax, all the way up and down the back.

Always allow time for coughing: it will start as the patient straightens up.

Using thorax compression can be lifesaving if the person in the chair is choking on sputum or food. During a workshop at GF Strong in Vancouver, a hospital attendant used lifesaving compression to dislodge a large amount of phlegm that was choking a patient. This patient happily recovered from the strongest compression ever. I have never administered that kind of force, but have successfully produced lots of expectoration with a combination of compression and cupping.

INHALATIONS BEFORE, DURING, OR AFTER RESPIRATORY MASSAGE

If a patient has a cold or cough, I usually give a steam-tent inhalation using drops of eucalyptus and other carminative oils to open up the breathing. This can be done by using a towel as a tent to trap the steam over a basin of hot water on the patient's eating tray, which I've rolled over their lap. I usually end the entire full body massage with a carminative lotion for a lasting effect.

Full Body Massage in Wheelchairs

Principles of Full Body Massage in Wheelchairs

1. Remember that all wheelchair users have neck issues for your massage focus, so I start at the neck working from the side or back of the chair while I collect information for my massage routine, timing, and focus.
2. Focus your massage on the pressure sites for seated posture of your wheelchair user.
3. Focus on the user's needs (i.e., if an arm mobility person, start on the arms and shoulders).
4. If the person has no strength in their arms or use of their arms, start with the legs to spend plenty of time reducing swelling, mobilizing the joints, and preventing pressure sores in the hips and heels.
5. If the person is fully dressed, work without oil (a common sense approach) and use lubricant where there is skin exposure (hands, feet and face).
6. Start your massage wherever the current issues lie. Constipation, for instance, requires massage to the back, abdomen, hips, and legs, and then leg pumping, so you can start in any of these areas for quicker relief. Respiratory focus for everyday cough, cold, or sinus problems would include more rib raking, tapotement, nasal root shaking, etc., so dedicating more time to the upper and lower respiratory systems is indicated during your full body massage routine. For rib raking, you might need to straddle the patient's knees, with your foot between the knees, in order to wrap way around the back to the ribs. I wedge myself up against the wheelchair when rib raking to get a good grip.
7. Adapt your hydrotherapy: put heating pads down the back of the chair, use hot water bottles for the abdomen and feet to keep the hands and feet warm. I use hot neck packs around the patient's neck while I am massaging elsewhere, and before and after the neck massage. For skin that is sensitive to cold, I also heat the massage oil. Remember that the Kneipp cold wash (with or without added witch hazel or rubbing alcohol) for each part of the body in a "clothes off" full body massage is excellent for stimulating the circulation, especially with wheelchair users' compromised lower extremities. Even a clothes-on, full body massage in the wheelchair can have a cold or contrasting hydrotherapy application for the feet with socks off!
8. Adapt the length of time for your massage to the setting, location, and activity. Sideline sports massage might last the length of a game intermission. With limited visitor hospital times, you can employ the whole family, one on each extremity, for a full body ten-minute massage.

FIGURE 3.15. Compression in the Wheelchair

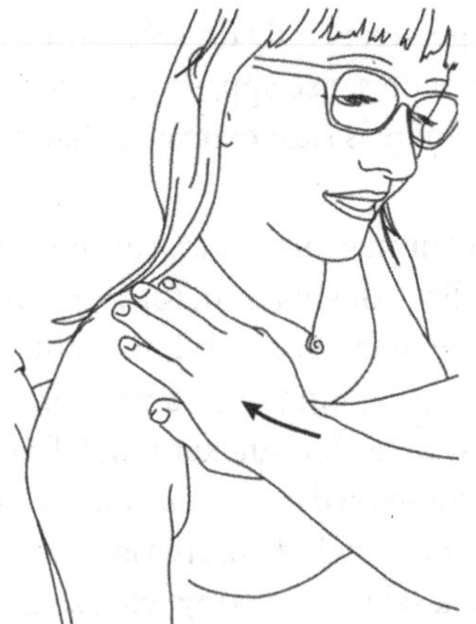

Reinforced palmar compression.

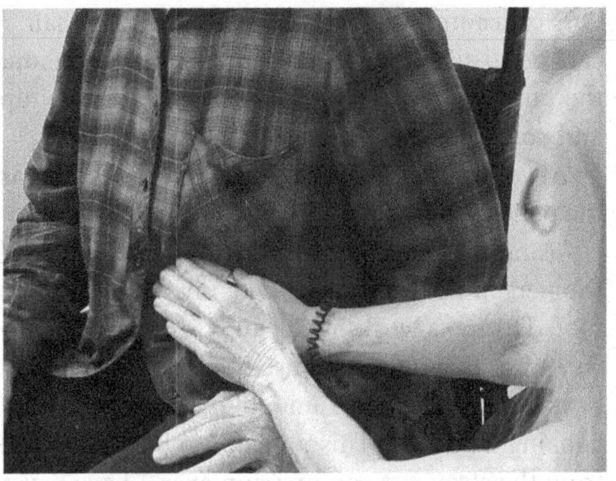

Reinforced palmar compression to lower lung lobe.

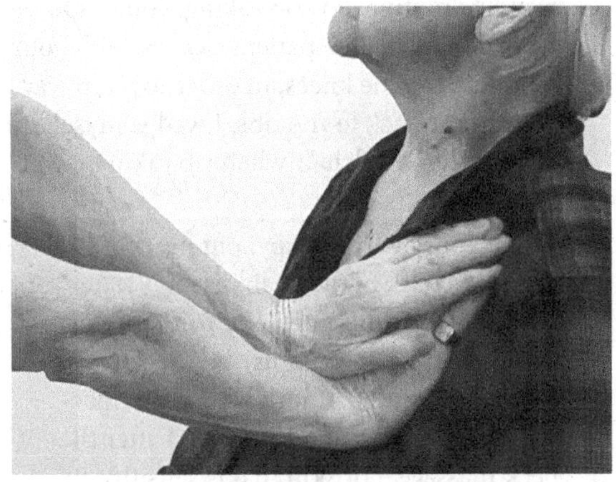

Reinforced palmar compression to upper lung lobe.

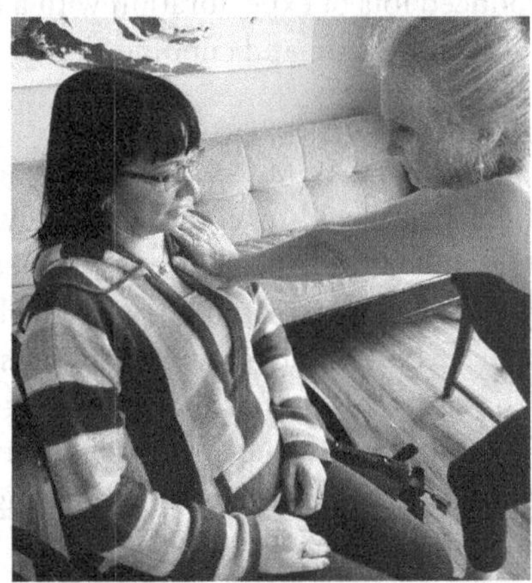

Reinforced palmar chest compression, stride stance.

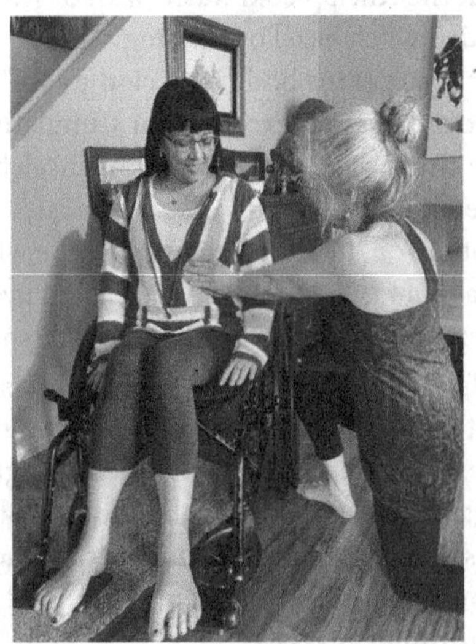

Reinforced palmar chest compression, half-kneeling stance.

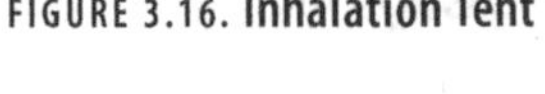

FIGURE 3.16. Inhalation Tent

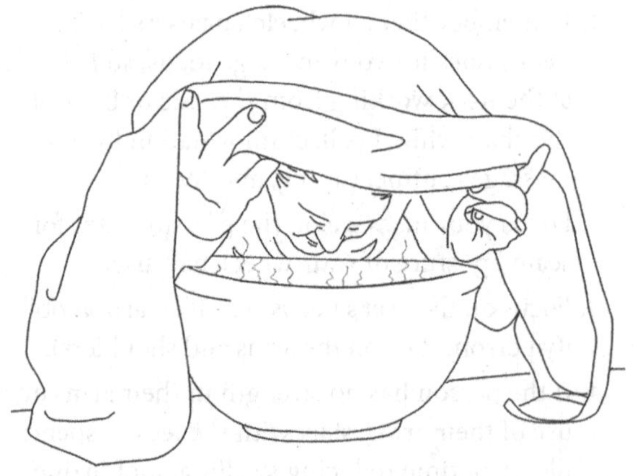

9. We are talking about massage in the wheelchair in this chapter, but you should practice your wheelchair transfers for situations where massaging out of the chair is best. Use massage to ease transfer preparations and completions, making both arrivals and departures a better experience. Pre-transfer massage gives people better flexibility in their body and a positive tactile message as you transfer them to the new location.

FIGURE 3.17. Sympathetic and Parasympathetic Nervous Systems

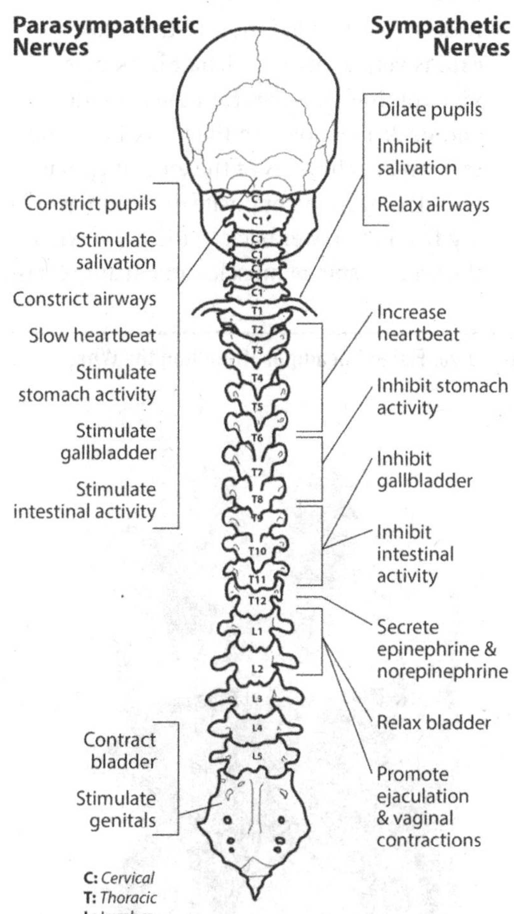

Massage works with the parasympathetic nervous system, which induces calm in the body. By contrast, the sympathetic nervous system helps the body respond to danger.

10. Most importantly, use the "f-word" constantly: feedback, feedback, feedback! Your massage will not be perfect unless the person on the receiving end is also your instructor!

Routines for Full Body Massage in Wheelchairs

The routines for full body wheelchair massage can be done in ten minutes or an hour, with one or more people. They can be done a number of times throughout the day (or night), in a variety of locations ranging from bed to desk, indoors to outdoors. You can give a wheelchair massage under the stars! Whether your wheelchair massage recipient is active, going to work every day, or on a wheelchair sports team, or nearing the end of their life, be sure to encourage them to rest for ten to twenty minutes after you finish the full body massage. This gives you time to run an Epsom salt bath, if that is an option, and also gives the receiver a chance to let the benefits of the massage settle in through relaxation.

BACK MASSAGE

Straddle the wheel of the wheelchair, so one foot is in stride position along the back of the chair.

1. With one arm, reach across the front of the patient and cup the far shoulder. This arm will prevent the person from tipping forward.
2. Slide your other hand between the chair back and the person's back. Bend your hand along the base of the fingers, keeping the fingers together, straight, and stiff so they can have the power to penetrate. Lift your fingertips into the patient's back muscles by pushing the back of your hand into the back of the chair and levering away from the chair. This levering motion is the key to getting the most power for depth. Be careful to check the pressure, as just a little levering gives deep penetration into the muscles.
   - Use single-handed fingertip kneading (levering from the back of the wheelchair), thumb kneading, palmar kneading, and fisted kneading intermittently on the lower back, between the shoulder blades, and

FIGURE 3.18. **Levering in Back Massage**

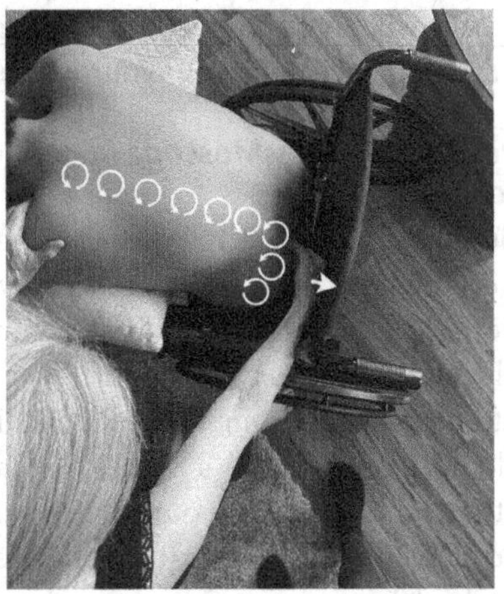

Push the back of your hand into the back of the chair and lever away from the chair into the muscles of the patient's back. To continue levering as you move up the back, have your patient sit up in their chair.

up and down along the spine between the erector spinae muscles that run parallel to the spine and the spine itself. There is a nice groove to fit into between the bony spine and the cord-like muscles of the erector spinae, which run from the sacrum to the base of the skull.

- Palmer stretching strokes, when done in the wheelchair, usually involve bunching up the clothing, which makes it a challenge. Do this slowly to allow all types of clothing to be accommodated. I often do the stroke in the most convenient clothing-bunching direction (i.e., palmar strokes down the back smooth clothing, palmar strokes up the back bunch clothing!).
- I use single-handed thumb stretching extensively in my wheelchair back massage routine, moving from the shoulders and neck area down to the lower back and sacrum attachments of the erector spinae muscles, or in the opposite direction, working from the lower back to the neck, where the erector spinae muscles attach at the base

FIGURE 3.19. **Fingertip Kneading, Straddling the Wheel**

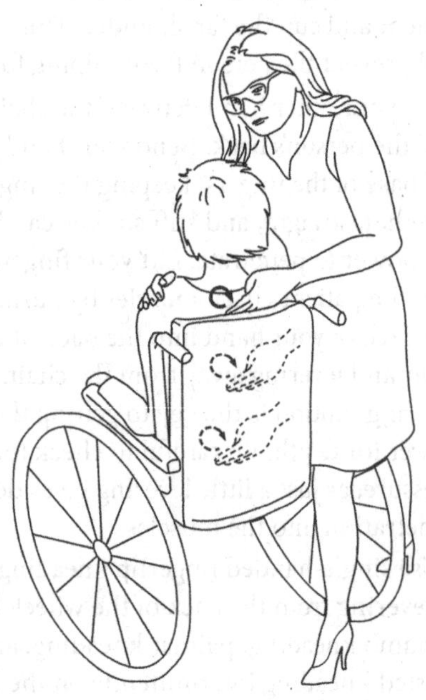

FIGURE 3.20. **Fisted Kneading, Straddling the Wheel**

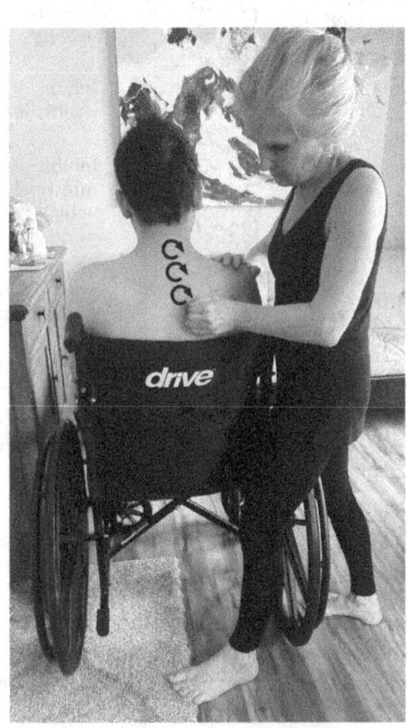

FIGURE 3.21. Tandem fisted rhomboid kneading

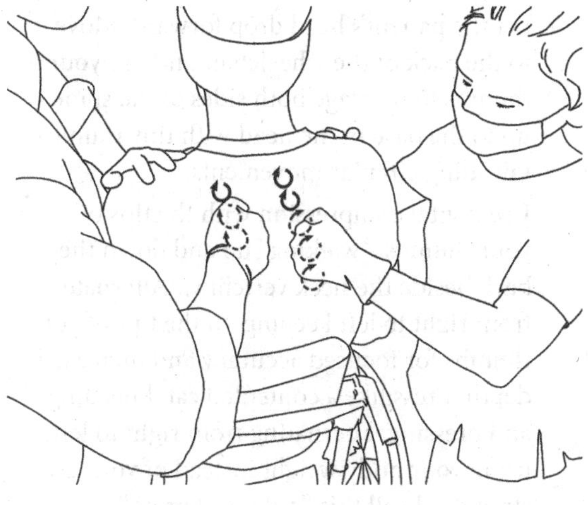

FIGURE 3.22. Levered bilateral two-handed fingertip kneading

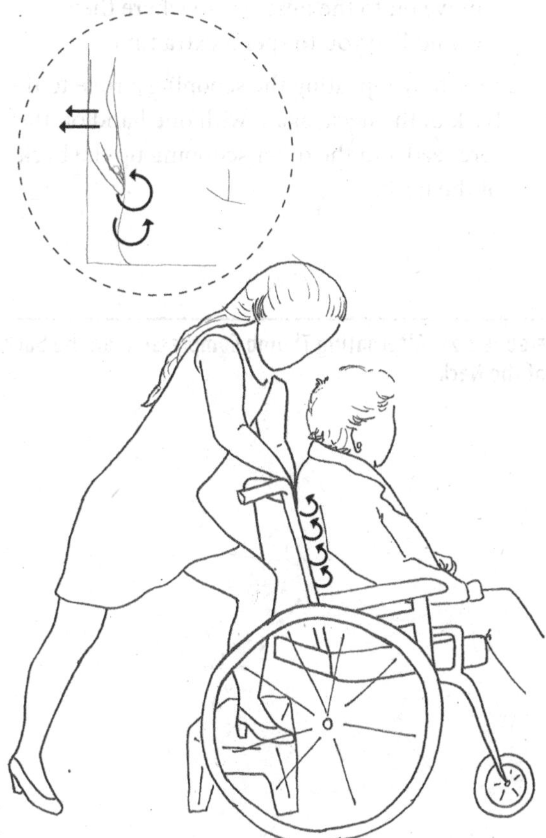

Stand on a stool, if that gives you better access.

of the skull. I find it easier when the person is in the chair to go from the top down. This can be done through pajamas and clothing, but is most easily done skin on skin.

3. Move to the other side of the chair to balance yourself and the massage experience for the person on the receiving end and repeat.

Bilateral Two-Handed Technique

Shorter people may want to stand on a stool for this technique.

1. Standing behind the chair, slide both hands down the back toward the seat of the wheelchair (between the chair back and the patient's back). Sliding hands down is easy if the patient is tiny or they are wearing slippery fabric. If your hands are sticking to their clothing or unable to slide downward, you must lift the person with one hand in order to slide the other hand down without getting stuck. When you arrive at the bottom of your reach or hit the chair seat, put your chin on the patient's shoulder, again striding back from the chair.
   - If you are tall, you might be whispering in their ear instead of resting a chin on the shoulder. Everyone is a different height and all patients are different heights in the wheelchair.
2. Then lift up with your fingertips on both hands at the same time, into the patient's back muscles under their hips or lower back and stay there for about two minutes, easing up the tension in the gluteal muscles and lower back and helping to prevent pressure sores in this area.
3. Work your way up the back very slowly with levered fingertip kneading. Ask the patient about their favorite spots to linger longer with your back massage.
   - You can also use compression on the lower back. I change my wheelchair user's posture to lean forward in the chair, elbows on knees and head dropped chin to chest, allowing the long spinal muscles to stretch.

If my wheelchair person is using a chair that has a removable back or removable sides, I can work all around the available hip and gluteal muscles for lower back relief and many other areas of the body, repeatedly compressing and releasing tight muscles.

NECK MASSAGE

1. Standing at the side of the wheelchair, put one hand on the person's forehead. With the other hand, massage their neck muscles in an upward scooping motion. Have a *C*-shape to the massage hand. Do this for three or four minutes before moving on.
2. Let the patient's head drop forward. Move to the back of the wheelchair and use your thumbs to massage both sides of the spine up to the base of the head with tiny thumb-kneading circular movements.
3. Use digital compression with the tips of your thumbs, "walking" up and down the back beside the neck vertebrae. Alternate from right to left keeping on the tips of your thumbs for focused accuracy and increased depth. Press like a contented cat, kneading and pressing, alternating from right to left, using your body weight instead of your arm strength. I call this "poke and press."
   - Your patient will have some favorite spots where they are hoping you will spend all your time massaging, so ask before you move on to the next stroke where they would like you to spend extra time.
4. Finish by repeating the scooping stroke to the back of the neck, again with one hand on the forehead and the other scooping up the back of the neck.

FIGURE 3.23. **Bilateral two-handed effleurage**

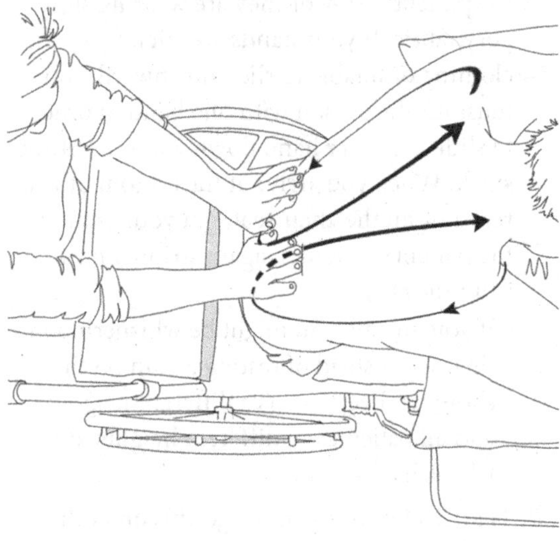

FIGURE 3.24. **Compression**

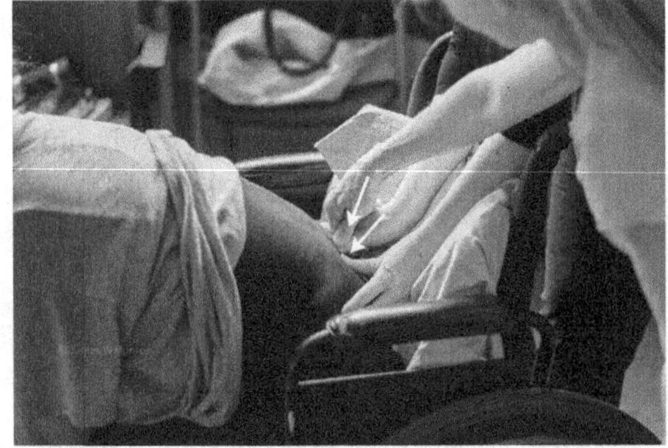

Compression eases the muscles of the lower back.

FIGURE 3.25. **Alternating Thumb Compression on the Back of the Neck**

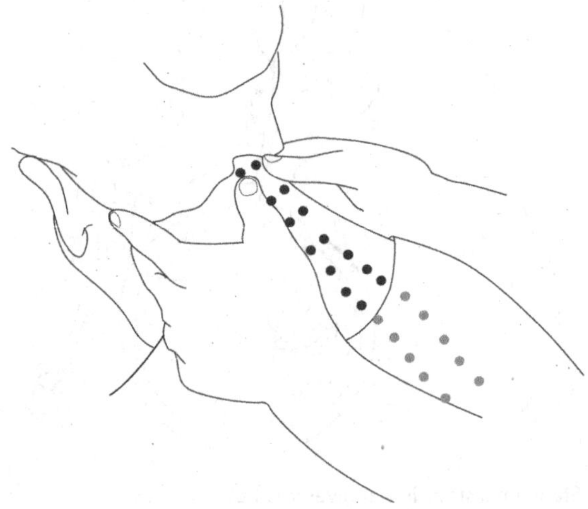

ARM AND HAND MASSAGE

1. Effleurage by placing both hands beside each other wrapped across the person's arm starting at their hand and moving upward to the top of the shoulder. Wrap your hands around the shoulder from front to back and then glide lightly back to the hands on either side of the arm without pressure. Never use pressure in a downward direction on the extremities. Move your effleurage three times up and down the arms.

FIGURE 3.26. Single-Handed Scooping Neck Massage

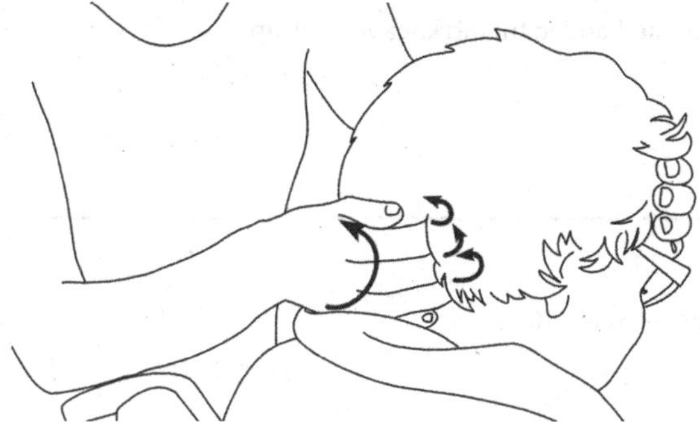

The head here is flexed forward with forehead support.

FIGURE 3.27. Arm Effleurage

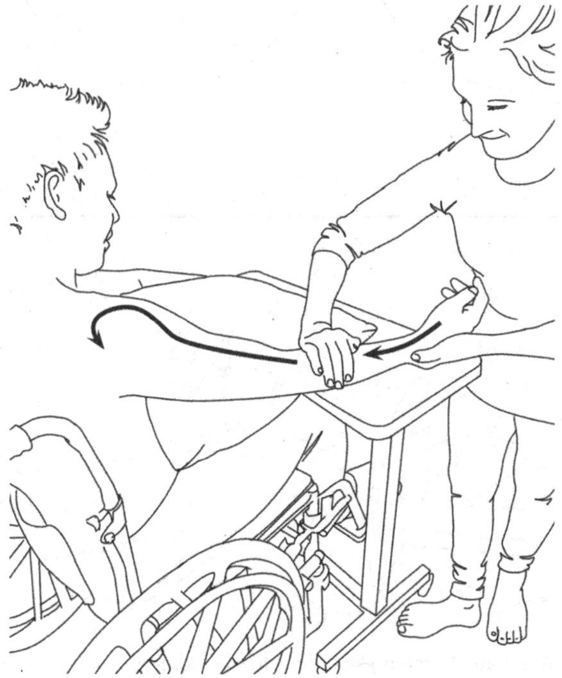

2. On the third up, stop at the shoulder with a reinforced palmer kneading to the deltoid shoulder muscle. This opens up the circulation to the whole arm.
3. Work your way down the arm with alternate thumb kneading, again always pushing the pressure up toward the heart. Massage the biceps with alternate thumb kneading, and the triceps with single-handed thumb kneading.
4. Cup the elbow and palmar knead the whole elbow joint. Use alternate thumb kneading all around the elbow joint thoroughly and focus extra time at the elbow where there are concentrations of muscle and tendon attachments.
   - The inner elbow is very sensitive and often a favorite spot for you to linger, especially for those who are strong enough to push their own chairs. For people who do not wheel themselves, massaging this area will prevent the elbow from becoming fixed and stiff. Similarly, massaging the forearm will help to prevent the hand from permanently contracting.
5. I use single-handed thumb kneading on the inner and outer aspects of the forearm. This is very relaxing for the person on the receiving end of the massage.
6. Focus on the wrist with tiny alternate thumb kneading. Your patient will think that they are in heaven!
7. The hand massage is a popular part of the wheelchair massage, especially for people who self-propel.
   - First massage the back of the hand with alternate thumb kneading.
   - Then massage individual fingers by corkscrewing them with a direction away from the center finger, which can be corkscrewed either or both ways. Massage each finger three times in this twisting motion. Don't

FIGURE 3.28. Alternate Thumb Kneading: Biceps, Triceps

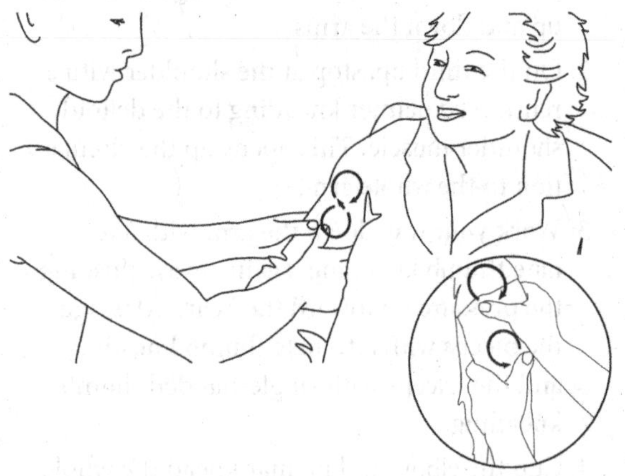

Alternate thumbing kneading, biceps.

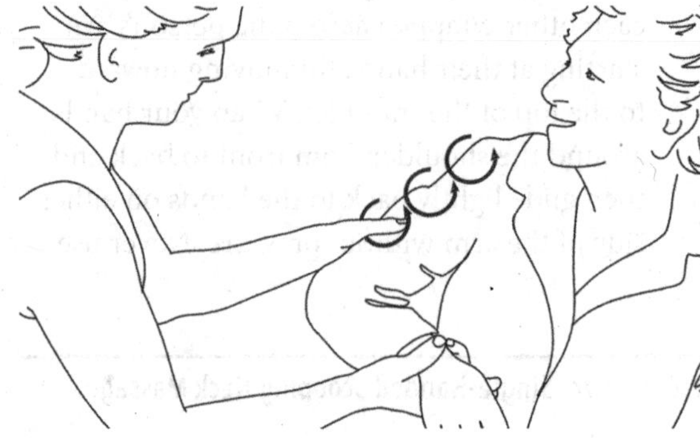

Single-handed thumb kneading, triceps.

FIGURE 3.29. Elbow Massage

SINGLE-HANDED PALMAR KNEADING

ALTERNATE THUMB KNEADING

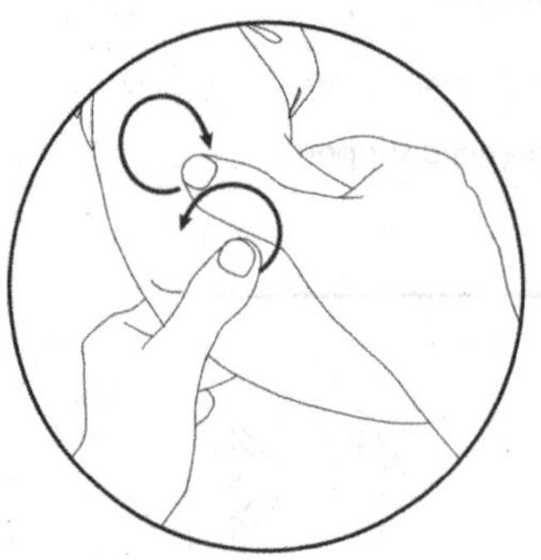

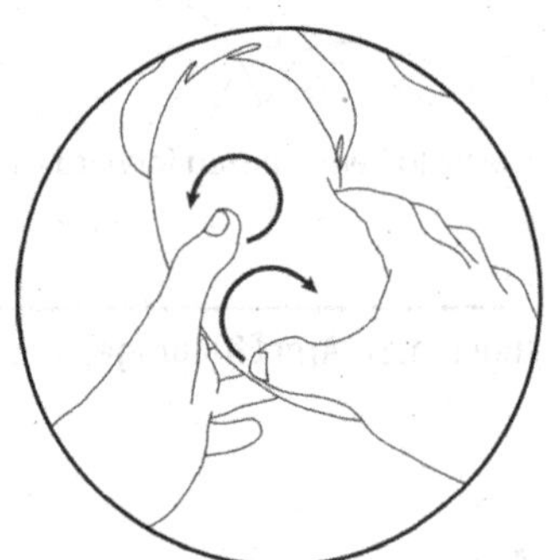

FIGURE 3.30. Forearm Massage

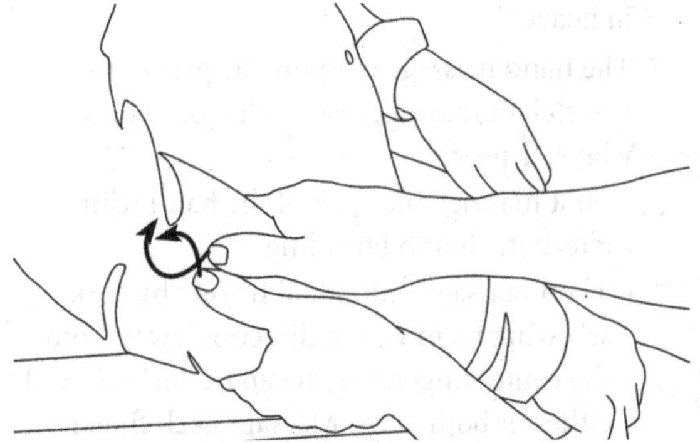

Alternate thumbing kneading, back of forearm.

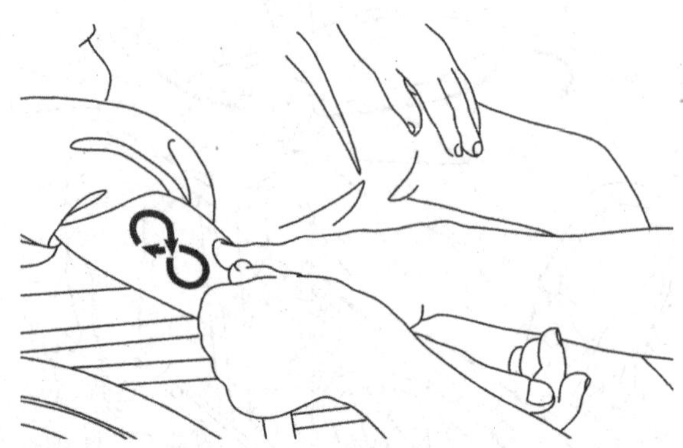

Alternate thumbing kneading, front of forearm.

worry: it will feel natural to do it in one direction and unnatural to do it in the wrong direction!

- The palm of the patient's hand requires a completely different direction of pressure. Although I have instructed all pressure to be upward toward the heart, for the hand I change things. Tilt the patient's hand so it is in a halt position. Grasp the wrist with both hands and, with your thumbs, massage the heel of the hand and work toward the base of each finger with teeny-weeny alternate thumb kneading. People just love this special hand massage.

8. At the end of the arm massage, I do some light reflex stroking, without any pressure, from the shoulder to the fingertips three times.

FIGURE 3.30. CONTINUED

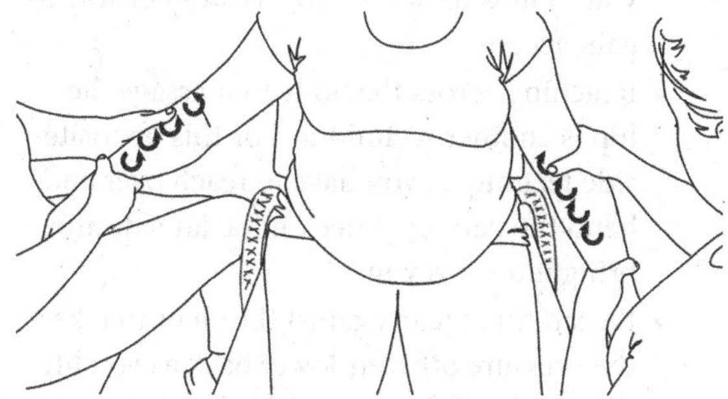

Tandem single-handed thumb kneading, forearm.

FIGURE 3.31. Wrist Massage

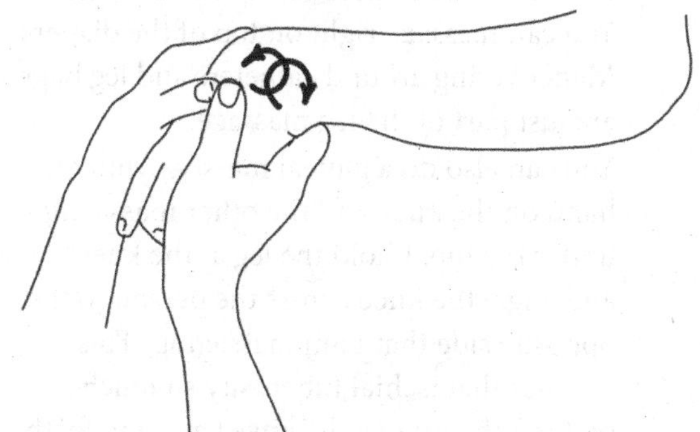

Alternate thumb kneading, wrist.

LEG MASSAGE

The entire leg massage can be done in the wheelchair with the person's legs elevated for comfort, to prevent swelling, and for therapeutic postural stretching.

The leg massage includes the hips, thighs, knees, lower legs, and feet.

At the beginning of a leg massage, I use a standing stride position for massaging the hip and thigh, then I squat or sit for the lower leg and kneecap rub. Then I get a stool and sit (you could also squat) for the lower leg work and foot massage, or I find a pillow so I can sit on the floor and spend a lot of time helping with the swelling and giving a longer foot massage.

Be sure to navigate around drains and tubes. Many people in wheelchairs have urinary pouches or catheter drains that run down the leg to a urinary reservoir strapped to the lower leg.

FIGURE 3.32. Hand Massage

ALTERNATE THUMB KNEADING: BACK OF HAND WITH HAND FISTED

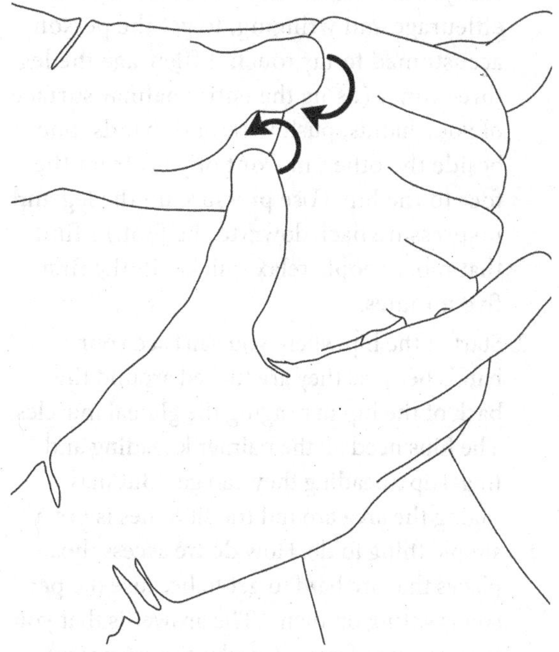

Note that this stroke goes opposite to the principle of massaging toward the heart.

FIGURE 3.32. CONTINUED

ALTERNATE THUMB KNEADING: PALM

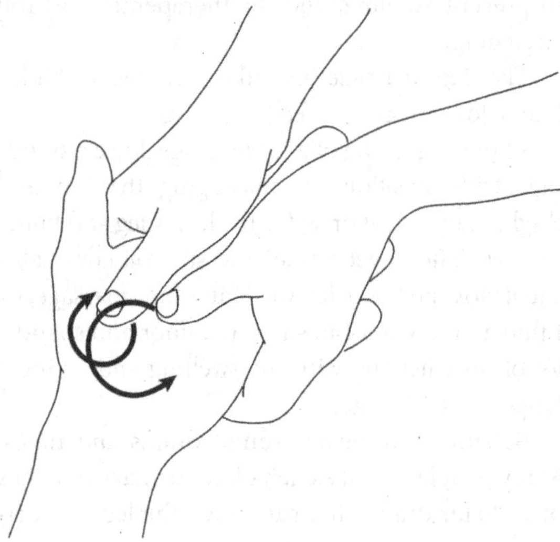

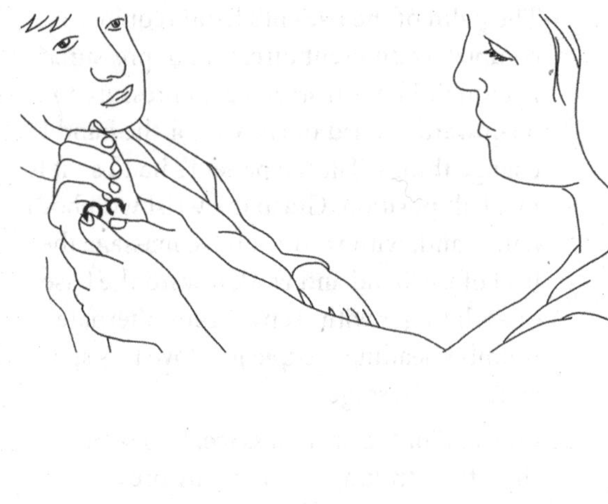

1. I always start massaging at the top of the leg to open up the circulation to the entire extremity. If you take the tension off the top of the leg, the contents will flow more easily. I use broad-based strokes, such as effleurage and wringing, to get the person accustomed to my touch. Effleurage the leg three times (using the entire palmar surface of your hands, push with both hands, one beside the other, in front of you) from the foot to the hip. (Use pressure up the leg and no pressure back down to the foot.) I find that most people relax quickly in the first five minutes.
2. Start at the hip where you can't see your hands because they are tucked around the back of the hip massaging the gluteal muscles. The hips need all the palmer kneading and fingertip kneading they can get. But massaging the area around the sit bones is not a simple thing to do. How do we access those places that are hard to get to because the person is sitting on them? The answer is that you have to work from all angles to gain access.
   - Slide both hands under the patient's hip and lift your fingertips.
   - You can also lift the patient's leg and slide your hands under the hip as another way to gain access.
   - Reaching across the body to massage the hip is another technique. For this opposite-side technique, you have to reach over and bend the patient's knee on the far side and bring it toward you.
   - Be careful to lean against the chair to take the pressure off your lower back as you lift the weight of the person's body onto your fingertips. The person usually has diapers on, and some have tubes and drains that can be a challenge. Experience teaches you to work around these common obstacles. You can massage right on top of the diapers. Maneuvering around catheters and leg bags are just part of the leg massage.
   - You can also do a gluteal massage with one hand on the knee and the other massaging under the hip. I hold the leg at the knee and angle the knee across the person to the opposite side that I am massaging. This exposes that ischial tuberosity so much better. I then move the knee back and forth across the person as I knead the gluteal

FIGURE 3.33. **Leg Effleurage**

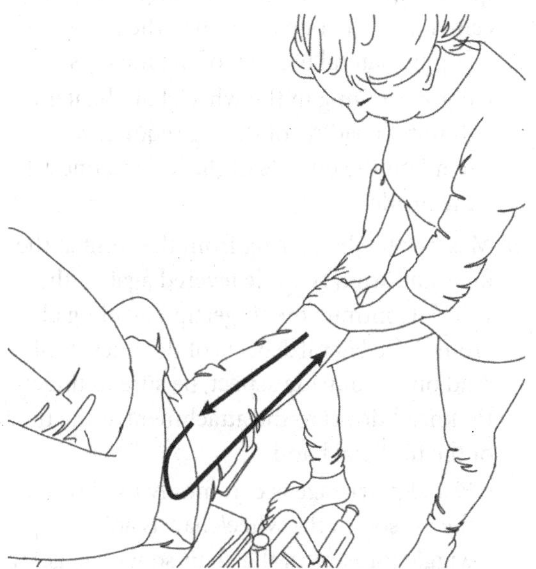

Put your foot on the patient's footrest and place the patient's leg across your bent knee.

muscles with my fingertips. This extra movement helps get deeper into the muscle group. Then add in the fingertip kneading and the hip is getting a double work out! Ask for feedback. Ask about the depth of pressure, as everyone is different. Ask about how deep to go with this stroke combo. Remember: the weight of the person is sitting on your fingertips!

3. Wring across the leg, wrapping your hands right under the leg to include the hamstrings. You can massage both legs from the same side of the chair or walk around the chair to the other side. Reach across and lean against the arm of the chair to prevent using your lower back, but to give you strength for your pull and push in this wringing to the thigh muscles.
   - For wheelchair users, wringing is easiest to do out of the chair, because you have good access to work up and down the entire

FIGURE 3.34. **Levered Fingertip Kneading: Sit Bones**

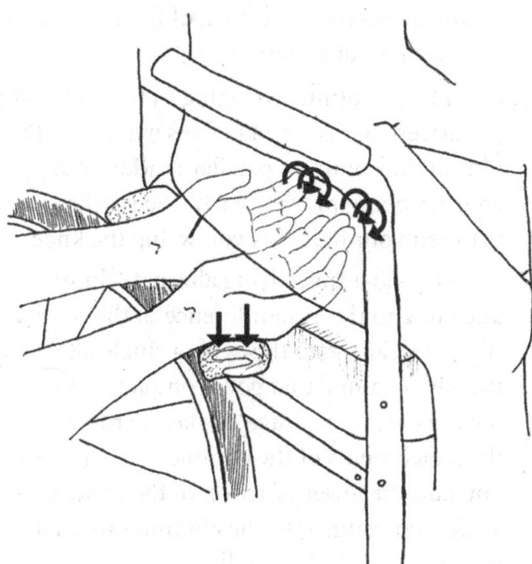

This shows the stroke from the side of the chair.

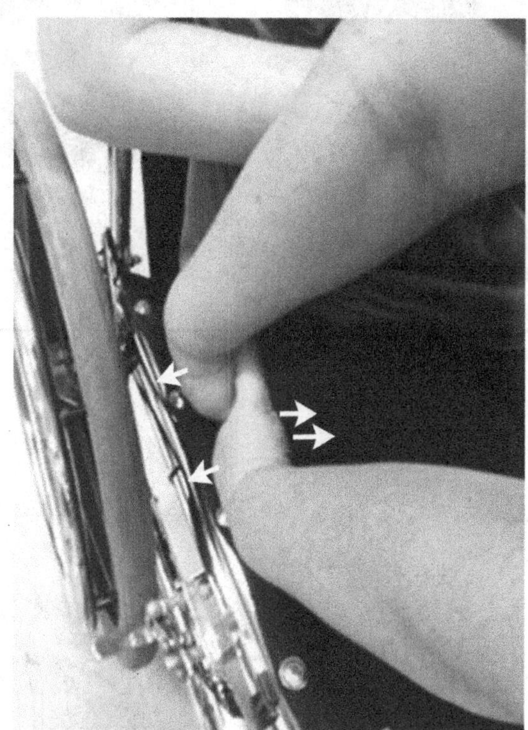

This shows reaching across the body to massage under the hip.

leg. When massaging in the chair, you can still wrap around to the back of the leg: it just takes practice. Lifting the foot up, with the knee bent, allows easier access: wrap your hands around the underside muscle for a more thorough wringing.

FIGURE 3.35. **Single-Handed Gluteal Massage**

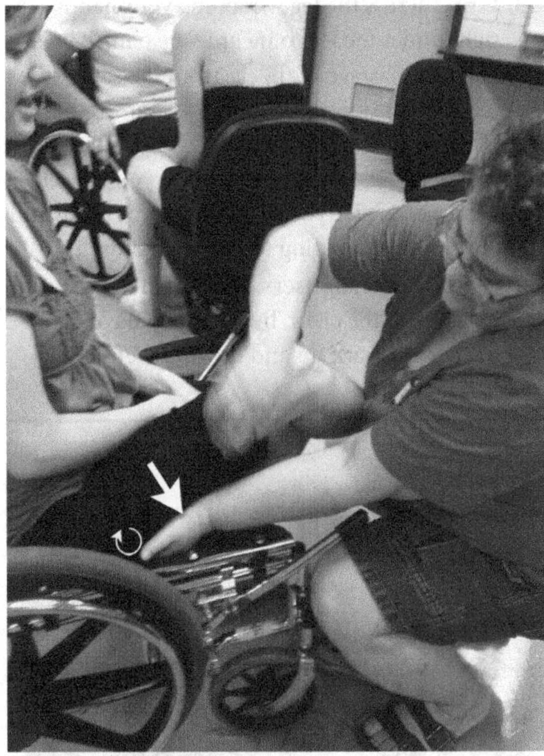

FIGURE 3.36. **Wringing the Lower Leg**

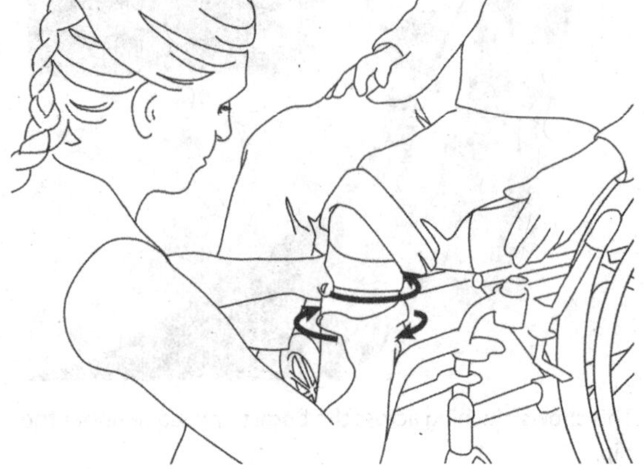

4. Use lots of alternate thumb kneading to the quadriceps on the top of the thigh down the center, and then up and down the two sides, along the lateral borders of the muscles.
   - For massaging in the wheelchair, bilateral thumb kneading of the leg requires one hand on the outside of the leg and one on the inside.
5. Massage the hamstring from the front at the knee and from the side levered against the wheel. Continue the fingertip kneading all around the lateral aspects of the knee itself. And on the outside aspect, be sure to fingertip knead down to the attachment at the tibia of the iliotibial band.
   - Fisted petrissage is commonly used when the person in the wheelchair is able to wiggle forward in the chair so we can get up and behind the back of the knee when the knee is bent in a seated position. I go as far as I can up the underside of the hamstrings by lifting the person's foot up onto my knee or my thigh, giving me better access to the hamstrings from the back of the knee up to the ischial tuberosity.
6. Be sure to continue wringing to the end of the quadriceps across the knee inserting into the tibia at the common patellar tendon. Adapt your wringing to "sandwich" the patella between your hands as you wring the knee.
7. I like to add a special, big alternate thumb kneading to the circumference of the patella (the kneecap). I do this with a single alternate thumb kneading that goes completely around the knee with one huge stroke. It crosses over the attachments of the common patellar tendon and the lower junction of the quadriceps as they converge into the common patellar tendon housing the patella.
   - Then I concentrate on the attachments of the hamstrings at either side of the knee, in the back at the outside edge, pulling toward myself with bilateral fingertip kneading, massaging both sides at the same time with focused fingertip kneading.

- If the person can move their legs, I get them to extend the lower leg so the muscle attachments on either side of the knee bounce out and identify themselves under my fingertips.

8. The lower leg gets a lot of focused alternate thumb kneading to the tibialis anterior, which is on the outside of the ridge of the tibia (shinbone). The massage goes from immediately below the knee to the toes, massaging up and down for three intervals.
9. The back of the lower leg is massaged in an upward "milking" motion with alternate palmer kneading, lifting up with each stroke from the Achilles tendon to the back of the knee. Anchor the patient's foot down with your foot or knee, so when you "milk" the calf muscle, you do not lift the foot each time. Massage in strong upward lifting strokes.
10. Squeeze the patient's foot firmly a number of times. Use wringing and alternate thumb kneading bilateral to the ankle.
    - Sometimes it is important to leave the patient's shoes on so their feet don't swell. If the foot is free, massage the heel of the foot with the heel of your hand in circular palmer kneading. Work the sole of the foot with alternate thumb kneading. Use two-handed calcaneus kneading to pressure sites, bilateral thumb kneading to the malleoli, alternate thumb kneading to the dorsal and plantar surfaces, and corkscrewing on the toes. Use overhanded stiff-fingered palmar percussive strokes to the soles.
    - You can lift the foot up so the sole of the foot is facing you and you can deliver some alternating digital thumb pressure (a poke and press). This is a favorite if the person can feel their feet.

FIGURE 3.37. **Alternate Thumb Kneading: Knee**

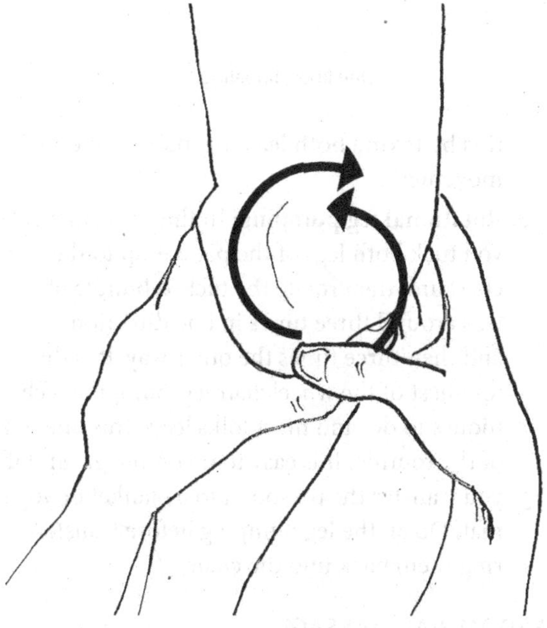

FIGURE 3.38. **Alternate Thumb Kneading: Tibialis Anterior**

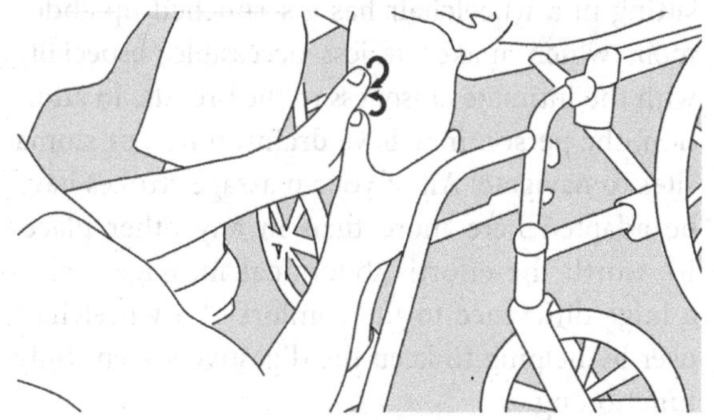

LEG PUMPING

Leg pumping can tip over a wheelchair. Make sure to have the brakes on, and back the wheelchair up against a wall or something solid.

The point of abdominal leg pumping is to press the knees to the chest and to mechanically move the digestive organs, pressing them down and releasing. As I explained earlier, leg pumping really helps the digestion start moving, so you might get sound effects! It can be done before the tummy massage or after the abdomen is finished.

I use all three styles of leg pumping with wheelchair patients: alternate, simultaneous, and rotational leg and hip movements. One person can do it alone, but it's ideal for two people to work together. This is a great opportunity to involve a member of the family who needs to feel useful.

1. **Alternate leg pumping with two people:** While I pump the leg I am holding, the other

FIGURE 3.39. Milking the Calf, Foot Anchored Three Ways

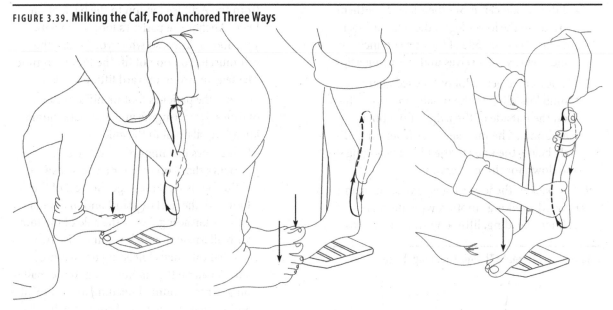

One foot, half kneeling. Both feet, standing. One knee, kneeling.

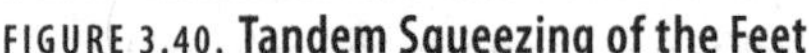

FIGURE 3.40. Tandem Squeezing of the Feet

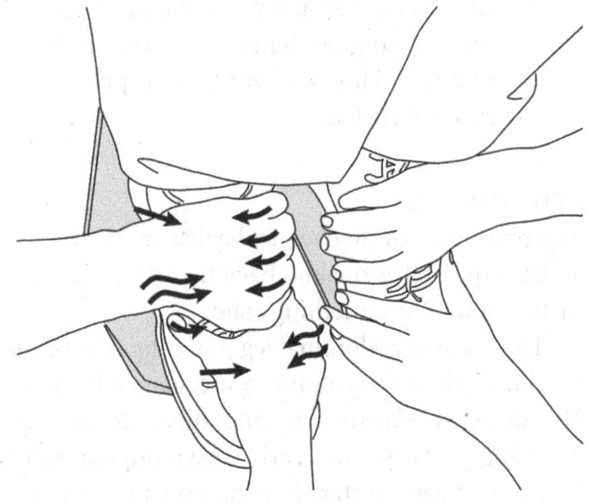

person holds the other leg and waits. When I finish pumping and straighten my leg out, they start bending the leg they are holding into the abdomen. We repeat this motion again and again in a continuous movement like walking.

2. **Simultaneous leg pumping with two people:** Together, we bend the patient's knees to their chest and then stretch out the legs. It is easier with two, but one person can perform this by taking both legs together in one movement.
3. **Rotational leg pumping:** In this movement, you tuck both legs of the patient up to the chest and then rotate the tucked bundle of legs around three times in one direction and then three times the other way. It is the toughest of the wheelchair leg-pumping techniques to do, and most folks leave this one out of the routine. It is easy to do on the ground if you transfer the person onto a blanket or yoga mat. Do all the leg pumping before transferring them back into the chair.

ABDOMINAL MASSAGE

The abdomen is an important focus for massage of wheelchair users and often gets left out. A person sitting in a wheelchair has a scrunched up abdomen, which makes it less accessible, especially with the intimate closeness of the breasts. In addition, the person may have drains, tubes, or stoma sites to navigate. All of your massage strokes have be adapted here more than in any other place. It's worth the effort! Abdominal massage makes a huge difference to the comfort of a wheelchair user by helping to keep the digestive system fully functioning.

1. Start with palmar kneading to the anterior (front) of the abdomen. Standing or sitting or kneeling at the side of the chair, use overhanded palmer kneading (or single-handed or reinforced palmar kneading) over the entire abdominal area. Start on the patient's right side in the lower corner near the hip and travel up to the ribs, then across to the left side and down.
2. Sandwich the abdomen, with one palm on the front of the abdomen and one hand on the person's back.
   - Standing to the side of the chair, move both hands in circles at the same speed and in the same direction. Then move them in alternating directions.
   - Do this at least three times slowly and firmly, getting feedback from the person about your pressure. Most people are too light with this stroke. It needs to be firm to help alleviate constipation.
3. Single-handed fingertip kneading is performed in the same direction, lingering in each of the four corners of the abdomen. The four corners are located in the lower and upper corners next to the hipbones and ribs. Alternate between big palmer strokes and tiny fingertip strokes.
4. Keeping your hands still in one place, continue with a palmar vibration on the abdomen. Use your palms one on top of the other or side by side on the tummy. I usually place one of my hands on the back of the person, between the chair and their back, as I use my other hand to do a single-handed vibration. I like to keep up the palmar vibrations for about three minutes so it can have a penetrating effect. This is very important for pain management. The longer you keep up this stroke, the more effective and far-reaching it is for reducing pain. It overrides the painful contracting of the abdominal muscles.
5. Finish with light reflex stroking in the same direction as digestive movement, using a very light touch and a continuous momentum. This stroking is like numbing the area so the person cannot feel the discomfort below the touch. Maintain this stroke for minutes, not seconds, for the best results.

FACE AND SCALP MASSAGE

Adapting the regular massage for face and scalp to the wheelchair is a matter of adjusting your posture and seeing how you can more easily get to all the places with the person sitting up. You can stand behind the person, or if that is not possible, in front of the person. Sometimes by standing at the back of the chair, the patient is too high up for you to reach around to the front of their face, so come around the front and massage them face to face. The following stroke sequence can be done in either position.

1. Start by bilaterally massaging the temples with your fingertips along the hairline. Ask for feedback about your pressure. Move your fingertips to the jaw and get the patient to wiggle their jaw from side to side so you can feel the ligaments move under your fingertip kneading. Use your pointer finger to massage in the little notch in front of the ears. You can tilt the person's head back so it is resting on you or on a small pillow that you can insert behind the head for support. Make sure the person can still swallow and their head is not too far back for comfort.
2. Do some firm thumb stroking to the forehead, starting on the bridge of the nose and moving your thumbs up the bridge of the nose and out along the eyebrows and upper ridge of the eye. Alternate one thumb coming up the nose and out the eyebrow to the temples and then the other. Move the same thumb stroking up the forehead in a bilateral movement with your thumbs starting in the center of the forehead and moving out at the same time to the temples. Each time, start a little higher on the forehead until you reach the hairline at the top. Then start again at the eyebrow level and repeat the sequence up to three times.

3. Work your fingertips into the scalp and hook onto the muscles underlying the scalp with firm pressure using the tips of your fingers. Use a gripping circular stroke to move the muscles. Do not rub across the scalp itself. Move to a new spot and cover the whole scalp by balancing your two hands across from each other. Get feedback about how firm you can be!
4. Then lighten up and use a shampoo stroke to massage the entire scalp. Wipe off your hands so you don't get hair all over your patient's face with the next stroke.
5. Finish with light stroking using the tips of your fingers, working from the center of the face and sweeping to the outside edge of the face. You can also stroke the face with the back of your hand, which is very soft, but you would never know that until you experience it!
6. Now rub your hands vigorously together and just let them rest on the face and radiate warmth as the finishing touch! (Do this at least twenty times!!)
7. For the finish, ask the person if they would like something repeated. Ask them where their favorite spots were now that you are all finished, and then spend a couple of minutes on those spots. Last call for favorites (usually the scalp).
8. For the finale, tilt back the chair, if you can, and cover the person with a blanket. Get a hot water bottle for their neck and for their abdomen. Place them in a great location—if indoors, looking out a window; if outdoors, looking at a garden.

POST-MASSAGE TREATMENTS

Ice water footbaths are an easily provided treatment for people in wheelchairs, and are good for both swelling and headaches. You don't have to wait for the end of the massage, either: you can provide them before, during, or after the massage.

If the chair is a tilt-back chair, I like to put a cool eye pack on the patient and tell them to rest for a few minutes. I coach them to keep breathing deeply, like in yoga class, and I'll just tiptoe out to my car, leaving them to drift off to sleep (making sure their brakes are on and their seatbelt is done up).

WHEELCHAIR MASSAGE: THE SHORT VERSION

Teaching massage to others, including friends and family, is an essential part of my massage practice. The bigger the massage team, the more massage the wheelchair user will receive, which will make for more comfortable wheeling and better health.

You can use this as a handout when you teach others.

1. **Brakes and seatbelt:** Lock the breaks and put on the seatbelt!
2. **Back:** Straddle the wheel and support the patient's shoulder. Use levered fingertip kneading to the erector spinae muscles. Standing in stride position, use bilateral thumb kneading to the neck and shoulders, and fingertip kneading and palmar kneading to the back.
3. **Neck:** Straddle the wheel. Use single-handed neck scooping, bilateral thumb kneading, and alternate digital compression (poke and press).
4. **Arms and hands:**
   - **Arms:** Effleurage the arms. Use alternate thumb kneading to the biceps, single-handed kneading to the triceps, palmar cupping to the outer elbow, fingertip kneading to the elbow pressure site, inner elbow kneading, and single-handed thumb kneading to the forearm.
   - **Hands:** On the dorsal side, use alternate thumb kneading. On the fingers, use cork-screwing. On the palms, use tiny alternate thumb kneading.
5. **Legs:** Elevate the legs, when possible, with the feet higher than the heart for postural drainage. Note that only wheelchairs that allow a patient to lie prone will accommodate this.
   - **Hips:** Use levered fingertip kneading to the gluteal muscles at the ischial tuberosity pressure site; from same side, lean across to massage the opposite side. From the front, use two-handed fingertip kneading. For single-handed levered fingertip kneading, lift the knee and thigh with one hand and slide one hand under the hip; lever the fingertips.

- **Thighs:** Use wringing and alternate thumb kneading.
- **Knees:** Use alternate thumb kneading.
- **Lower legs:** Use alternate thumb kneading to the tibialis anterior, scooping to the calf, with wringing and mini-effleurages to reduce swelling.
- **Feet:** Use wringing and alternate thumb kneading bilateral to the ankle, single-handed heel of your hand to heel of the patient, two-handed calcaneus kneading to pressure sites, bilateral thumb kneading to the malleoli, alternate thumb kneading to the dorsal and plantar surfaces, and corkscrewing on the toes. Use overhanded stiff-fingered palmar percussive strokes to the soles. Finish with light reflex stroking, ten times.

6. **Leg pumping:** Use alternate, simultaneous, single rotational, and double rotational pumping.
7. **Abdomen:** Use overhanded, single-handed, and reinforced palmar kneading; single-handed fingertip kneading; palmar alternating sandwich kneading (one hand on the abdomen, one hand on the back); running, static, fine, and course vibrations; scooping; bilateral lifting; mini-effleurage; and light reflex stroking.
8. **Face and scalp:**
   - **Face:** Use temporal fingertip kneading, temporal mandibular fingertip kneading, thumb stroking to the forehead, fingertip kneading around the ear attachments, and fingertip stroking to the contours midline up to the ear. Finish with reflex stroking with fingertips and the back of the hands, ten times.
   - **Scalp:** Using a clawlike fingertip grip, massage the scalp muscles with firm pressure. Be sure to work the pressure site at the back of the head where it touches the headrest. Use single-handed and bilateral fingertip kneading. Finish with a brisk shampoo stroke.
9. **Full body finale:** Use reflex stroking from head to toes. Add a hot water bottle to the neck, and one to the abdomen with the patient's hands on top.

VIDEO LIBRARY

Visit brusheducation.ca/wheeling-in-good-hands to watch these videos:

First steps checklist: Put the brakes on with Sylvia

First steps checklist: Checking the brakes and position of the leg rests with Jo

Negotiating clothing: Massaging the foot through the shoes – in the classroom

Adaptive postures for massaging in the wheelchair: How not to tip the wheelchair back with Molly and Fernanda

Adaptive postures for massaging in the wheelchair: Sitting on a stool for a face-to-face massage with Sylvia

Wheelchair massage for the digestive system: Sandwich stroke with costal angle massage with Jo

Wheelchair massage for the digestive system: Abdominal massage with Doady

Wheelchair massage for the digestive system: Leg pumping – modification for leg injury with Jo

Wheelchair massage for the circulatory system: Common sites of pressure ulcers – fingertip levering to the ischial tuberosity

Wheelchair massage for the circulatory system: Common sites of pressure ulcers – levered massage to the hips

Wheelchair massage for the respiratory system: Upper respiratory – neck and facial massage including rib raking with Doady

Wheelchair massage for the respiratory system: Fingertip kneading to the pectoral attachments with Jo

Wheelchair massage for the respiratory system: Percussive cupping including compression with Jo

Back massage routine: Single-handed and bilateral levering with Sylvia

Back massage routine: Fingertip kneading and fisted kneading to the rhomboids and erector spinae with Bo

Neck massage routine: Bilateral alternating digital compression to the erector spinae with Barbara

Head, neck, and shoulder massage routine: Thumb kneading with fingertip kneading and scooping to the occipital ridge

Arm massage: Routine with Sylvia

Arm massage: Routine with tremors and absence of sensation with Barbara

Arm and hand massage: Routine with variations of sensation with wheelchair Athlete, Ed

Arm massage in tandem: Routine with Bo

Hand massage: Routine for spinal cord injury with palmar aspect with Molly and Fernanda

Leg massage: Accessing the hip with sling with Dixie

Leg massage: Accessing the hip with short-term injury with Jo

Leg massage: Routine for spinal cord injury with Barbara

Leg massage: routine for multiple sclerosis with pressure stockings with Dixie

Leg massage for supine position in chair with Molly and Kyrie

Leg massage: Mobilizing the knee with alternate thumb kneading with Warren

Leg massage: Lower leg massage and mobilizing the hip – in the classroom

Abdominal massage with Sylvia

Face and scalp massage: Routine with Barbara

Face and scalp massage: Routine with Dixie

Face massage: Fingertip kneading and upward strokes to the face with Sylvia

Scalp massage Working your fingertips into the scalp with Doady

Favorite massage: Sylvia's favorite

Review: Arm massage in tandem with Dixie

Review: Leg massage with Sylvia

George

George Coletti seemed peaceful and excited in a calm way about his approaching one-hundredth birthday. I had met George, hands-on, twenty years earlier in Nelson, when he asked me to massage his wife, Kay, who had ALS. Some years later, I began to massage his daughter-in-law, Mary, who also had ALS. Now, in 2021, he had his own aches and pains.

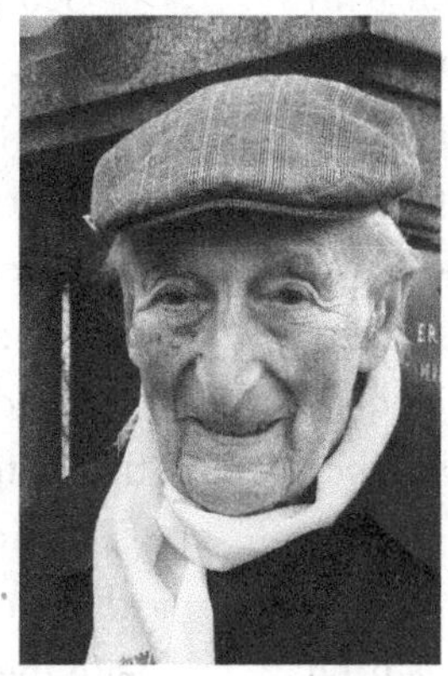

George Coletti.

They say that real life is stranger than fiction. The experience of having two people in the same family, unrelated to each other, with ALS was for me an example of the unimaginable.

I knew ALS well from my life with Brian Carpendale, my mentor in the 1970s. He died of ALS ten years after being diagnosed, and in his last five years was speechless and immobile. Kay Coletti was different from my ALS experience with Brian. She could use her voice, and she always welcomed me and my offers to teach her family to massage her. I loved massaging her and teaching her two grandchildren to massage her.

George was well aware of his age, turning 100, and his vulnerability in a summer of Covid shutdown. So, I assured George that I would always be wearing a mask and gloves when handling him.

George Coletti was a very straightforward man, always strong in his opinions about family values. He wasted no words, starting with our first massage lesson with his lovely wife, to my last lesson in his driveway and garage, where we taught my students via Zoom about reducing his extremely swollen ankles!

At the edge of his garage, there was room to put a chair and wheelchair. I set up my laptop computer and put my camera phone on a tripod to record and Zoom the leg massage session with George. This was my first time doing a Zoom class outdoors.

Years earlier, with help from my colleagues Melissa and Sonia, I had filmed a wheelchair massage tutorial with Mary Coletti on George's lawn, down by the lake. The place between the Coletti family's two houses, where over the years I massaged first Kay and then Mary, is full of good memories for me.

Today, I was bringing a world of students via Zoom to George's garage and driveway. I teased George about finally getting the privilege of massaging him. For several years, I had parked my canoe and paddleboard on George's beach. As a thank-you, each year I had given George a massage gift certificate, and each year he had given it to one of his friends. So, over the years, I had met lots of George's substitute massage friends!

But now in his final desperation to see if he could get out of his wheelchair and walk again, he was asking for my professional help. His ankles were unrecognizable. They were the most swollen ankles I had ever seen. The only ankles to compete with George's were those of a palliative patient with failing kidneys. George was far from failing. He was lively, in perfect health from the knees up!

George was used to being my video subject. He had been the star, along with his son Lou and his grandson Mike, when I was filming Mary.

In the Zoom class, I tried to make a therapeutic impression on George's swollen ankles that would last until the next day. I showed his daughter-in-law, Tamara, how to massage his ankles to keep reducing the extreme swelling. George was in all his glory as he regaled the Zoom classroom with stories of our times together, and with a precision my memory couldn't match. I used ice to massage his ankles, demonstrating ways to keep these newly found ankles moving. Tamara was enthusiastic about her job of helping me to keep him happy and moving. She was the best student to teach—eager to learn, and so good with her hands-on skills.

Now, George was able to put his feet on the ground and steady himself with his walker, getting out of the wheelchair that had been his security seat. His ankles were now reduced to a more normal size and he was feeling very proud of his willingness to finally try massage therapy.

I showed George some of the film clips from the session we had just concluded, so he could see how he would continue to help me teach. I knew that I had captured the session the right way when George approved of what he saw and gave me the go-ahead to keep using it to train others. This wheelchair massage session was very special for me. I realized that I could keep George close in my teaching life with our film about massaging his swollen ankles!

From George's driveway, I raced to the clinic to continue the Zoom class, while my remote students watched *Massaging Mary: Hands On with ALS* on my YouTube channel. This film was the perfect follow-up to the Zoom session we had just had with George. It is a film about Mary in the last couple of years of her life. George is in the film talking about how massage had helped Kay, and how it was now helping Mary.

George was my authenticity barometer. If George endorsed my work, then my work was good. I had the stamp of approval.

George had given my Zoom class a great experience! Seeing his ankles for the first time in months, and giving him relief for hours from the skin tension and ache of the extremity, was a good feeling that lasted throughout the weekend of the class.

I think back to the session with George and what we talked about. I feel like I had an audience with the pope of Kootenay Lake! The condition of his legs was life-threatening, and we talked about the inevitability of his life ending, and how to end it as comfortably as possible.

Now George is gone. He died and left me many gifts.

George knew about the magic of touch. I will always be grateful for the years of early morning paddleboarding, canoeing, and kayaking from his beach, and finally, for the opportunity to help George get on his feet.

4

Massage Routines for Specific Issues of Wheelchair Users

This chapter presents massage routines for specific problems arising from wheelchair use. Some routines can be performed in the chair or out of the chair. Some routines, though, are best performed out of the chair.

So the first part of this chapter focuses on transfers. Knowing how to transfer a patient properly to and from a wheelchair protects them and you.

Transfers

Massaging before Transfers

I've encouraged wheelchair users to build a team of hands-on caregivers to give day-to-day massages that make it easier to move their limbs before transferring from bed to wheelchair after a long night's sleep, and before transferring from wheelchair back to bed at the end of the day. Pre-transfer mini-massages make that physical transition easier, by making limbs more mobile and at the same time creating a positive emotional reinforcement for sometimes an awkward or uncomfortable change.

Transfer Techniques

I am the first to ask others to help me transfer a wheelchair user. Many people who don't expect to help, or haven't been asked to help, are educated when they assist me.

Even if you are not a massage therapist—maybe you have a family member in a wheelchair—I hope you can envision yourself as a wheelchair transfer helper. The ability to transfer someone is useful and important knowledge. The ability to save your own back in the process is equally important. I learned by making lots of mistakes over the years and I'm hoping that these illustrations will help you avoid my mistakes.

The diagrams of transfer sequences in Figure 4.1 show you how to transfer safely in several common situations. The situations are broader than what you might need for the massage routines presented in this chapter—I cover wheelchair-to-car transfers here, for example. But I want you to have lots of opportunities to take your loved ones out on the streets of our towns and cities, no matter what the season or event.

Figure 4.1 shows transfers in "one direction," from wheelchair to another location. To transfer back to the wheelchair, do the steps in reverse!

BASIC SEQUENCE FOR ONE-TO-ONE TRANSFERS

1. Position the wheelchair beside the transfer location. If you are transferring to a bed, the wheelchair should be parallel to the bed. If you are transferring to a standard chair, the wheelchair should be at an angle to the chair.
2. Put on the brakes!
3. Face the wheelchair user and position your legs outside their legs.
4. Get ready to lift with your legs, not your back! Plant your feet a shoulder width apart, bend your knees, and lean toward your patient with a straight back.
5. Ask your patient to put their arms around your neck, like they are giving you a hug.

Position your hands to give you the best purchase for lifting your patient—under their arms, or gripping the waistband of their pants (even better, use a transfer belt).

6. Lift. As you lift, adjust your arms and hands to fully embrace and stabilize your patient.
7. Pivot to the new location.
8. Using your legs, ease the patient down into a sitting position. I squeeze their knees with my legs.

Massage Treatments for Specific Wheelchair Conditions

This section outlines specific massage treatments for some of the most common conditions of wheelchair users.

The main factor at play here is the use of the chair, how long someone stays in the chair every day, and what led them to be in the chair in the first place. For example, if they have a high-level spinal cord injury, they may have contractures in all their extremities. If they have use of their arms, there will be issues in the upper body and possible overuse injuries from self-propelling in the chair.

Other issues arise for short-term versus long-term wheelchair users. Short-term users—for example, people recovering from stroke or surgery—often have issues related to compensating for weak or sore parts of the body. Long-term users—for example, people with spinal cord injury or neurological conditions such as ALS or MS—often develop spinal problems.

FIGURE 4.1. **Wheelchair Transfers**

STARTING POSITION

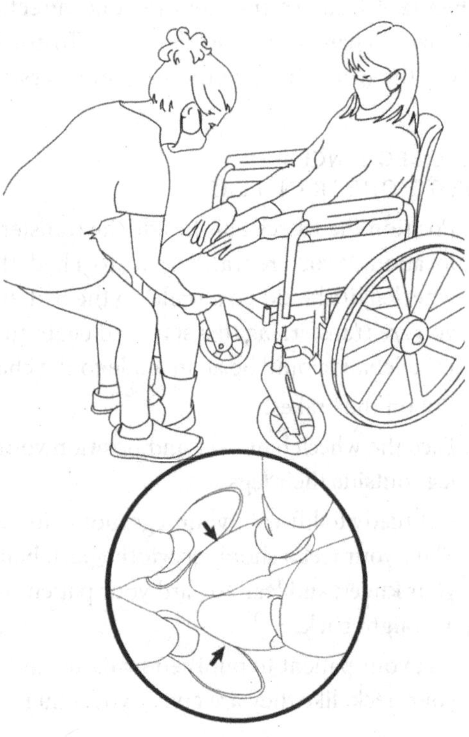

Face your patient. Position your legs outside their legs.

continued next page

FIGURE 4.1. CONTINUED

WHEELCHAIR TO BED OR TABLE

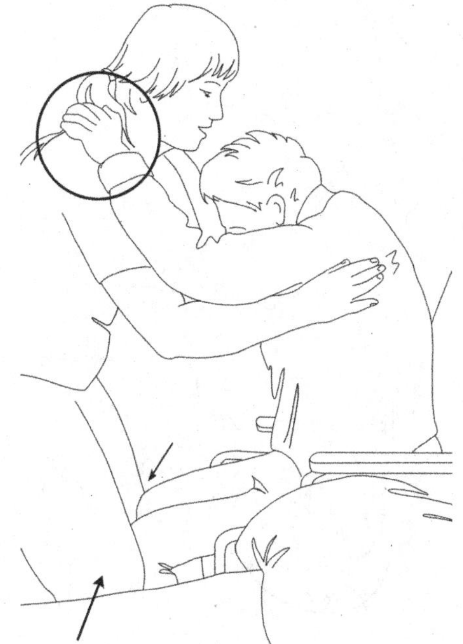

a. Get ready to lift.

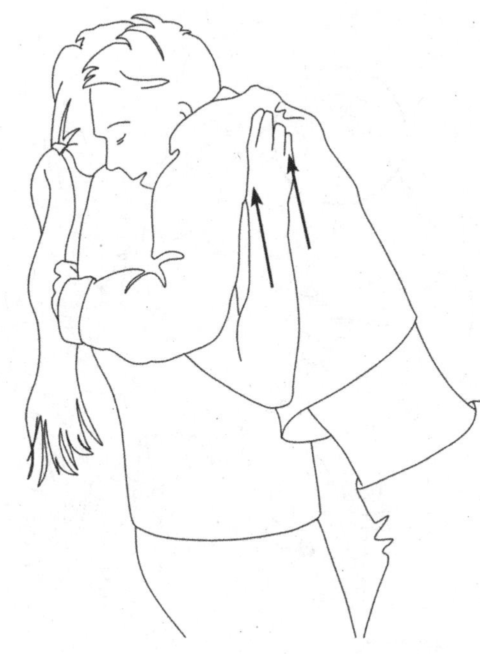

b. Lift and pivot.

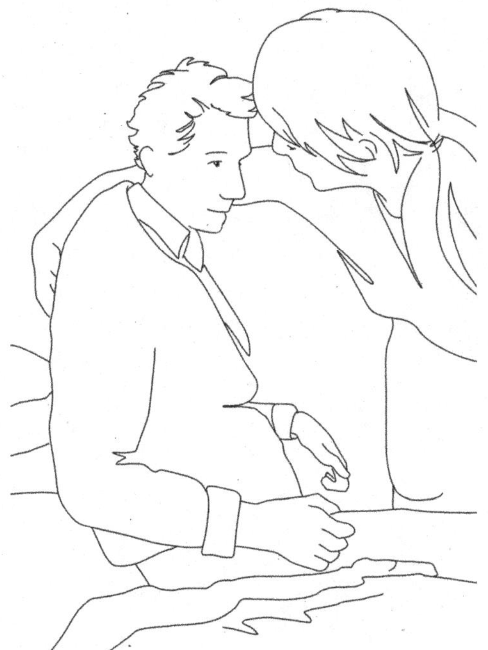

c. Ease the patient into a sitting position.

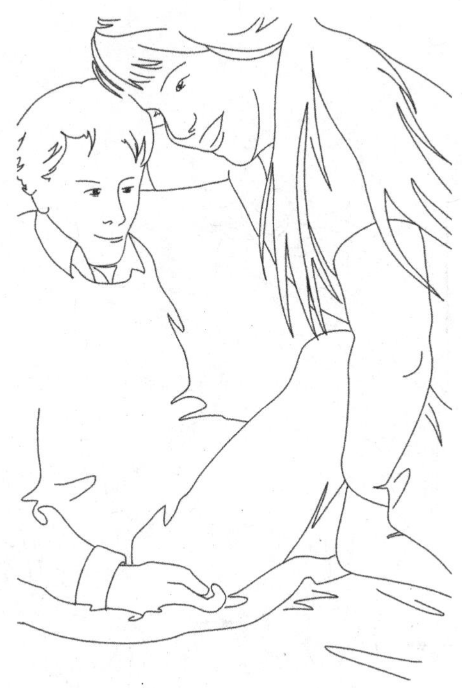

d. Swing the legs up.

FIGURE 4.1. CONTINUED

WHEELCHAIR TO CHAIR

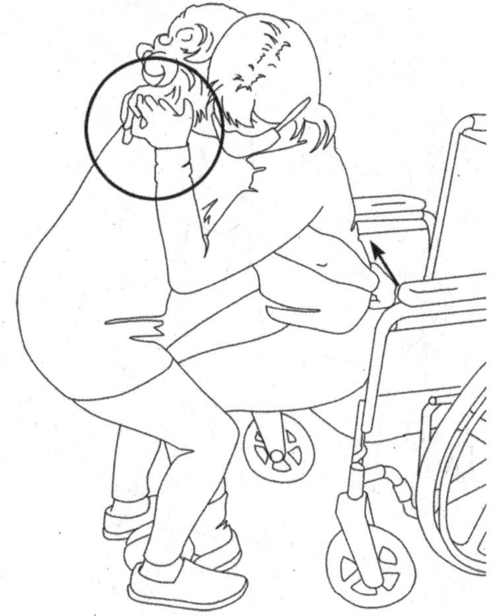

a. Get ready to lift.

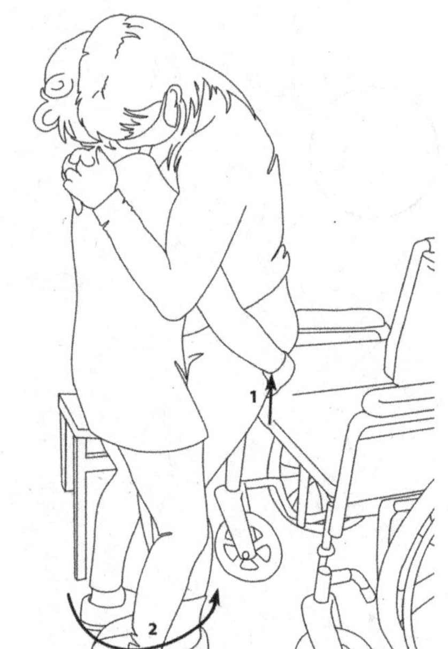

b. Lift and pivot.

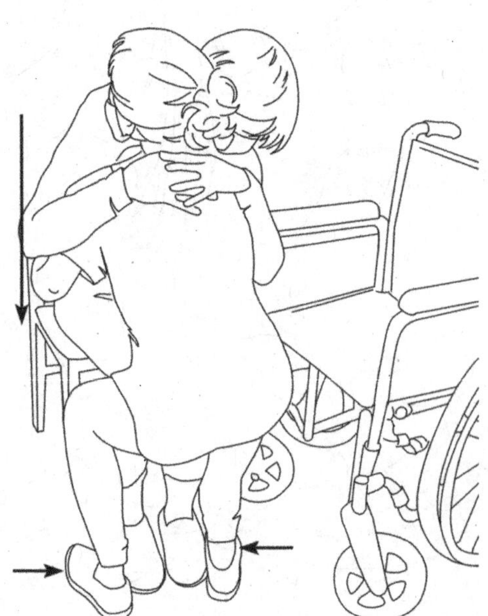

c. Ease the patient into a sitting position.

FIGURE 4.1. CONTINUED

WHEELCHAIR TO CHAIR WITH TRANSFER BOARD

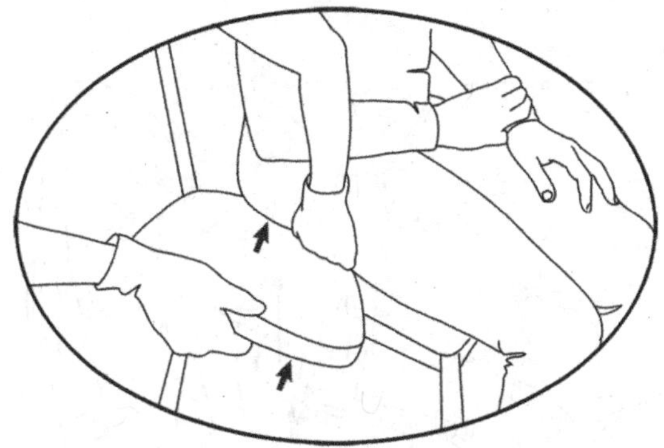

Remove one arm of the wheelchair. Position one edge of the transfer board securely under the patient.

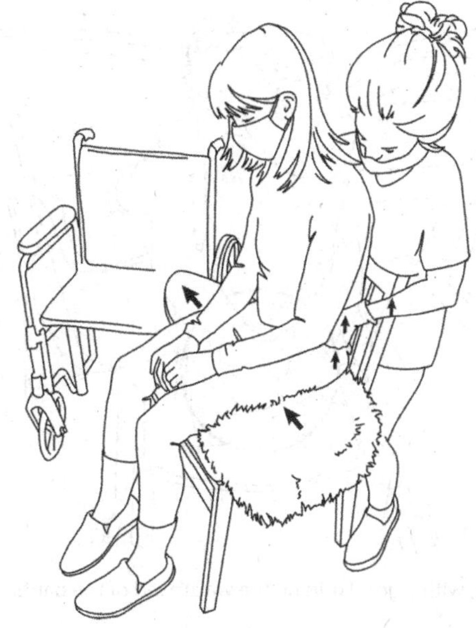

The board forms a bridge that you slide the patient across. Working from behind the patient, grip the waistband of the pants and slide the patient across the board to the new location.

WHEELCHAIR TO CAR, ONE TO ONE

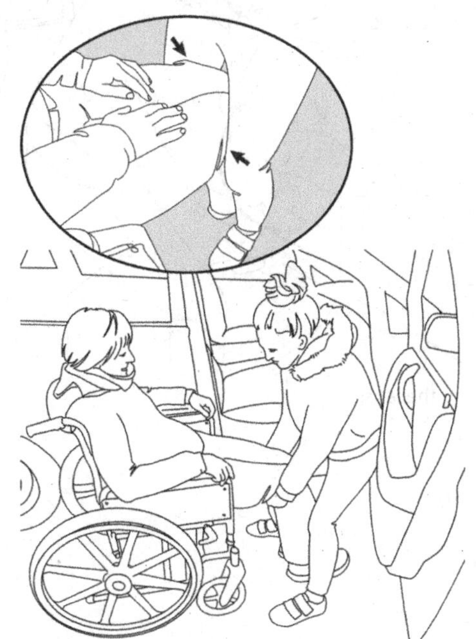

a. Position your legs outside your patient's legs.

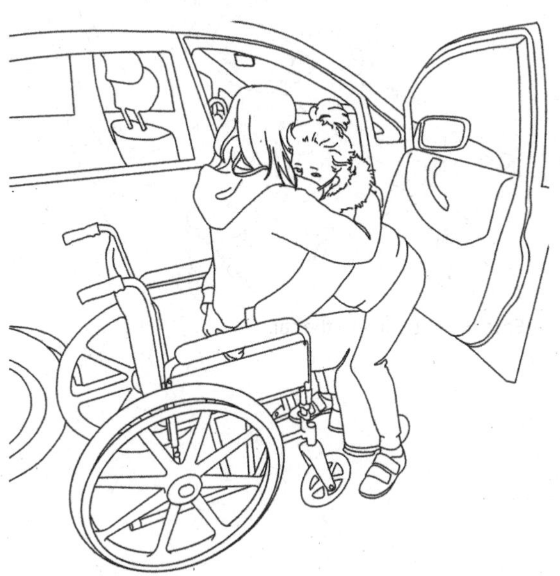

b. Get ready to lift.

FIGURE 4.1. CONTINUED

WHEELCHAIR TO CAR, ONE TO ONE

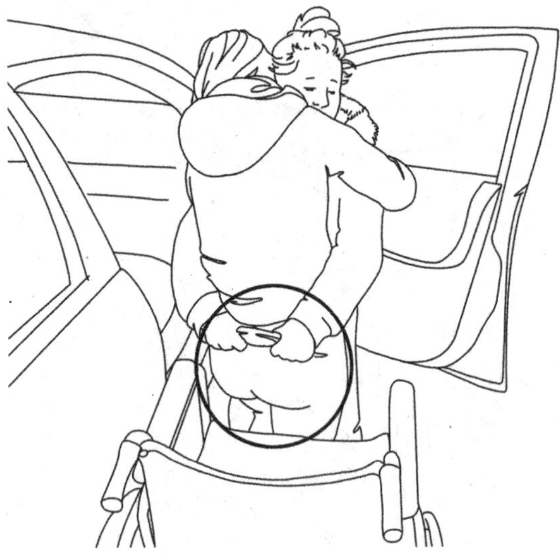

c. Lift, with a good grip on the waistband of the pants.

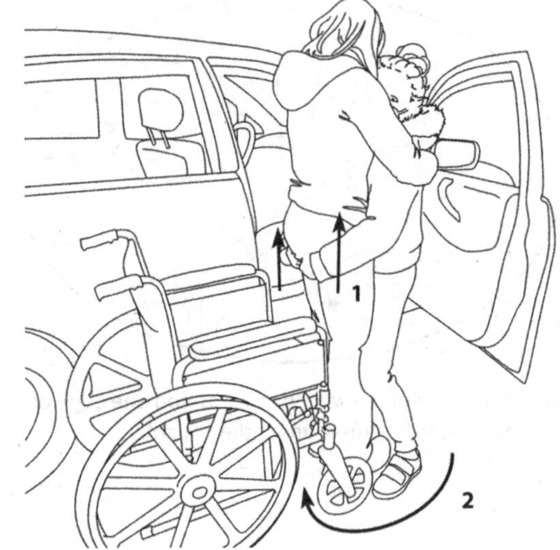

d. Get a good grip under the patient's glutes and pivot.

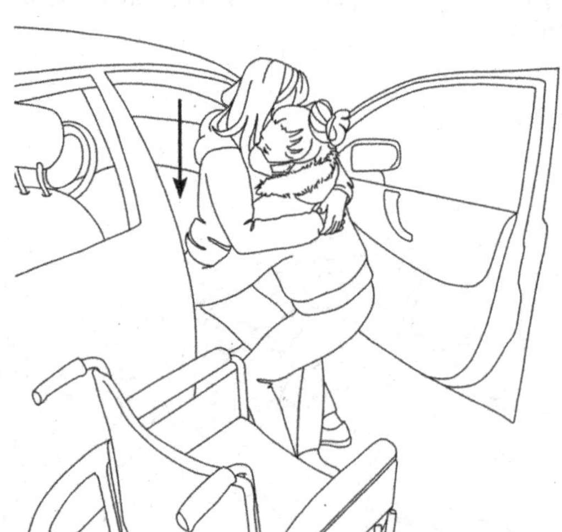

e. Ease the patient into the car.

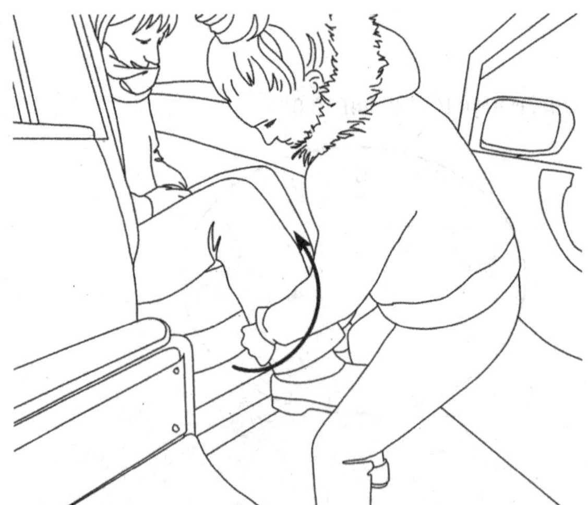

f. Swing the legs.

FIGURE 4.1. CONTINUED

WHEELCHAIR TO CAR, TANDEM

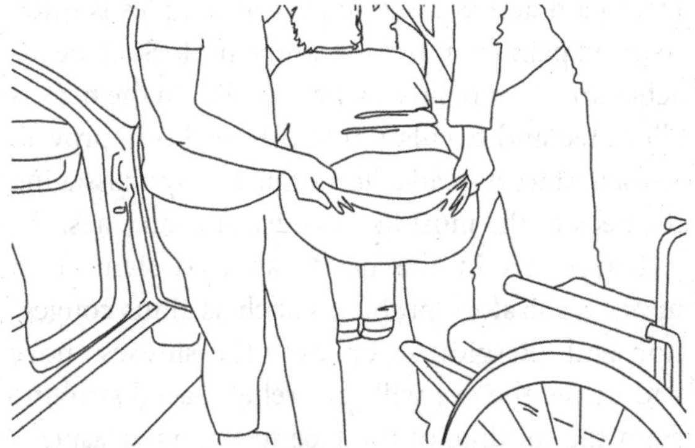

a. A tandem transfer to a car requires more room to maneuver than a one-on-one transfer, so don't place the wheelchair too close to the car. Lift: this view from behind shows a good grip on the waistband of the pants.

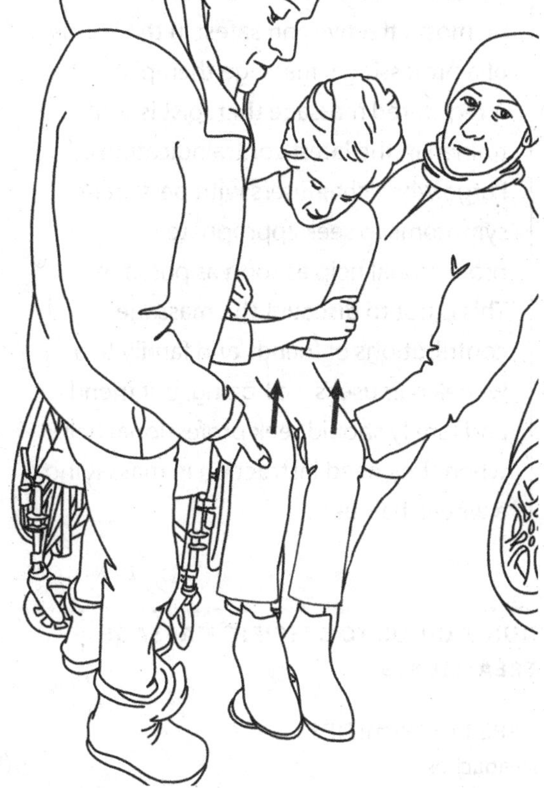

b. Lift: this view from in front shows how hands under the knees balance the waistband grip at the back.

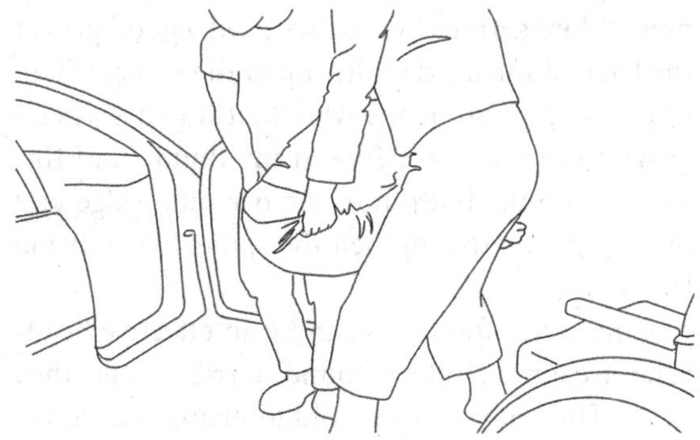

c. Pivot.

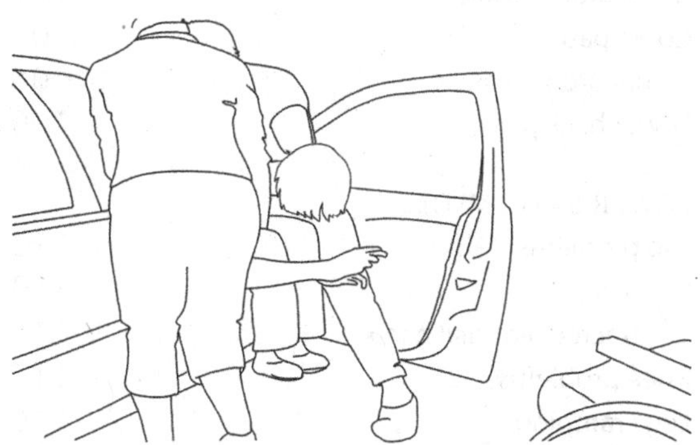

d. Ease the patient into the car.

An important caution: massage treatments for some of the complex conditions discussed in this chapter will be most effective and safest in the hands of a professional massage therapist. A registered massage therapist is well trained in the latest contraindications. I urge wheelchair users with persistent symptoms to seek appropriate professional help as soon as possible. This is not to discount the massage contributions of friends and family to a wheelchair user's well-being, but friends and family should seek professional help when they need instruction in massaging a wheelchair user.

QUICK GUIDE TO SPECIFIC MASSAGE TREATMENTS

Headaches

Many headaches are caused by changing shoulder and neck pressure due to wheeling those wheels. Even pain across the forehead or temples is often referred pain from tension in the neck. Such headaches are often relieved when tension in the neck is alleviated and circulation to the head is improved. Always start a headache treatment by massaging the neck as the most likely cause of headaches.

Symptoms in the head can also stem from upper respiratory problems such as sinus congestion and allergies, so opening the sinuses above and below the eye will give relief. Facial stroking from the midline of the face to the outer aspects can often relieve a headache, especially a sinus headache.

Fluid retention due to immobility or palliative shutdown of the kidneys can be experienced not only in the arms and legs, but also in the head (as the fifth extremity). Often, as the swelling is addressed through massage of the extremities, headaches also diminish.

Other headaches can result from the daily stressors of being a wheelchair user. These can also be helped with massage.

Light headaches caused by stress or lack of sleep are often helped by massaging the temples and the occipital ridge at the back of the head and base of the skull. The temples are easily massaged with stiff fingertip kneading at the hypersensitive area right on the hairline where the skin and scalp meet. More serious headaches need a good grip at the back of the head at the top of the spine. When I'm massaging someone who is sitting in a wheelchair, I use the web between my thumb and fingers to cup the bottom of the occipital ridge and pull up gently to lengthen the spine, like a lifting traction.

Cold water footbaths can be an effective headache treatment—they sound terrible, but they work! The body sees the cold footbath as a "counterirritant" and goes looking to address the issue at the feet, giving the head a neurological rest. This isn't a perfect treatment of all headaches, but it works well for many—combined with your relieving massage treatment, of course!

IN-CHAIR HEADACHE TREATMENT

This "kitchen table" head, neck, and shoulder massage is great for headaches. It is intended for people in wheelchairs, but it's useful in many other situations, too—for example, for people sitting at the kitchen table, or on the couch watching television, or in a deck chair on the back porch.

Ask for feedback and use it as your guide. For example, you might spend more time around the eyes or temples or jaw if that seems to be the area that elicits the most relief.

MESSAGE MENU FOR HEADACHES

1. **Natural squeeze to the shoulders and arms:** Place both hands on the shoulders and give a squeeze to develop a rapport and accustom the person to your touch. Work down each arm, alternately squeezing and releasing.
2. **Trapezius scoop:** Develop the squeeze, giving scoops of the trapezius with the heels of your hands. Lift the shoulder muscle up like a mother cat lifts up her kittens. Hold the muscle, coaching the patient through a couple of deep breaths, and then let go of the muscle on the last out breath. This is my pressure gauge stroke. Be sure to ask for the "f-word" (feedback), using questions such as "Can I be firmer? Should I be lighter?"

FIGURE 4.2. **Headaches: Natural Squeeze**

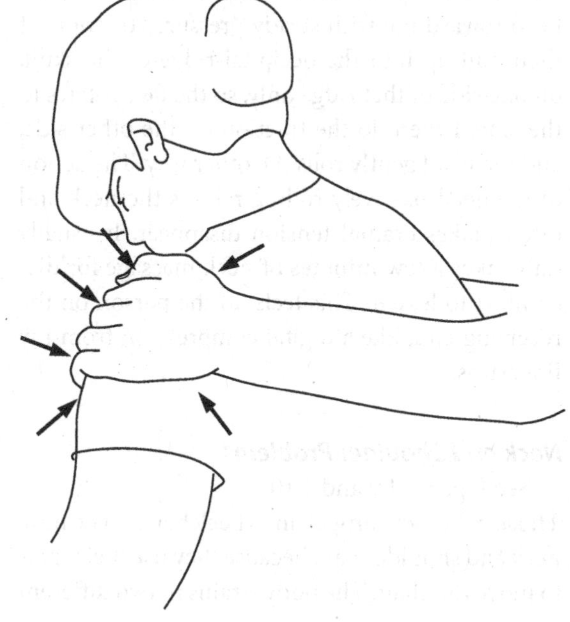

3. **Digital compression on the rhomboids:** Move from the trapezius squeeze to digital compression with your thumbs. Wrap your fingers lightly around the throat to position your thumbs on either side of the spine just under the occipital ridge. Taking care not to squeeze the throat with your fingers, and alternating between your thumbs as you work, poke and press, like walking with the tips of your thumbs on either side of the spine on the erector spinae muscles from the occipital ridge to the top of the rhomboids. Once you get to the rhomboids, slow down and work your static digital compression deeply as you move to the bottom of the scapula. This area can be quite tight. Be sure to check with your patient that your pressure is right. Keep your thumbs at the same speed and rhythm as they alternate to work down both sides of the body.
4. **Head tilts:** Always keep the nose pointing forward during this sequence. Have your patient in a sitting position. Move to the patient's side and place one hand on the forehead, and one at the base of the skull using the web of your hand between the thumb and fingers. Lift and slowly tilt the head three times in each direction, pivoting the head on the top of the spine. Be sure your movements are slow and careful. Sometimes I use these head tilts at the start of a headache treatment to see how stiff the person's neck is since this is a common origin of headaches.
5. **Temporal kneading:** Move to the back of your patient and place your fingertips on the temples right at the hairline. Slowly knead all around the jaw and the temple area. Have the person release his or her jaw by relaxing the mouth open slightly.
6. **Percussive tapotement to the upper back:** For the trapezius, deltoids, and rhomboids, give a percussive tapotement massage.
7. **Percussive tapotement to the lower back:** Have your patient lean forward, with their

FIGURE 4.3. **Headaches: Trapezius Scoop**

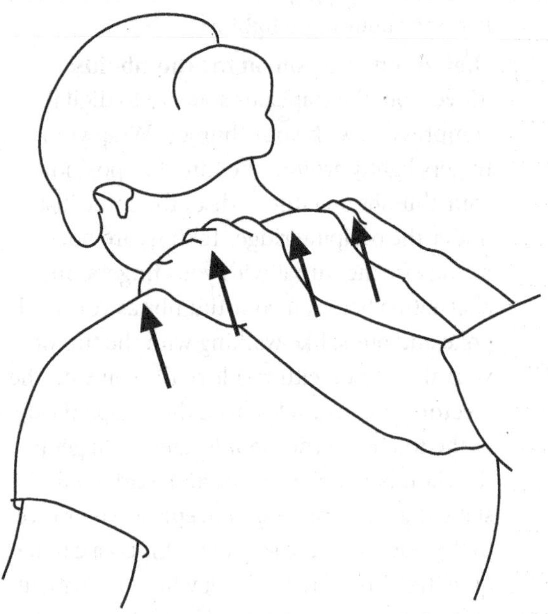

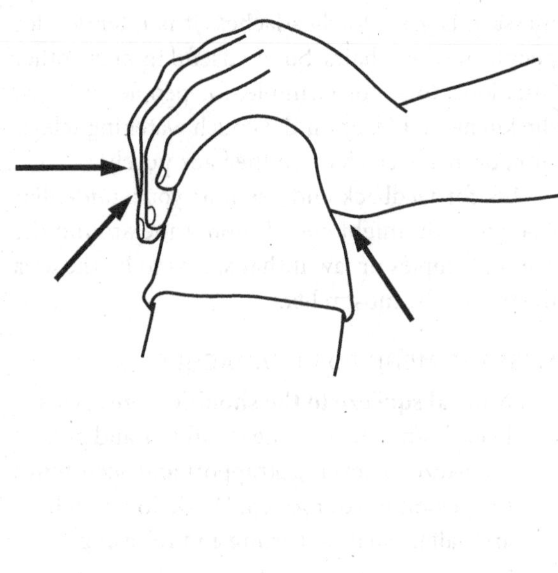

FIGURE 4.4. **Headaches: Digital Compression, Rhomboids**

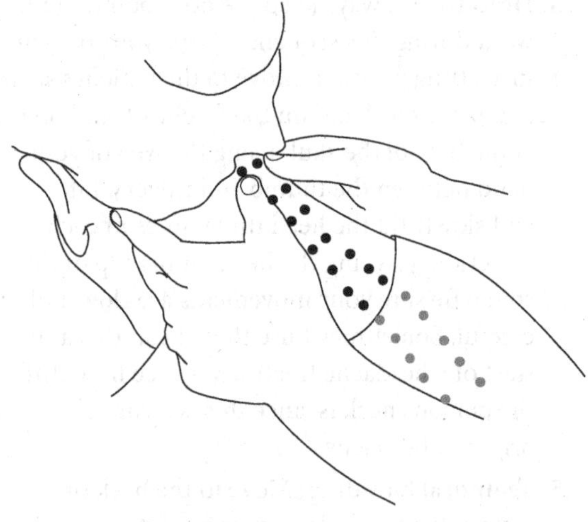

elbows on their knees or leaning onto pillows on their lap, with their head dropped down. Alternatively, they could wheel to a desk or tabletop and rest on it. Stand to the side and perform this percussion over the the back, being careful not to thump on the spine itself.

8. **Shoulder squeeze (repeat).**
9. **Head tilts (repeat).**
10. **Light reflex stroking:** Stroke lightly with your fingertips from the top of the head and out to the shoulders and arms, and from the top of the head down the spine.

RELIEVING NECK TENSION TO RELIEVE HEADACHES (SUPINE, FACE-UP)

When I am treating someone lying supine, I hold the head along the base of the skull, pulling the head toward me with steady pressure (traction). I then pull up into the occipital ridge of the skull, on one side of that ridge only, so the face rotates to the side. I then do the traction on the other side, and the head gently rolls the other way. The action of the head passively rolling relaxes the neck and often makes cranial tension disappear. It usually only takes a few minutes of neck massage for discomfort to lessen. This feels, to the person on the receiving end, like a digital compression from my fingertips.

Neck and Shoulder Problems

See Figures 4.9 and 4.10.

Those who self-propel in wheelchairs may have neck and shoulder pain because they use their arms to move the chair. The body strains in two different

FIGURE 4.5. Headaches: Head Tilts

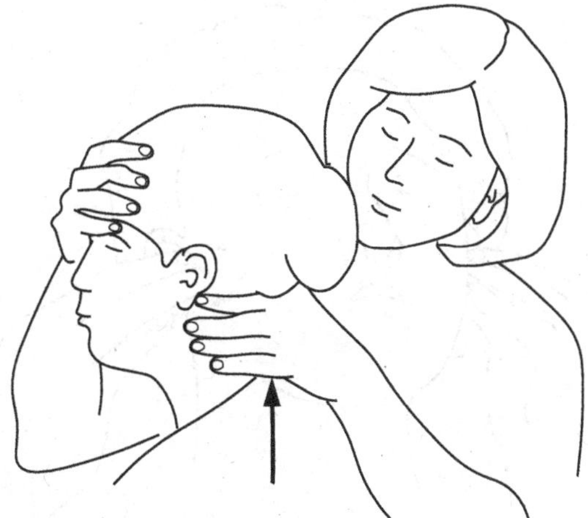

a. With a scooping action, lift at the back of the head under the occipital ridge to give traction.

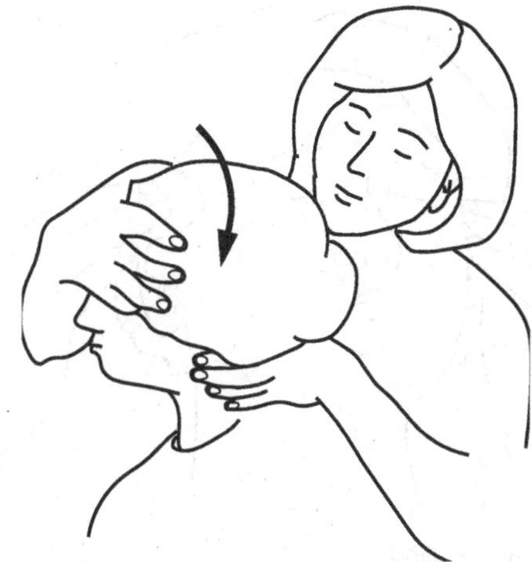

b. Gently move the ear to the shoulder.

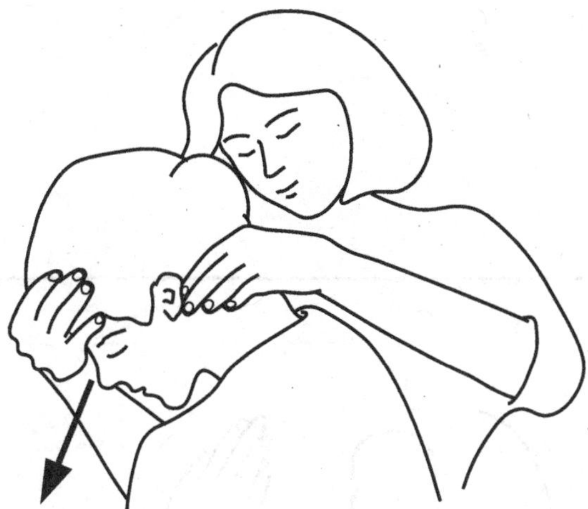

c. Drop the chin to the chest.

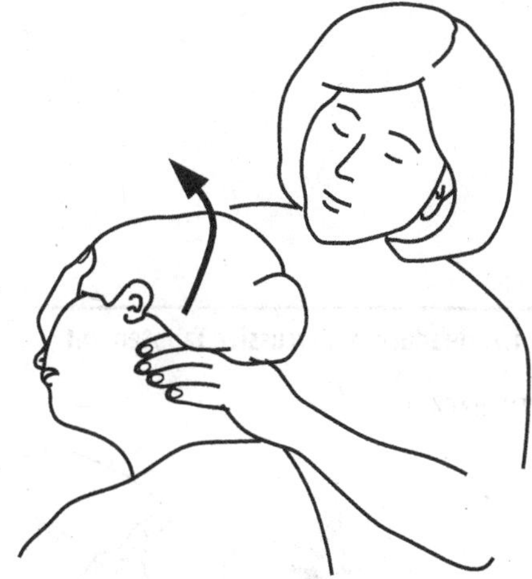

d. Gently move the ear to the opposite shoulder.

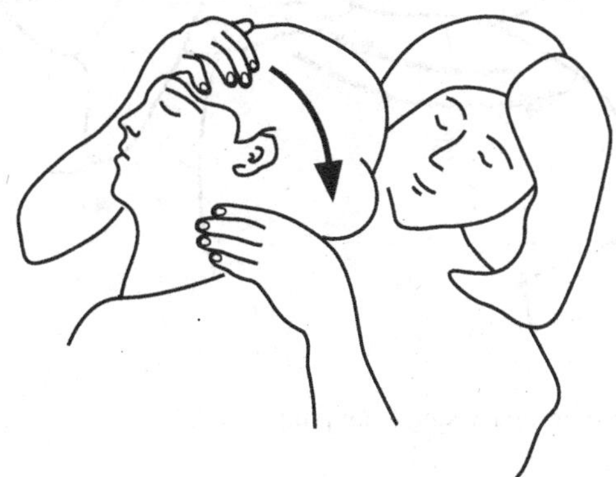

e. Tilt the head backward.

FIGURE 4.6. Headaches: Temporal Kneading

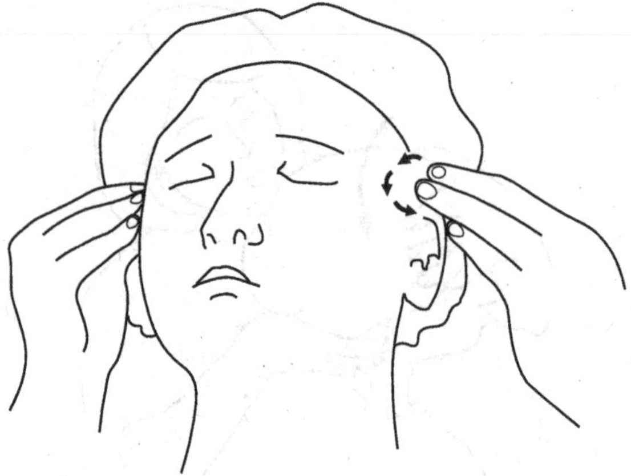

Temporal kneading.

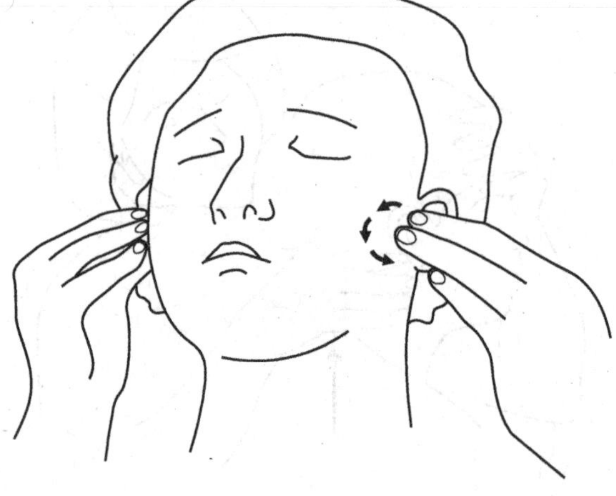

Temporal mandibular kneading on the chin bone below the zygomatic arch.

FIGURE 4.7. Headaches: Percussive Tapotement

FINGERTIP HACKING

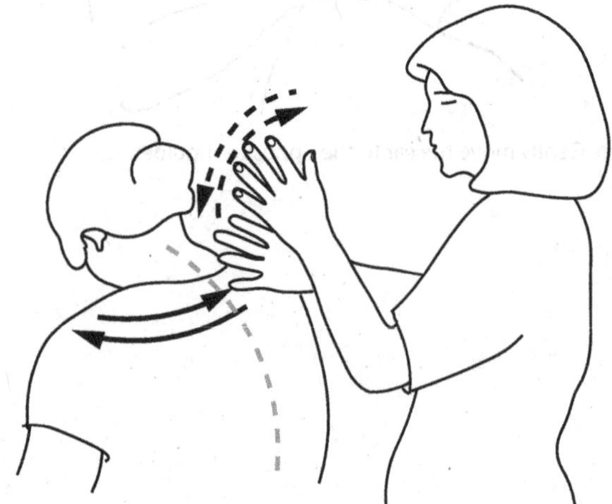

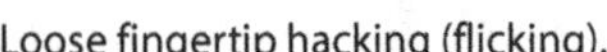

Loose fingertip hacking (flicking).

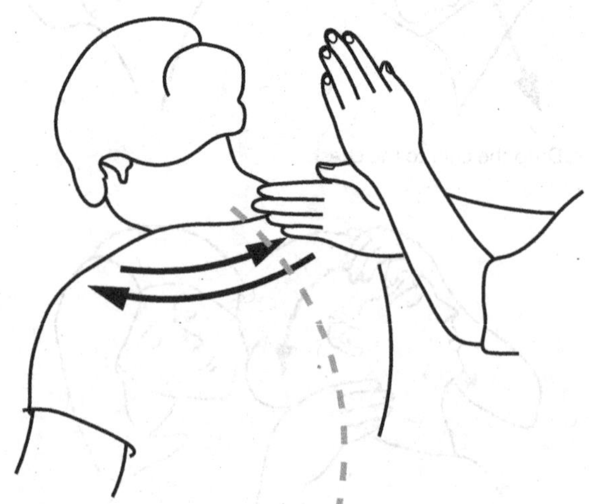

Stiff fingertip hacking (chopping).

FIGURE 4.7. CONTINUED

CUPPING

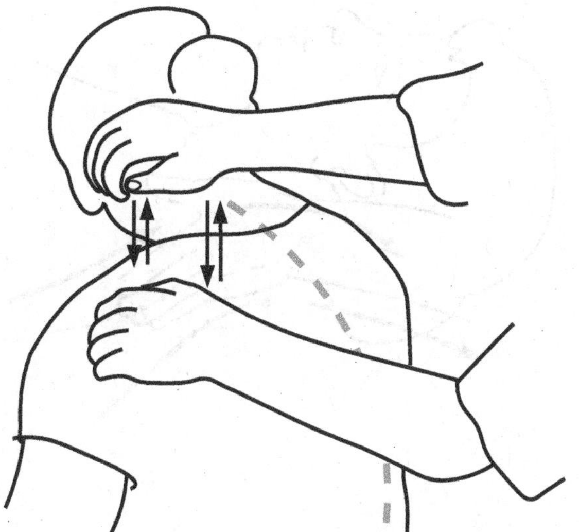

Be sure you get a hollow sound, not a slapping sound.

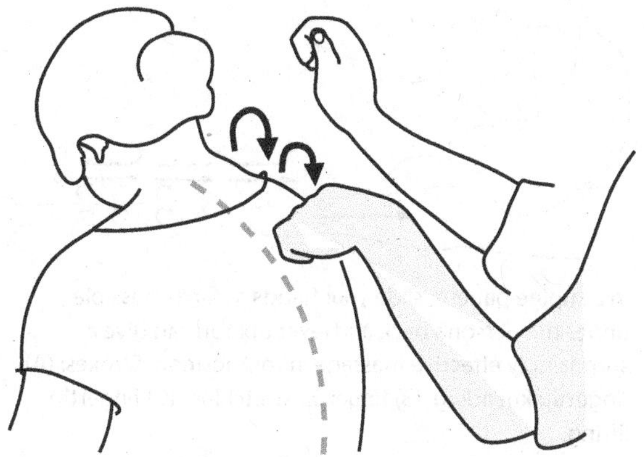

Use a "monkey paw" with a flip-flop wrist.

POUNDING

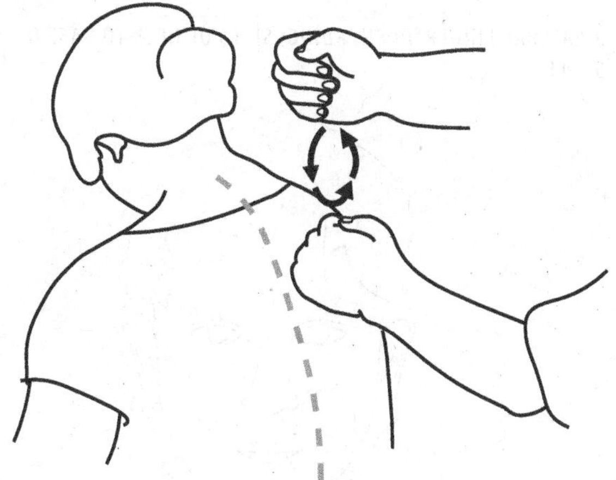

Pounding: roll your fists toward your body in a "Ferris wheel" motion.

FIGURE 4.8. Headaches: Relieving Neck Tension

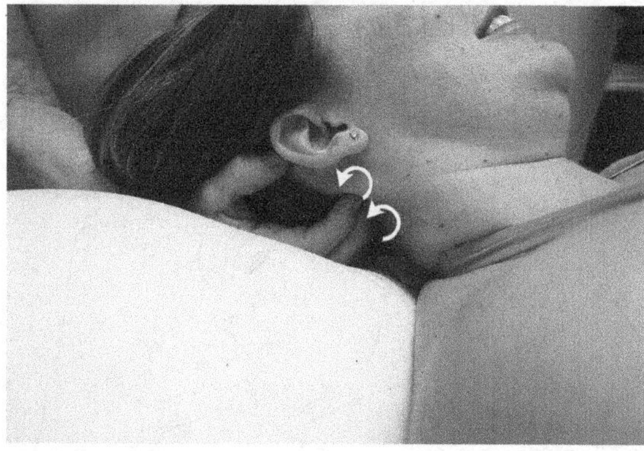

While doing the alternating traction, I add in some fingertip kneading to those tight muscle attachments at the base of the skull at the occipital ridge. The combination of traction and massage works wonders. This is one of my patients' favorite massage routines.

FIGURE 4.9. Massage for Neck and Shoulder Problems

FINGERTIP STROKES DOWN THE BACK

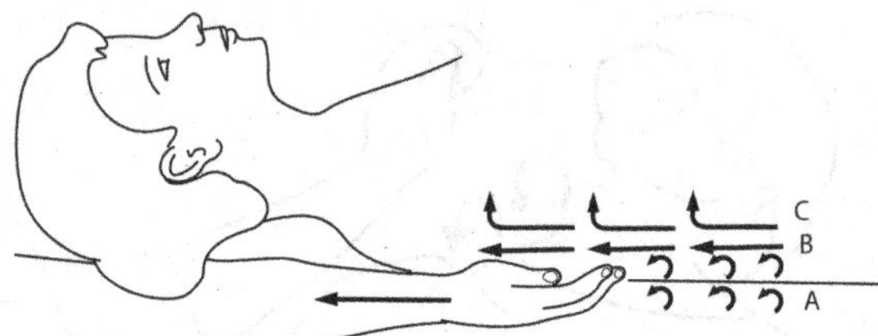

In a supine patient, slide your hands as far as possible under the person's back and lever up. You can give a surprisingly effective massage in this position. Strokes: (A) fingertip kneading; (B) fingertip stretching; (C) fingertip lifting.

REFLEX STROKING TO THE NECK MUSCLES

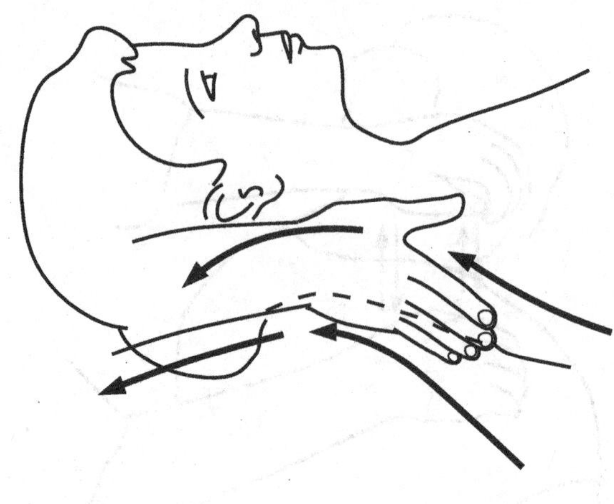

MODIFIED EFFLEURAGE TO THE NECK

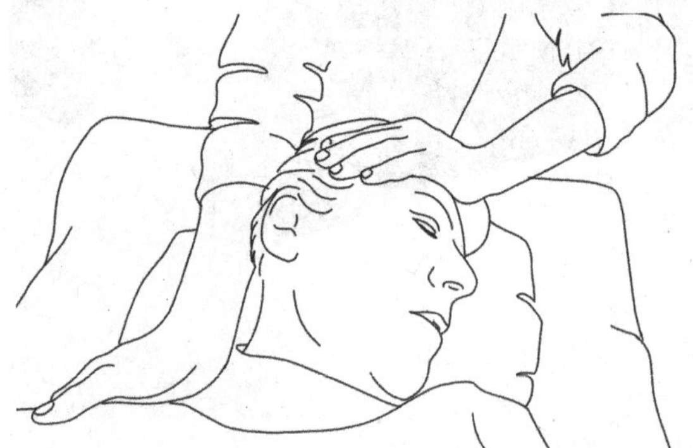

Use one hand to press the head gently to the side to give a little more space for the effleurage.

BILATERAL FINGERTIP KNEADING, SIDES OF NECK TO BASE OF SKULL

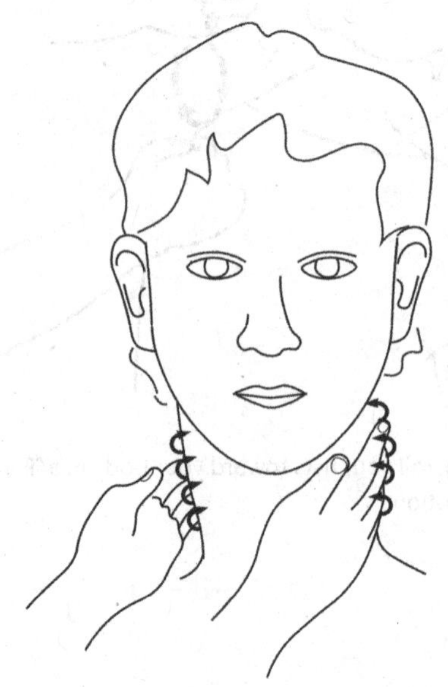

FIGURE 4.9. CONTINUED

DEEP FINGERTIP KNEADING, TRAPEZIUS AND NECK MUSCLES TO BASE OF SKULL

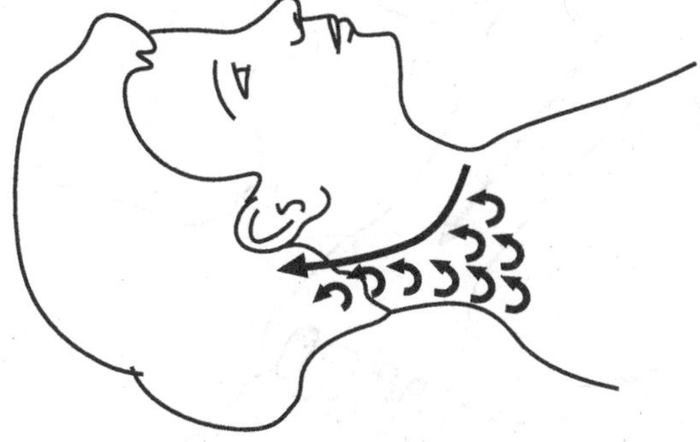

LIGHT FINGER STROKING, PRESSURE FROM THE HEAD DOWN

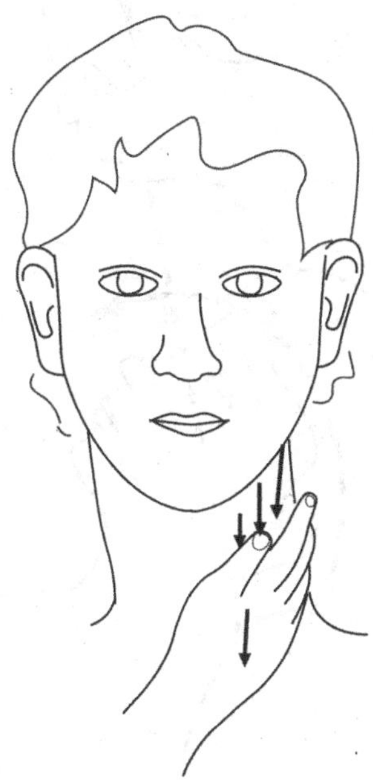

This stroke can help with lymphatic drainage.

SCOOPING THE RHOMBOIDS, ERECTOR SPINAE MUSCLES, AND TRAPEZIUS MUSCLES

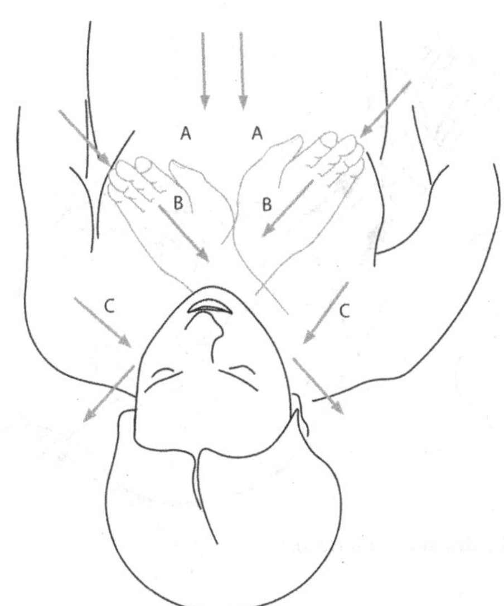

Slide your hands under the patient's body and scoop them toward you to work the erector spinae muscles (A), rhomboids (B), and trapezius muscles (C). Alternate your hands scooping diagonally across the person's back as you pull toward you. Be sure to avoid any pressure on the spinal column itself.

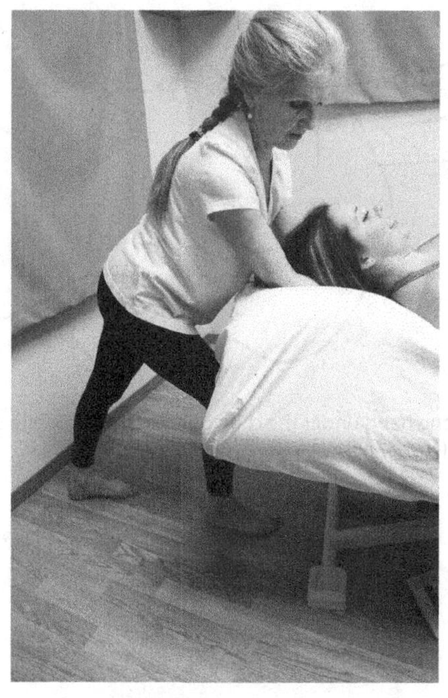

To get your body in the right position for this scooping stroke, be sure to use the stride position.

FIGURE 4.10. Methods to Relieve Neck Tension

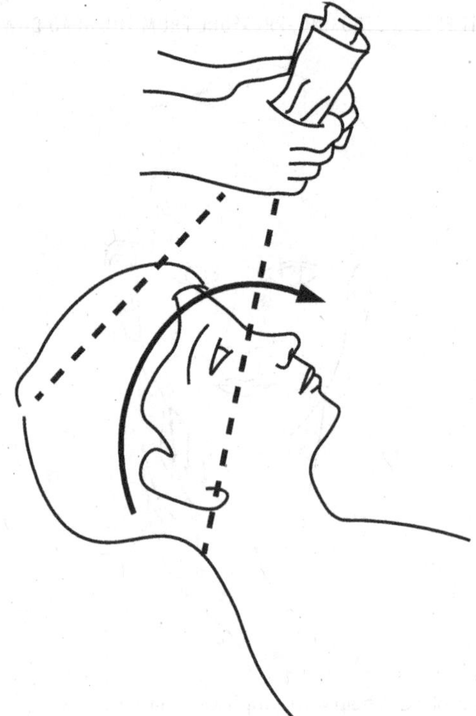

Towel flexion lifting both sides of the towel together.

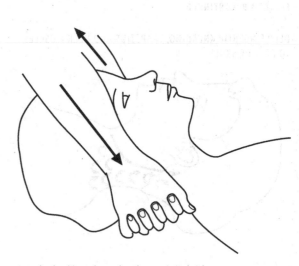

Interlocked hands under the occipital ridge.

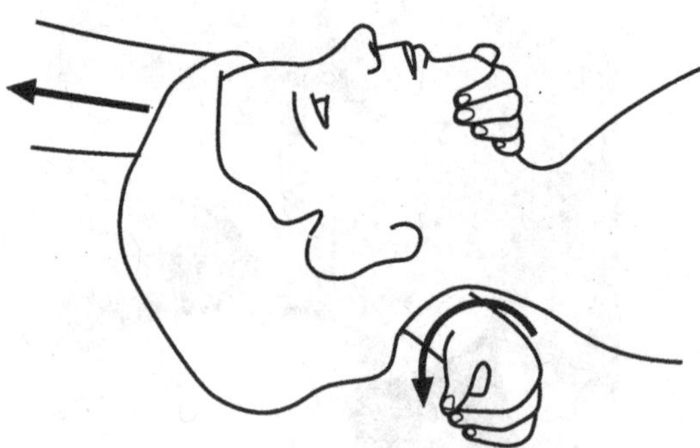

With one hand under the chin, pull toward you while the other hand rolls under the occipital ridge.

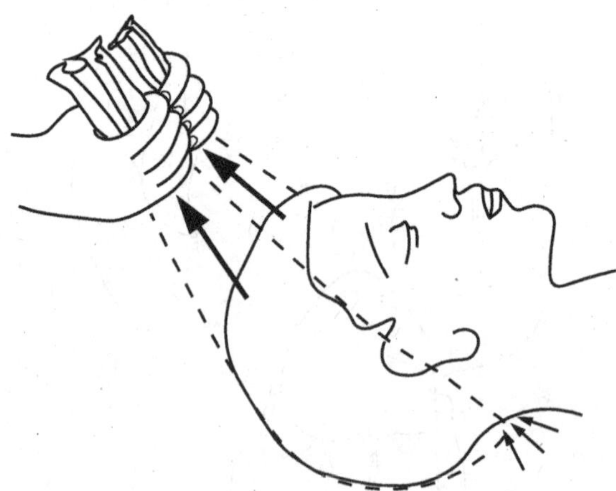

Towel extension (traction).

FIGURE 4.10. CONTINUED

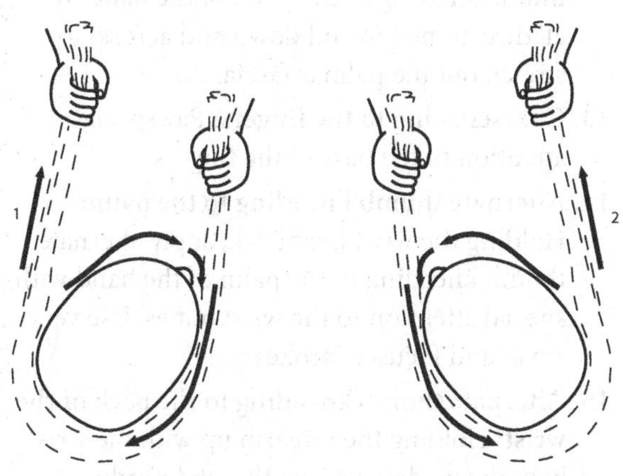

Face rolls: pull straight up on one side of the towel and then the other, so the head gently rotates from side to side.

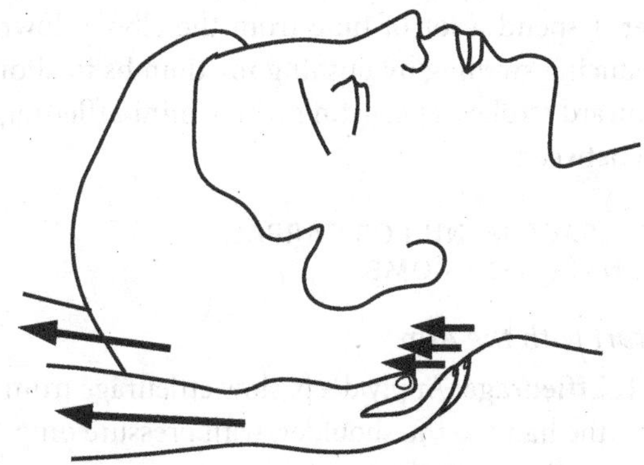

Fingertip traction from the occipital ridge.

ways: arms and shoulders as well as head and neck. Arms and shoulders need massage because of the grip of the hands on the wheels. The unusual use of the forearms, upper arms, and shoulders, from the combination of sitting for hours paired with the mobilization, result in the forward flexing of the trunk and the shortening of the chest muscles attached to the shoulder girdle.

The strokes illustrated for neck and shoulder massage are all to be performed with the patient in a supine, face-up position (on their back). The head is rotated or stretched (ear to shoulder) when necessary to accommodate strokes along the side of the neck.

Carpal Tunnel Syndrome

Carpal tunnel syndrome is caused by a pinching of the median nerve, which runs from the neck down the arm to the hand. It causes pain, numbness, or tingling in the wrist and hand where the nerve supplies the sensations for the half of the hand that houses the middle finger, pointer finger, and thumb.

Because wheelchair users who self-propel use their hands to grip the wheels, they are prime candidates for carpal tunnel syndrome. This is especially true of wheelchair athletes, who go hard with a lot of starting and stopping that relies on their hands.

Carpal tunnel syndrome is often caused by swelling. The swelling of the body, especially at the ends of the extremities (hands and feet), causes a variety of problems, such as not being able to wheel comfortably or not being able to pick things up or have a strong, confident grip on the wheelchair. Swelling in the arms and hands can also cause the carpal bones of the wrist to get jammed together, pinching the median nerve.

Carpal tunnel syndrome, when severe, is usually treated by splinting the wrists overnight. Although discomfort is felt primarily in the wrists, massage helps to diminish pain and restore circulation by reducing edema (swelling) throughout the entire arm.

First massage the head, neck, and shoulders to open up circulation to the arm. People with rounded shoulders can have tight muscles that clamp down on the median nerve where it exits the neck vertebrae. A squeezing of the nerve anywhere along its route gives rise to pain farther along the arm. Sometimes, simply loosening up the top of the arm and neck area will help dissipate the problem. Use firm pressure with all your strokes to work the tension out of the shoulders. Doing the backstroke in the pool can also help loosen up this area for those wheelchair users who can swim.

Then move to an arm and hand massage. Use our basic routine for the arm. For all strokes, use firm pressure and small strokes, especially at the wrist, on the palm, and for each individual finger. I spend a lot of time from the elbow down, reducing swelling by pushing my thumbs in short upward strokes, alternating with a mini-effleurage in between.

MASSAGE MENU FOR CARPAL TUNNEL SYNDROME

Start with the Arm

1. **Effleurage:** Apply deep, slow effleurage from the hand to the shoulder, with pressure only on the up stroke.
2. **Palmar kneading to the upper arm and deltoid:** Use deep, slow strokes.
3. **Alternate thumb kneading to the upper arm:** Use alternate thumb kneading on the deltoid, the biceps, and the triceps. Knead the inner elbow at least six times.
4. **Wringing to the forearm:** With open-handed, C-shaped hands, wring from the inner elbow down the forearm and back up to the elbow.
5. **Effleurage to the forearm:** Use deep, slow effleurage from the wrist up to the elbow. Ask if your pressure should be firmer or softer.
6. **Thumb kneading to the forearm:** If there is muscle definition in the forearm, follow the contours of the muscles with your thumb strokes, keeping them penetrating and deep.
7. **Palmar kneading to the forearm:** Use the flat of your hand to smooth out the deep, grooving thumb kneading with deep palmar kneading.
8. **Frictioning:** Apply frictioning to any knotted or sensitive areas with fingertips, thumbs, or ice. Use ice frictioning liberally.
9. **Wringing to the forearm:** Move up and down with the stroke at least three times (but you can never do too much wringing).
10. **Repeat steps 6 to 9 three times.**

Move to the Hand

11. **Digital compression to the palm:** Move slowly and firmly. Focus on the heel of the hand, where the muscles may be pinching the nerve.
12. **Thumb stroking to the palm:** Use deep thumb stroking to the palm of the hand in all directions (up and down and across) to stretch out the palmar fascia.
13. **Corkscrewing to the fingers:** Pay special attention to the base of the fingers.
14. **Alternate thumb kneading to the palm:** Holding the wrist bent back, apply alternate thumb kneading to the palm of the hand with special attention to the wrist bones. Use very small and focused strokes.
15. **Alternate thumb kneading to the back of the wrist:** Holding the forearm up with the wrist bent down, do alternate thumb kneading to the top of the carpal bones at the wrist (again using small, focused, and firm strokes).
16. **Thumb stroking to the forearm:** Using short, deep, slow thumb strokes, move from the base of the hand halfway up the forearm. Make the strokes shorter and more concentrated near the wrist. Ask for feedback about tolerance for the pressure of this stroke.
17. **Finish:** Finish with wringing and then effleurage to the whole arm, followed by light reflex stroking.

As I work on the forearm with thumb and palmar kneading, I move the hand slowly between flexion and extension. This stretching movement maximizes effectiveness of the therapeutic strokes.

You may also want to add hydrotherapy contrast (cold and warm) arm bathing.

I find each patient distinctly different in the nature of their symptoms, which can range from complete numbness to partial tingling. The treatment is still basically the same. Work the head, neck, and shoulders, and then work down the arm to the wrist and hand. Find the person's particular areas of tension and develop a treatment plan that yields the best results.

The more you can loosen up the head, neck, and shoulders, and work the elbow, the better the hand feels. Lessening any pressure or edema in the arms, even if it is just for a few hours, gives a feeling of relief and ease of movement. This condition is like a headache in the arm, but one that for some people doesn't go away. The massage routine outlined above can be done several times each day for at least twenty minutes each time (minimum ten minutes per arm).

The best times for massaging anybody with carpal tunnel syndrome, or just swelling in the arms, are first thing in the morning and last thing at night. At the end of the day, people's arms are swollen due to gravity. A similar problem occurs at night, when the arms remain still during sleep. Massaging first thing in the morning helps get the circulation moving and relieves any pain or swelling that may have built up during the night.

Respiratory Problems

There are usually two types of wheelchair users, and they tend to experience different types of respiratory problems. Those who can propel themselves are more likely to have viral complaints such as chest and sinus congestion. Those who cannot propel themselves tend to have more longstanding problems that require full body respiratory massage. This level of immobilization can be due to conditions such as high spinal cord injury, geriatric frailty, or debilitating diseases such as ALS and MS.

Begin with a general massage for the back (pages 65 to 68) to help the nerves run smoothly out of the spine to the organs. The nerves that exit the thoracic area (upper and middle back) work the lungs, and the nerves from the lumbar area (lower back) work the digestive system. So massage the back thoroughly, knowing that you are helping problems such as digestive and respiratory dysfunction.

Then provide the respiratory massage your patient needs. No matter what kind of respiratory problem the wheelchair user has, your goal is to help them breathe better.

MASSAGE TO EASE CHEST OR SINUS CONGESTION

If the user has chest congestion that makes breathing difficult, begin your massage with a steam bath, which will help loosen some of the mucus. Pour boiling water and a few drops of eucalyptus oil into a bowl. Have the person sit in front of the bowl with their face in the vapor. Cover the head with a towel to make a steam tent and ask them to breathe slowly and deeply. Then apply cupping and other tapotement strokes to the back and chest to help loosen up any congestion.

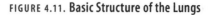

FIGURE 4.11. **Basic Structure of the Lungs**

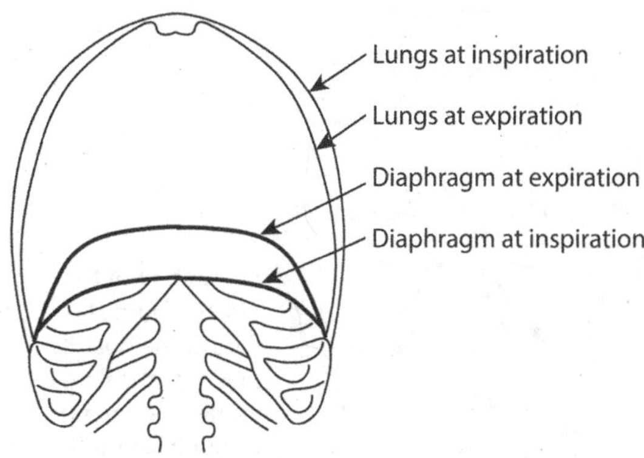

For upper respiratory congestion, shaking strokes to the nose and throat can also help ease breathing. For shaking strokes, make a *C*-shape with the hand and move your fingertips back and forth from side to side in a fast, but gentle, fluttering motion. Use a large *C*-shape to fit the front of the neck and a smaller fingertip *C*-shape to run up and down the nose where it attaches to the face.

MASSAGE MENU FOR FULL BODY RESPIRATORY MASSAGE

1. **Wringing to the trunk:** Start with wringing to both sides of the trunk of the body.
2. **Costal border scooping:** The sides of the person are also a great place to ease up breathing with a scooping massage along the costal angle of the ribs.
3. **Kneading and thumb stroking to the diaphragm:** Use fingertip kneading and bilateral thumb stroking to the attachments of the diaphragm to the ribs. Kneading along the edge of the ribs may give some extra release to help breathing. Your fingers should roll over the edge of the costal angle (bottom rib) to get the diaphragm attachments.

FIGURE 4.12. **Respiratory Shaking**

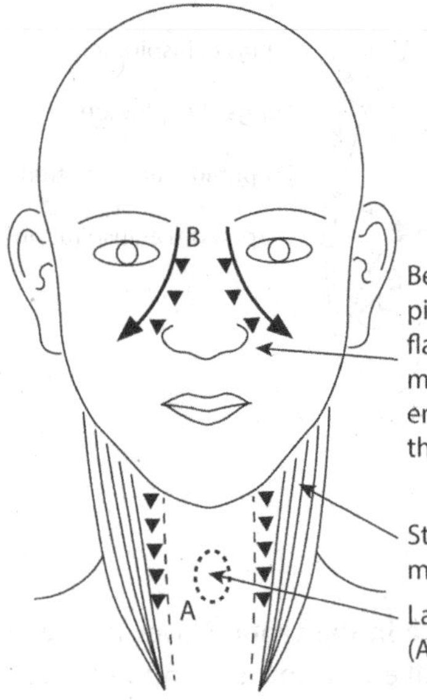
B
A
Be careful not to pinch inward at the flare of the nostrils: maintain the flare entrance opening throughout the stroke.
Sternocleidomastoid muscle
Laryngeal prominence (Adam's apple)

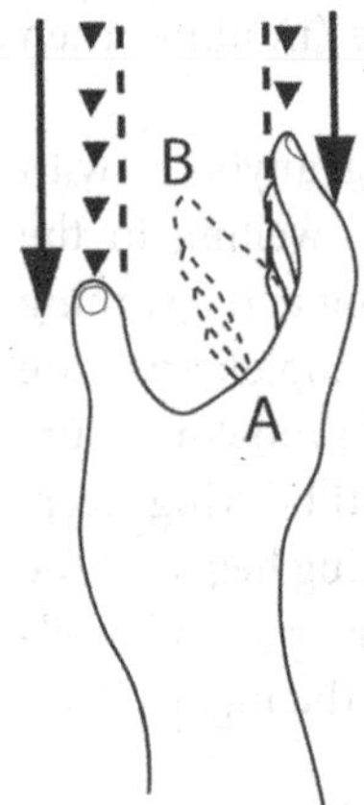
B
A
A. Hand grip for laryngeal shaking
B. Hand grip for nasal root shaking

FIGURE 4.13. **Respiratory Massage: Costal Border Scooping**

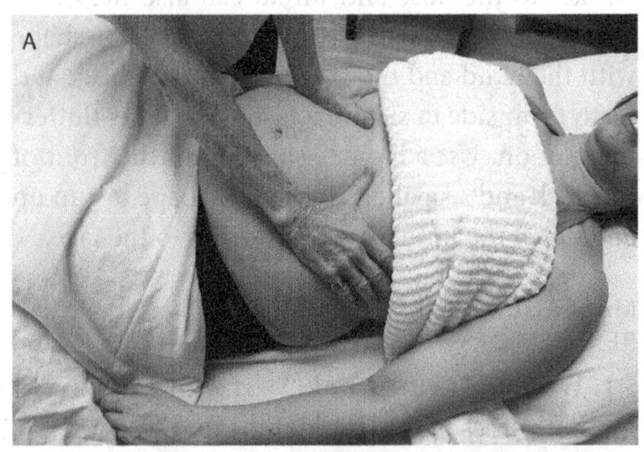
A

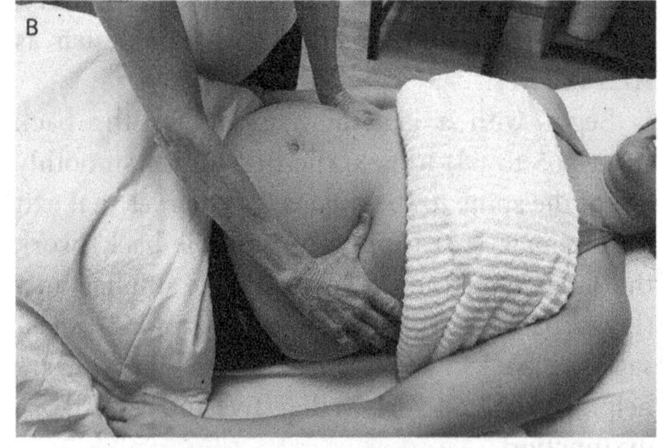
B

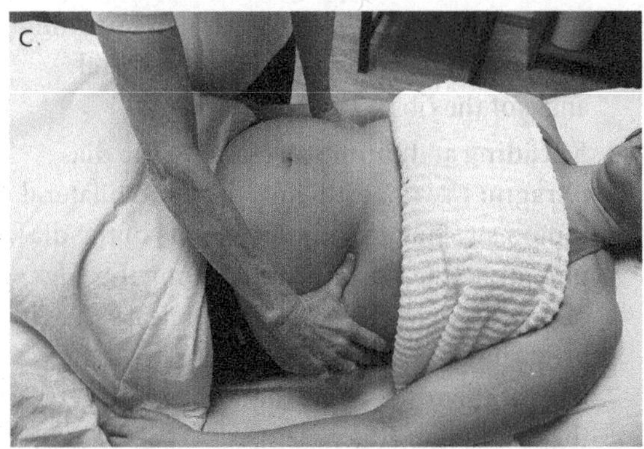
C

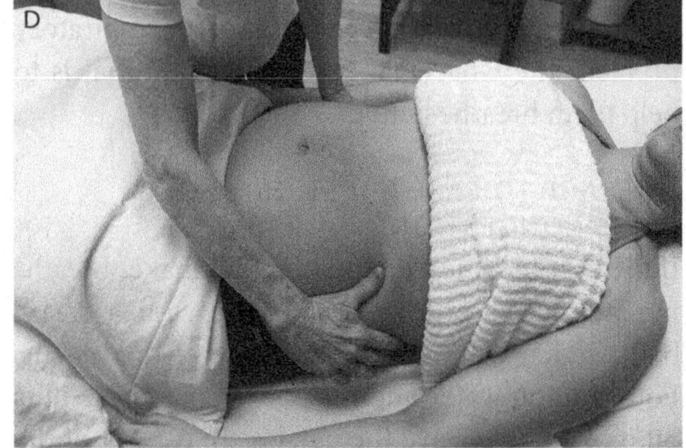
D

FIGURE 4.14. Respiratory Massage: Diaphragm Strokes

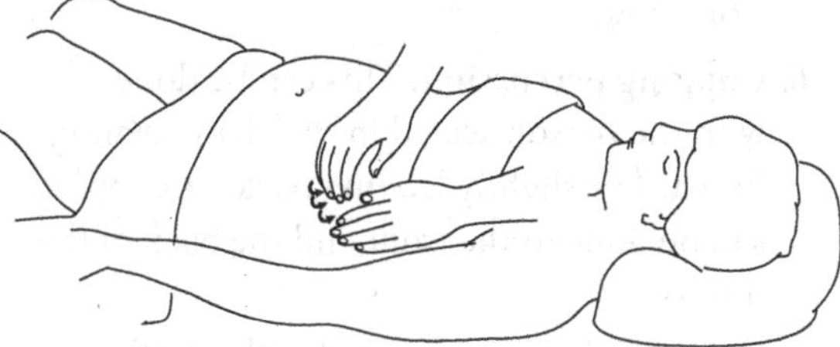

Kneading along the edge of the ribs.

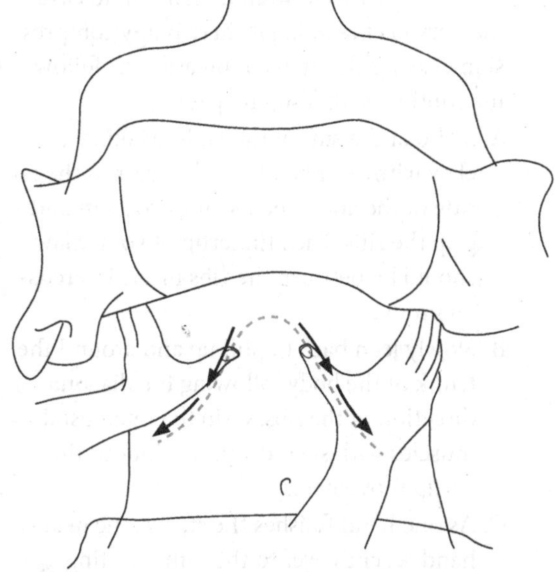

Bilateral thumb stretching under the costal angle.

FIGURE 4.15. Respiratory Massage: Rib Raking

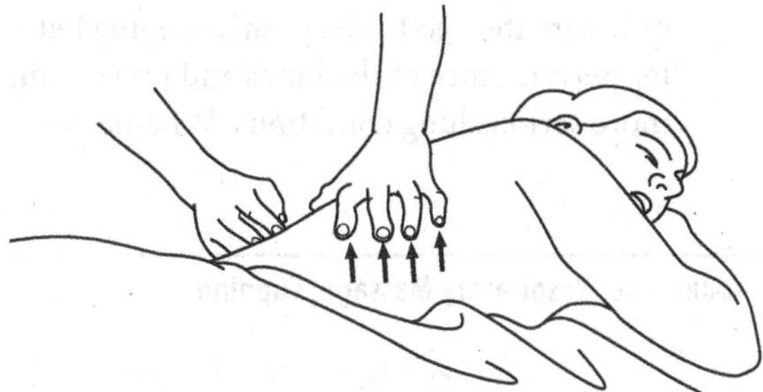

Fit your fingers between the ribs and pull to help stretch the intercostal muscles.

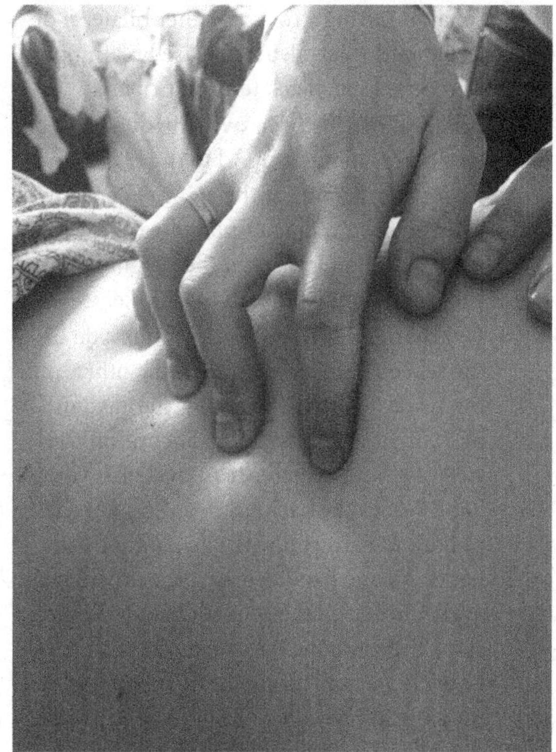

Use a clawlike hand for rib raking.

4. **Overhanded rib raking:** Rib raking draws the fingers across the tiny intercostal muscles between the ribs to stretch them out to ease the person's breathing if there is any compression causing shortness of breath. The following routine is for a supine patient.
   A. Stand at the side of the table. Making a claw with your hand, reach across to the far side of the abdomen as far as you can and grip the ribs. Each fingertip of your "claw" should be between the ribs in the intercostal grooves.
   B. Slowly lean back to pull up and around the trunk of the body following the diagonal direction of the ribs. Grip the intercostal muscles with slow, deep, continuous fingertip movements.
   C. As one hand finishes the stroke, the next hand reaches over to the same starting point and begins. Do this until there is a significant change in breathing, usually after five to ten strokes.
5. **Lifting to the thoracic and lumbar (in or out of chair):** Lifting strokes—either bilateral or overhanded—can also help ease breathing and relieve lower back tension or pain.
   - **Bilateral lifting:** Lean over the person and circle your hands around to the back, your fingertips meeting at the spine. Then slowly, very slowly, lift up and pull toward the front until your hands meet at the sternum, with very light contact to end the stroke.
   - **Overhanded lifting:** Work on one side of the wheelchair user and then the other, pulling toward yourself with alternating hands like you are bringing in an anchor off the side of a boat. Reach across and tuck your hand under the back toward the spine. Then pull up toward you with the palm of your hand. As one hand finishes, the other starts. Walk around to the other side and do the same lifting to the far side of the person's body. If you can't walk to the other side, it's possible to do both sides of the body from one side. The lifting on the near side won't be "overhanded," but it will still balance both sides and relieve that lower back pain or tension.
6. **Cupping percussion:** This can be done with the person seated in the chair, leaning forward or slightly leaning back, or cupping can be done to the front and the back of the thorax.
7. **Compression:** This is used with breathing, pressing in a pumping action to help elicit a stronger coughing reflex, aiding in expectoration.
   - A gentle mini-massage to finish off will leave a positive tactile experience as some of these movements may cause discomfort. If the person is suffering from lung congestion, remember that these strokes can be done as often as every hour to keep the lungs clear.
   - Whether the person is in or out of the chair, you can use these techniques at the beginning of the day, in the middle of their workday, on the sidelines of their sports match, or before they go to sleep, encouraging better performance of the lungs and preventing more serious lung conditions. Whether you

FIGURE 4.16. Respiratory Massage: Cupping

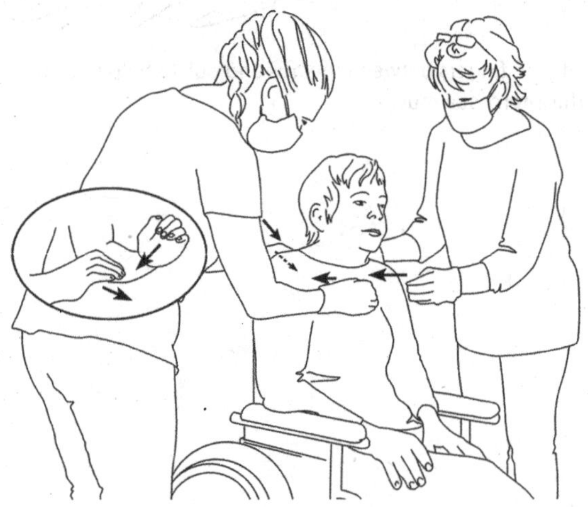

Tandem cupping, upper chest, front and back.

FIGURE 4.17. Respiratory Massage: Compression

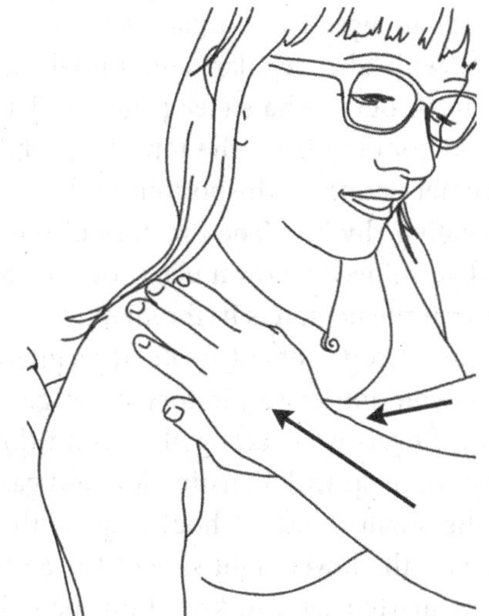

Reinforced compression, upper chest.

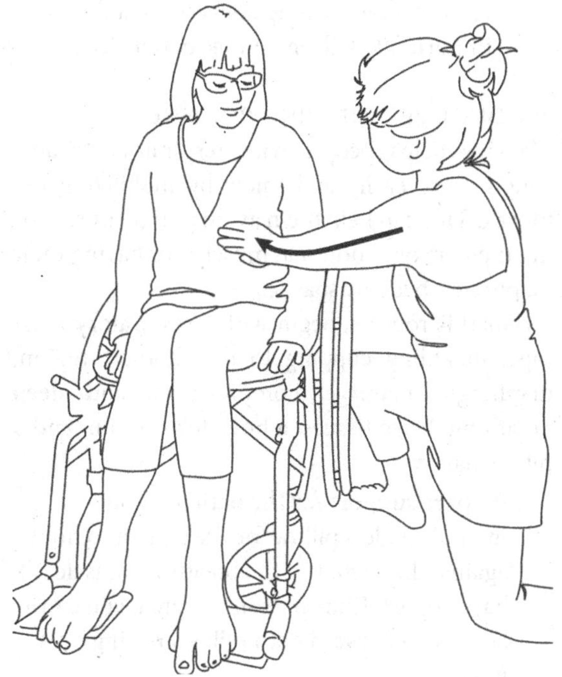

Reinforced diaphragmatic compression.

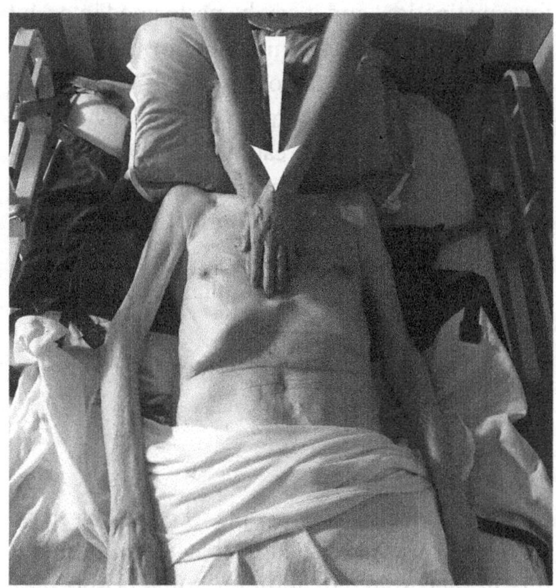

Reinforced sternal compression.

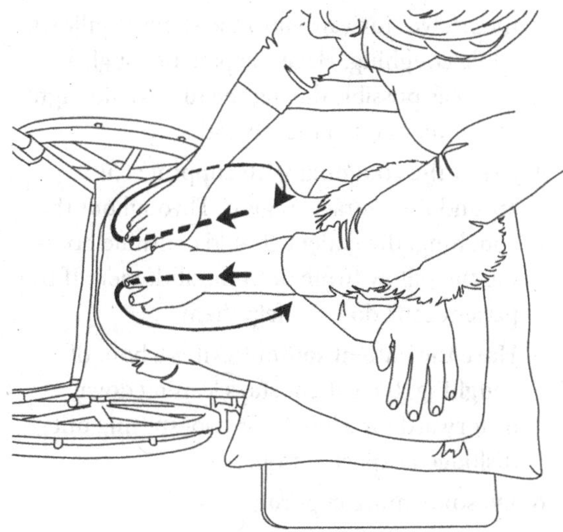

Two-handed compression, lower back.

take five minutes for a mini-massage or give a full body treatment, anything you have to offer will relieve lung congestion and more importantly will encourage better sleep.

PRODUCTIVE COUGHING ROUTINE

Massage helps people with respiratory trouble cough more easily and safely by mobilizing the thorax. This can help them avoid pulling or straining their rib or abdominal muscles, or having their diaphragm become spastic.

For this routine, begin with a respiratory massage, including cupping to the thoracic region, diaphragm massage, compressions, and deep breathing. Have tissues, a bowl for sputum, and a pillow handy.

1. **Prepare support for the patient's abdomen:** Provide a pillow for the patient to hold against their front so the breathing muscle has support. If the person is seated, you can lean them forward onto pillows resting on a table.
2. **Rotate the arms in both directions.**
3. **Get the patient coughing:** Have the patient take deep breaths and, if they can, throw themselves forward onto the support pillows while coughing. Have the patient cough as much as possible during the full exhale, right to the very end of their breath.
4. **Assist the coughing with cupping:** Cup around the thoracic region. Throughout the coughing, the patient should continue holding the pillow firmly into the abdomen. If the patient can't do this, help them.
5. **Have the patient spit out:** After a bout of coughing, the patient stays leaning down or forward for a breath or two, spitting out dislodged expectoration.
6. **Do some more cupping.**
7. **Have the patient slowly rise up with an inward breath.**
8. **Repeat three or more times:** Continue the process until the patient's lungs are clear.
9. **Massage the entire back.**
10. **Rest.**

Constipation

The massage routine for relieving constipation can be used for all digestive complaints.

Begin with the regular abdominal massage routine in or out of chair (see page 76). Do open *C*-shaped scooping from the top of the abdomen to the center and from the bottom to the center in an alternating rhythm. The pressure of the stroke will be determined by how much room you have to maneuver if the person is in the chair.

You can also do lots of bilateral wringing and lifting, as you did for respiratory massage. Vibrations and fingertip kneading all around the large intestine will help with constipation and gas. Start where the small intestine hooks up to the large intestine on the lower right side of the abdomen. It is particularly useful to knead on the descending colon, especially on the lower left side of the abdomen. Follow the path of the digestive system, remembering to linger in the corners (flexures) of the large intestine. When you reach the lower left corner, you can glide across the bottom, where the bladder is, to start the circle again. For a diagram of the digestive tract, see Figure 3.6.

Leg pumping is an important part of massage for constipation, and it can be performed in or out of the chair. The best stimulation for the digestive system is movement, not massage strokes. Leg pumping unwinds the digestive system. This is the same routine I use for treating anybody with constipation or digestive complaints: abdominal massage, then leg pumping, abdominal massage, then leg pumping.

You can pump the legs simultaneously or one at a time (alternate leg pumping).

For steps on leg pumping in a wheelchair, see page 55.

Spinal Problems

In my experience, most people who are long-term wheelchair users experience changes in the curvature of their spine. In addition, some people have preexisting back problems before they become wheelchair users. For example, if someone has scoliosis (a lateral curve of the spine)—whether a simple *C*-curve or a compound *S*-curve—that

FIGURE 4.18. **Leg Pumping to Relieve Constipation**

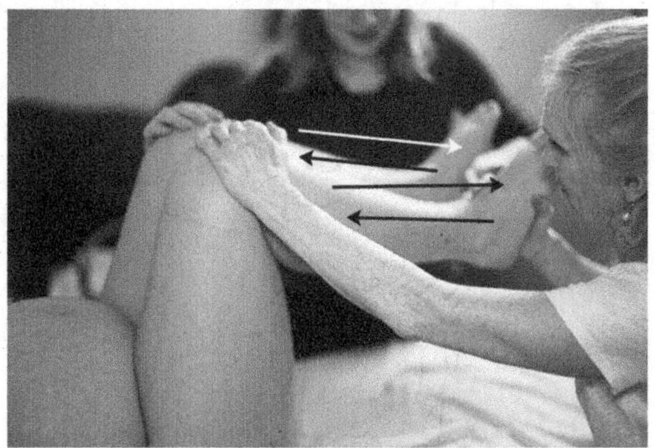

Simultaneous leg pumping: use your hand or forearm to press against the knees to help you bend your patient's legs.

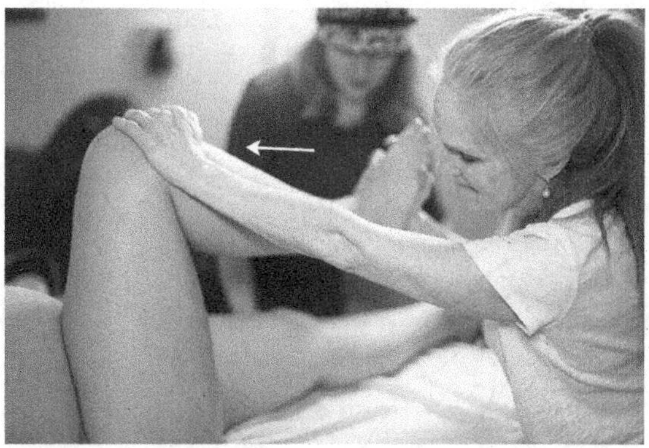

Alternate leg pumping: you can do this alone, but it is easier if you have a partner to work the other leg.

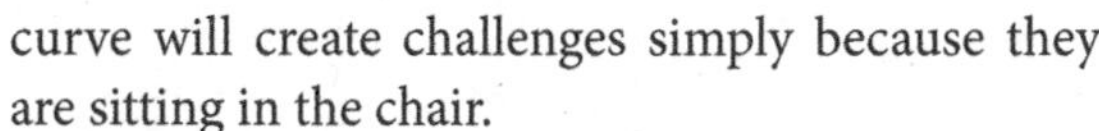

curve will create challenges simply because they are sitting in the chair.

You can try to mitigate the extra pressure on the spine with massage, working the muscles along the spine to stretch the contracted muscles and stimulate the overly stretched muscles to contract. Both contracted and stretched muscles need attention so they can recover from the daily strain of an immobilized back resulting from hours in the chair.

The more acute problems of kyphosis (humpback) and lordosis (swayback) often give rise to sacroiliac strain as the lumbar area gets pulled. Kyphosis includes highly rounded shoulders, tight, shortened pectoral muscles, and stretched, weak back muscles; lordosis is an excessive inward curve of the spine at the lower back.

Daily massage is what works, if not twice a day, to keep the back and spine healthy.

A spinal massage is best done out of the chair: on a bed or table, or on the floor. Start with the person in face-up position to stretch out the contracted pectoral muscles, and then with them face-down or side-lying (both sides) to work on tightness and adhesions in the back muscles.

In the starting position (face-up), position towels to help counteract kyphosis and lordosis. Place a rolled towel under the entire length of the spine. Then flex the patient's legs at the hips and knees, and support the flexed legs with a stack of towels. Make the stack high enough that the person's feet are slightly higher than their knees.

SPINAL MASSAGE MENU

Get the person to raise their arms and put their hands behind their head.

1. **Effleurage to the head, neck, shoulders, and abdomen.**
2. **Palmar stretching to the pectorals.**
3. **Thumb stretching to the pectorals.**
4. **Frictioning to pressure points:** Use your thumbs, fingertips, or palms.
5. **Palmar stretching/palmar kneading (repeat).**
6. **Scooping to the pectorals.**
7. **Frictioning to the muscle attachments on the sternum.**
8. **Scooping to the armpit:** This encourages lymphatic drainage (optional).
9. **Arm massage:** Apply the basic full arm treatment, focusing on the shoulders, elbows, and wrists with additional emphasis on the hands.
10. **Lower thoracic massage:** Apply rib-raking and diaphragmatic scooping, fingertip kneading, and costal angle massage.
11. **Neck twists:** This is like wringing. With one hand on the forehead and one reaching over the body to the far side of the neck, lift the

FIGURE 4.19. Spinal Massage: Palmar Stretching

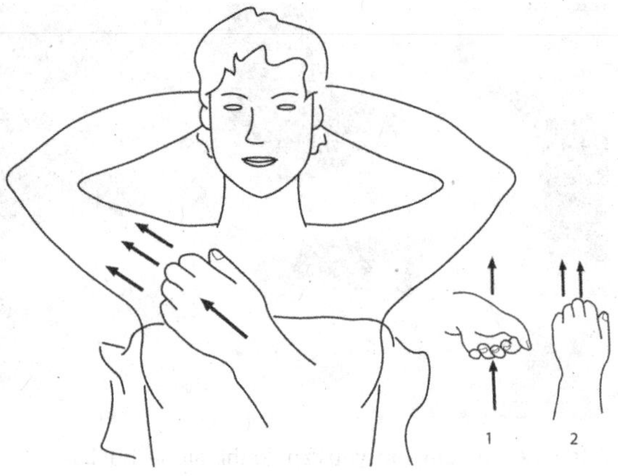

a. Palmar stretching to the pectorals. Use the backs of your fingers to roll across the muscle.

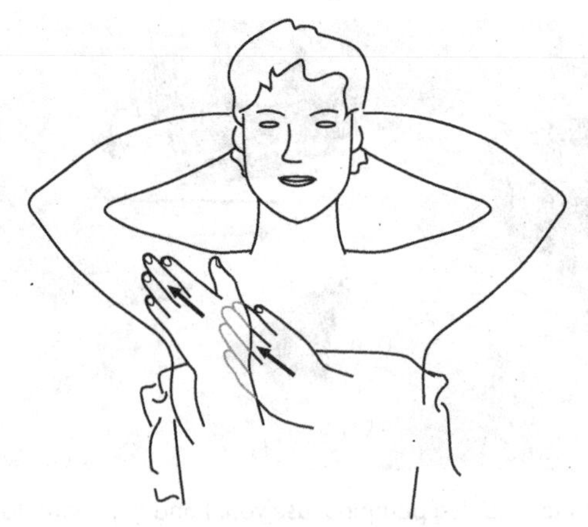

b. Overhanded palmar stretching to the pectorals: pushing away from yourself at the pectoral attachment at the sternum (chest bone).

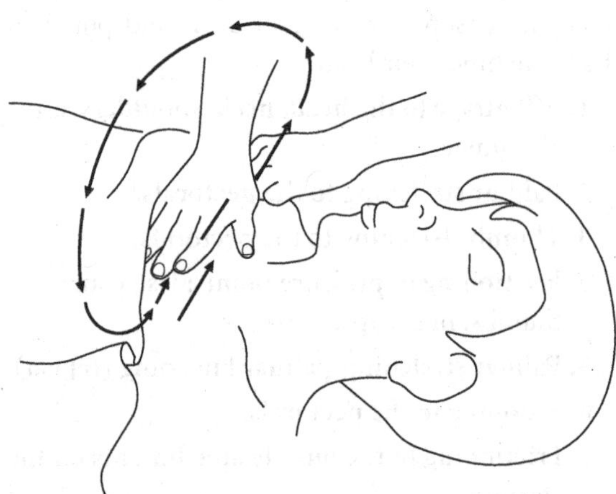

c. Overhanded palmar stretching to the pectorals: pulling toward yourself.

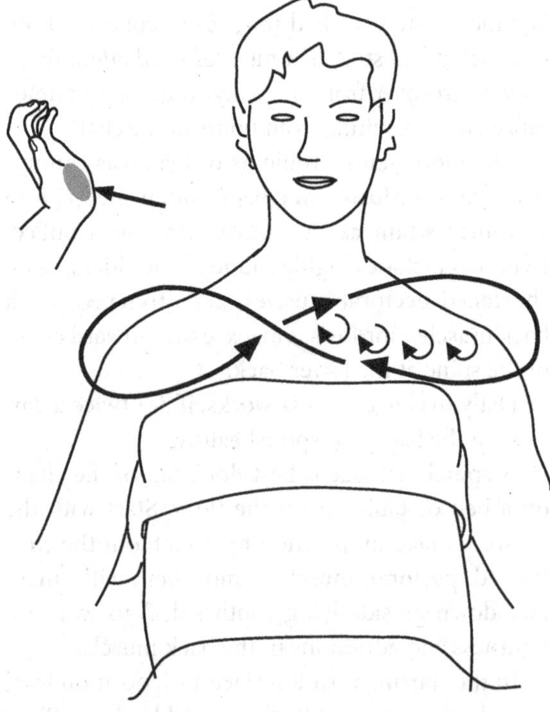

d. As a finishing or beginning pectoral stretch, use your palms to do a figure eight across the chest. Use the thenar eminence at the base of the thumb to knead circles around this path.

FIGURE 4.20. Spinal Massage: Frictioning Points along the Pectorals

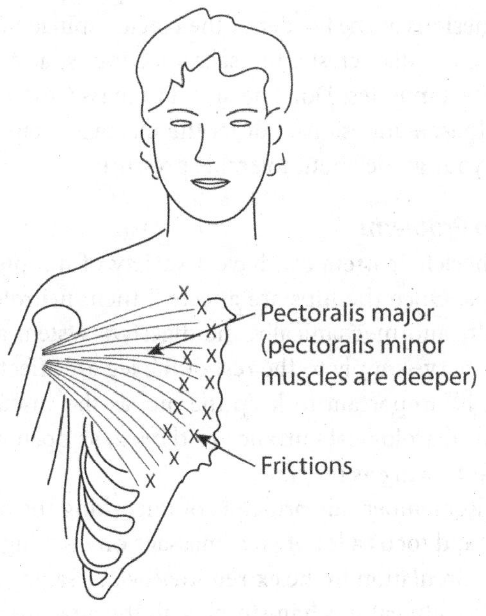

FIGURE 4.21. Spinal Massage: Scooping to the Lateral Pectoral with Alternating Hands

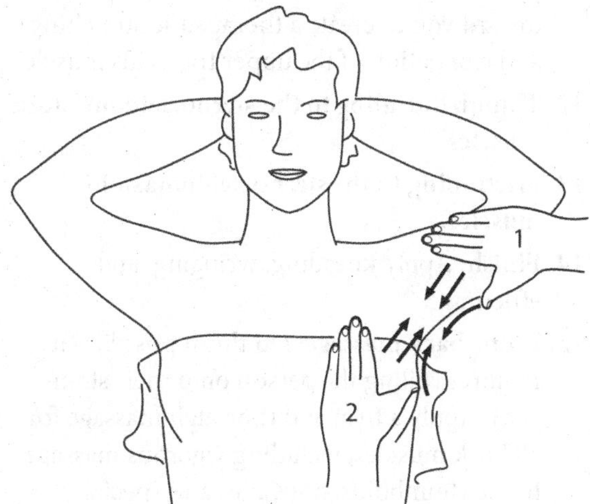

Axilla (armpit) scooping with the arm turned upward. Scoop with one hand, then the other.

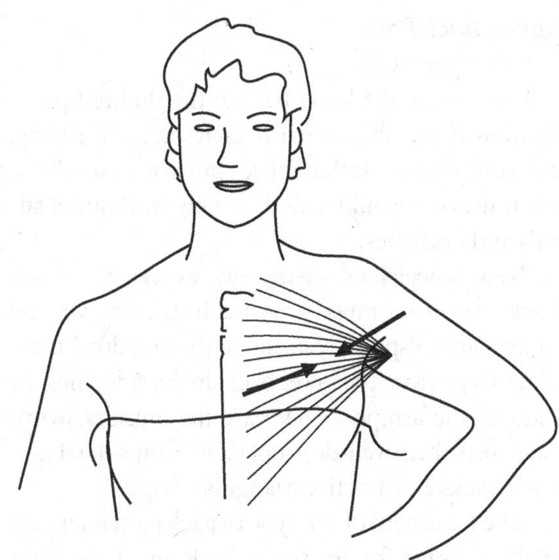

Scooping the pectoralis major with the arm turned downward.

FIGURE 4.22. Spinal Massage: Neck Twist

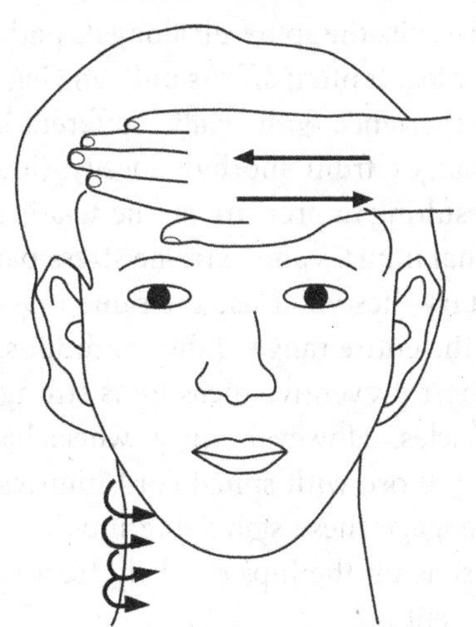

neck and pull the head so the face rotates toward you. As you push the face away from you, lift up from behind the neck and rotate it toward you to create a therapeutic stretching and elongation of the upper trapezius muscle.

12. **Thumb kneading to the sternocleidomastoid muscles.**
13. **Frictioning to the sternocleidomastoid muscles.**
14. **Finish:** Apply kneading, wringing, and effleurage.
15. **Prone back massage:** Do this if possible (it requires rolling the person onto their stomach). Apply a firm and thorough massage for all back muscles, including vigorous massage to the rhomboids, trapezius, and special attention to the lower back muscles to loosen them up.

Lower Back Pain

See Figure 4.23.

Pain moves to the lower back at the slightest provocation if the abdominal muscles are not strong. If I could have a training program for new wheelchair users, it would include a daily workout of sit-ups and crunches.

New wheelchair users may experience lower back pain from muscle spasms in the lumbar and gluteal area, especially in the latissimus dorsi muscles that go from the lower back up the sides into the back of the armpits. These are the muscles swimmers use: their well-developed latissimus dorsi give their backs a distinctive triangular shape.

The treatment of this type of back pain is an easy daily massage for the lower back and hips. Your aim is to relax the contracted muscles to improve mobility and to strengthen the lumbar flexors, lateral flexors, and trunk rotators to provide stability. Focus on massaging adhesions at the attachments of the erector spinae muscles, the iliac crests, the sacroiliac joints, and the gluteal muscles. Then use additional kneading and effleurage to soothe pain and increase relaxation.

Since it may be too painful to massage the area most affected, focus your attention on the areas above and below the focus of pain. Apply heat, and use effleurage and kneading strokes to encourage general stretching. Build the wheelchair user's tolerance for frictioning for any trigger points or adhesions at the border of the erector spinae muscles, the iliac crests, the sacroiliac joints, and the gluteal muscles. Don't be afraid to massage deeply to loosen adhesions, but let the massage recipient be your guide about tolerable pressure.

Hip Problems

Wheelchair users can have a variety of hip problems. Once the hips are affected, then, neurologically and mechanically, the digestive system and the nerve supply to the rest of the leg are affected. So, it's important to keep the hip, as the vascular and neurological entrance to the leg, as open and free-flowing as possible.

Remember our principle of uncorking the bottle, and focus a lot of your massage on opening up the circulation to the extremities by massaging the entire gluteal mechanism plus all the attachments to the ischial tuberosity and the iliac crest. You can do this out of the chair or, with levering techniques, in the chair.

Some people use wheelchairs after surgery for a short term. These people can experience unilateral symptoms because of measures the body will inevitably take to compensate for whatever immobility has been caused by the surgery.

Sciatica

Sciatica is described as a gnawing, tingling, or burning sensation in the lower back, where the sciatic nerve exits the spine, all along its path down to the lower leg. It often affects only one leg.

My experience with sciatic sufferers in wheelchairs ranges from morbid obesity (lower back issues resulting in pressure on the sciatic nerve) to non-spinal injuries and extreme stress paired with a sedentary lifestyle. I use the same massage routine for the entire range of the conditions.

The best preventive measure is strong abdominal muscles. However, most wheelchair users, especially those with spinal cord injuries, are not able to engage these stabilizing muscles. Massage that loosens up the hips can help treat sciatica or even prevent it.

FIGURE 4.23. Lower Back Massage

ERECTOR SPINAE STRETCH

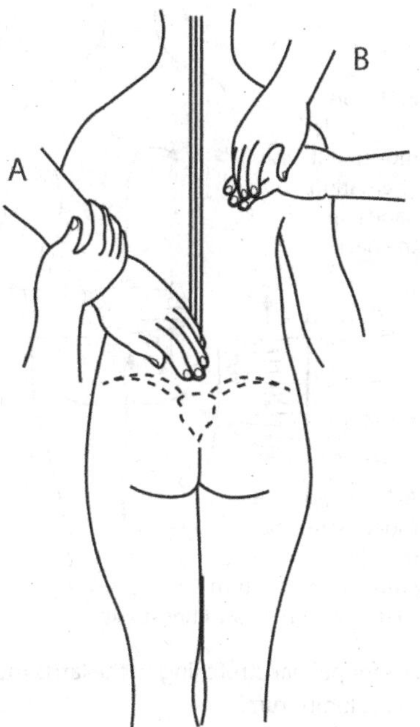

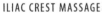

Stretch the erector spinae muscles with one or both of these two-handed variations: (A) wrist locked with other hand; (B) reinforced palms.

ICE MASSAGE

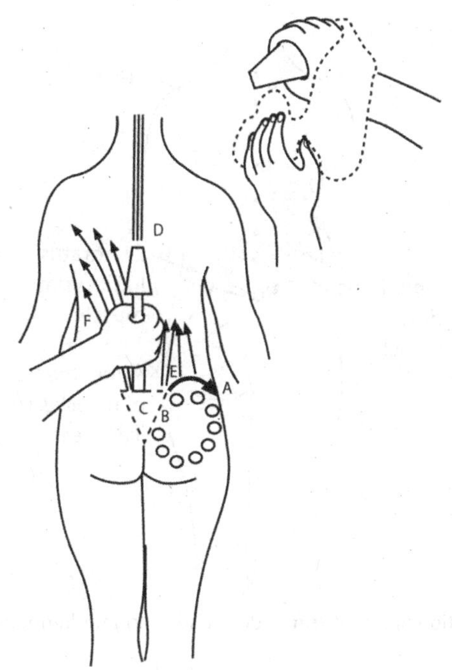

Keep a towel handy to mop up melting water. Strokes: (A) fan stroke to iliac crest; (B) gluteal kneading; (C) sacrum kneading; (D) erector spinae stretch; (E) quadratus lumborum stretch (F) latissimus dorsi stretch.

ILIAC CREST MASSAGE

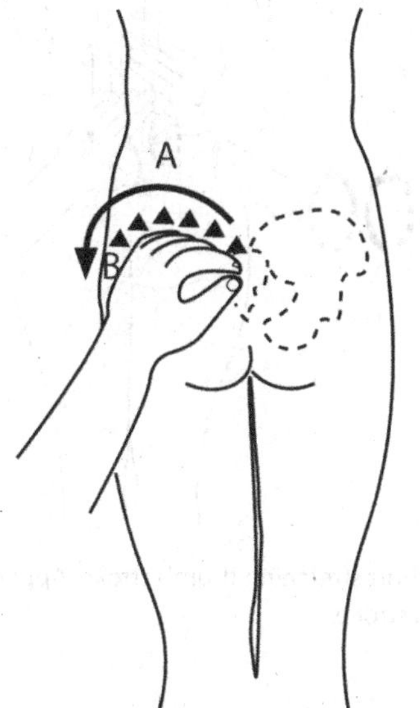

Strokes for the iliac crest: (A) fan stroke with all your fingers lined up next to each other; (B) fingertip kneading.

SACRUM KNEADING

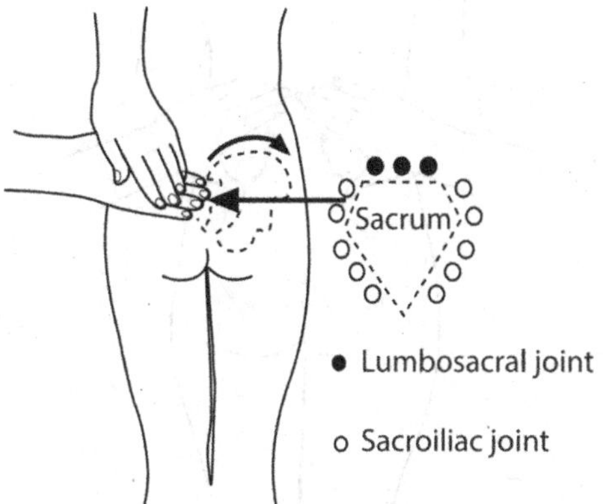

Reinforced or single-handed fingertip kneading to the sacrum is useful for any kind of sacroiliac joint pain (usually felt in the lower back and gluteals).

FIGURE 4.23. CONTINUED

PALM STRETCHING TO THE LATISSIMUS DORSI AND QUADRATUS LUMBORUM

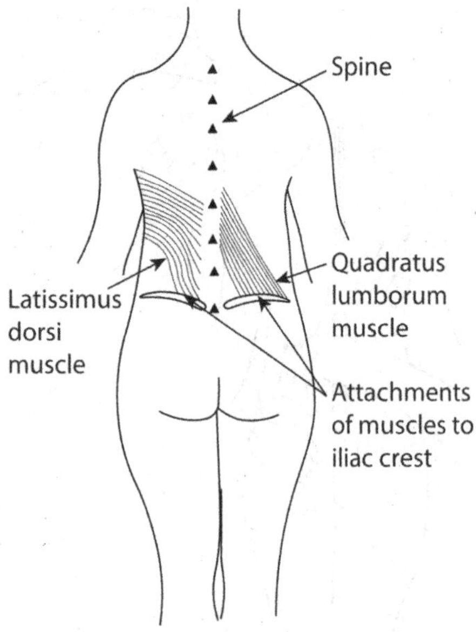

Location of the latissimus dorsi and quadratus lumborum.

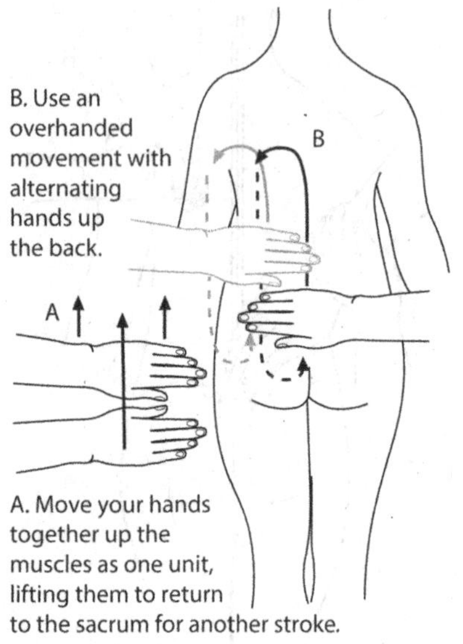

Two options for palmar stretching to the latissimus dorsi and quadratus lumborum.

THUMB STROKES

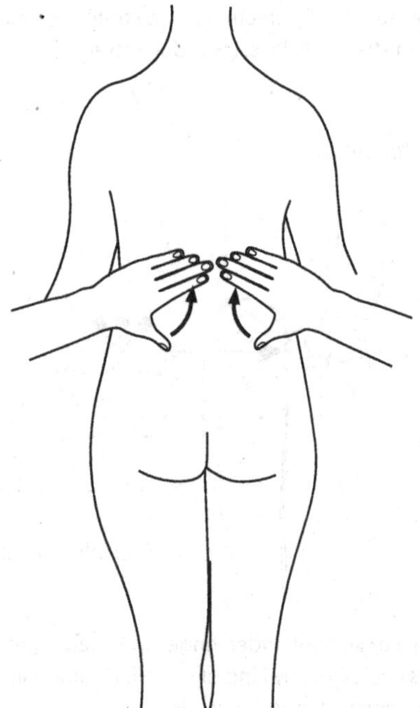

Thumb stretching to the quadratus lumborum. Move the thumbs toward the fingers, stretching the muscle underneath. Use both hands at the same time.

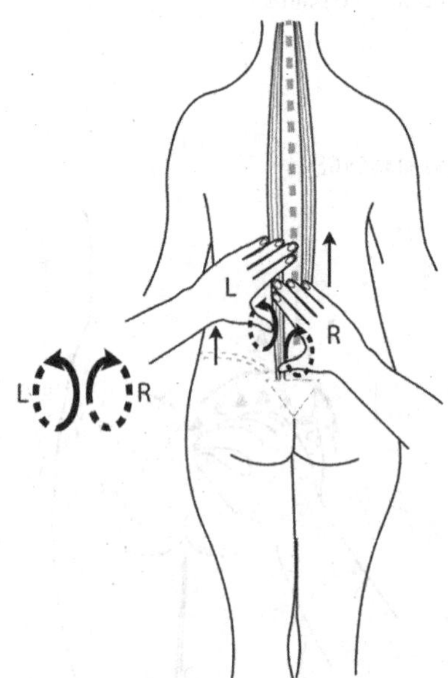

Alternate, short stretching thumb stroke. Apply pressure on the upward stroke.

FIGURE 4.23. CONTINUED

THUMB STROKES

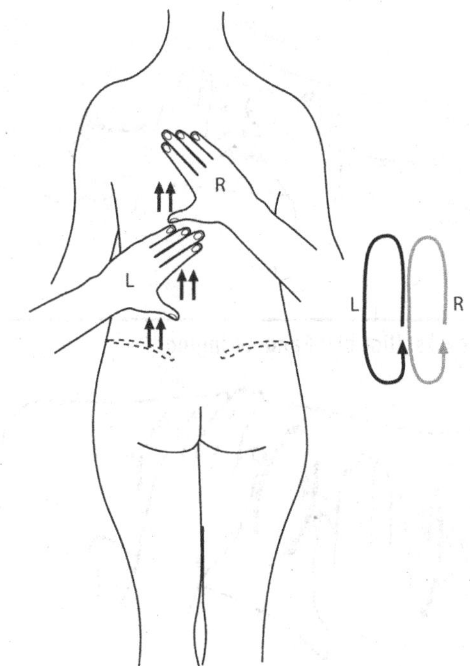

Alternate, long stretching thumb stroke to the quadratus lumborum and latissimus dorsi.

The side-lying massage position is perfect to get the whole hip loosened up, which makes the sciatic nerve happier. I always hope that wheelchair users can exit their chairs for a stretch, or use a standing chair, or that the chair itself can stretch out!

I often start on the unaffected leg to see what the real feel of my patient's leg is. I once started on the affected side and thought I had the treatment well covered, only to discover that the unaffected side was identical, although it had not exhibited any sciatica symptoms. My other rationale for starting my sciatica massage on the unaffected side is that people favor the painful side when moving or lying down. The unaffected side compensates for the painful side and does more than its share of the work of both legs.

SCIATICA MASSAGE MENU (SIDE-LYING)

1. **Overhanded palmar kneading to the hip:** Warm the hip up thoroughly, usually with palmar overhanded kneading to the hip and gluteals.
2. **Fisted kneading to the hip:** Make fists and use them in the same motions over the hip for a deeper kneading sensation.
3. **Alternate thumb kneading to the iliotibial band:** Move on to alternate thumb kneading along the iliotibial band.
4. **Whole leg massage:** Do all the deep massage strokes (wringing, alternate thumb kneading, and thumb stretching) for the whole leg—including the lower back and knees—as you would even without sciatica.
5. **Ice frictioning:** If the wheelchair user has a full-blown case of sciatica, use ice frictioning with the pointed end of an popsicle on the lower back lumbar area and the lumbosacral and sacroiliac joints. Use a facecloth or towel to catch the runoff of melting ice.
6. **Hydrotherapy:** A person with sciatica deserves an overdose of massage and hydrotherapy. Use Epsom salt baths, ice massage, and alternating cold and hot water bottles to provide relief and stimulation.

Contracted Iliotibial Band

The iliotibial band is a band of fascia extending down the outside of the leg from the ilium (or pelvis) to the tibial attachment at the top of the outer side of the lower leg. A serious case of contracted iliotibial band is painful and restricts movement. This condition often arises with wheelchair users who have had previous leg injuries or had contracted iliotibial bands before being in a chair. Whether this is a precondition or one that arises from being in the chair, your job is to keep this structure as supple as possible. This elasticity does not come easily. The iliotibial band is designed to be inflexible: it's made of fascia instead of red, meaty, elastic muscle.

The route of the band is usually very tender. Use effleurage, wringing, alternate thumb kneading, thumb wringing, and digital compression directly on the band. Repeat long effleurage strokes to "erase" the biting pain of the focused strokes so you can work into the area again.

MASSAGE MENU FOR CONTRACTED ILIOTIBIAL BAND

1. **Effleurage:** Apply this to the entire leg, three times.
2. **Reinforced palmar kneading to the hip.**
3. **Single-handed palmar kneading to the head of the femur.**
4. **Fingertip kneading to the attachments of the iliotibial band at the top of the thigh.**
5. **Alternate thumb kneading along the whole iliotibial band:** Begin where the band originates in the tensor fascia lata and gluteals and run down to where it attaches to the lower leg below the knee.
6. **Wringing across the iliotibial band:** Include the quadriceps. Use open-handed *C*-shaped wringing if you prefer.
7. **Deep palmar transverse frictions:** Use the thenar eminence (base of the thumb). Tuck your thumb into your fist and friction across the iliotibial band using your thenar eminence.
8. **Long strokes:** Stroke along the length of the thigh going up to the hip, like a mini-effleurage, first with the thenar eminence and then with the thumbs.
9. **Short strokes:** Move your thumbs forward and back in short strokes up the length of the thigh, always with pressure applied only toward the heart and just light contact on the way back.
10. **Transverse skin rolling:** Draw fingers toward stationary thumbs like a big pinch of the iliotibial band.
11. **Transverse stroke with the heel of the hand.**
12. **Transverse stroke with the thumbs:** Wring the tract slowly and deliberately.
13. **Reinforced palmar kneading.**
14. **Wringing to the leg from the femur to the toes.**
15. **Finish:** Apply effleurage and light reflex stroking.

Be sure to work the wringing and kneading strokes all the way down the iliotibial band to the attachment at the tibia past the knee joint. Linger at this lower attachment. This is where there is little elasticity because the iliotibial band likes to keep things inflexible and strong. For wheelchair users who have spinal cord injuries, there can be little sensation below the waist, so pain associated with a contracted iliotibial band won't be sensed, so you must be careful with deeper strokes.

FIGURE 4.24. **Iliotibial Band: Alternate Thumb Kneading**

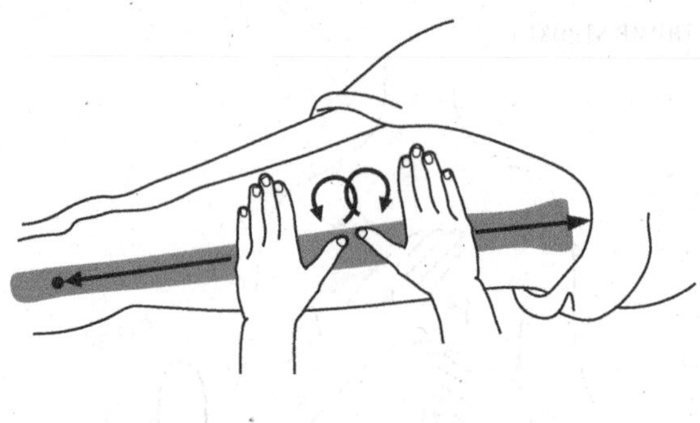

FIGURE 4.25. **Iliotibial Band: Wringing**

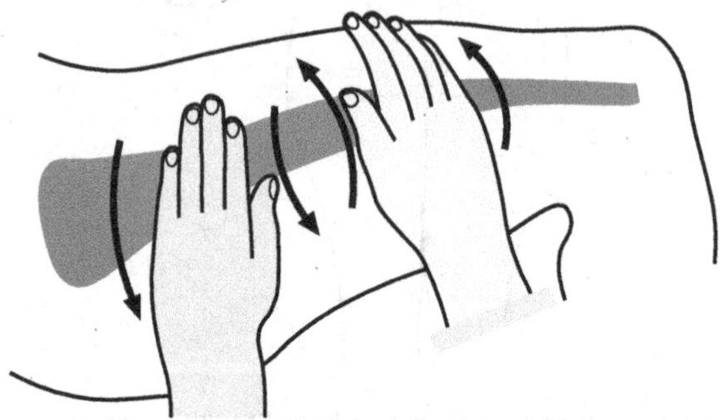

Wring across the iliotibial band, including the quadriceps.

FIGURE 4.26. **Iliotibial Band: Deep Palmar Transverse Frictions**

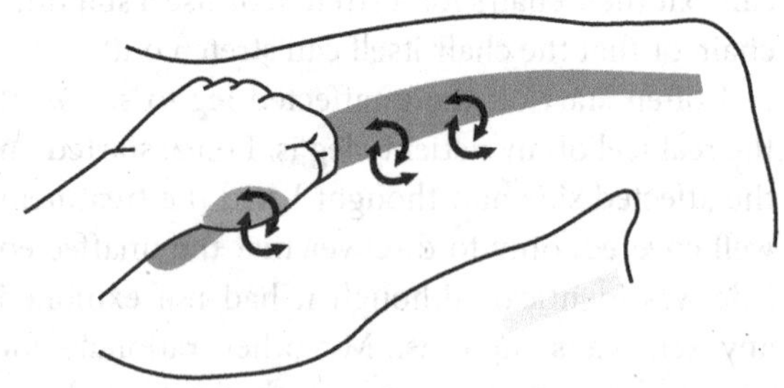

FIGURE 4.27. Iliotibial Band: Long and Short Strokes

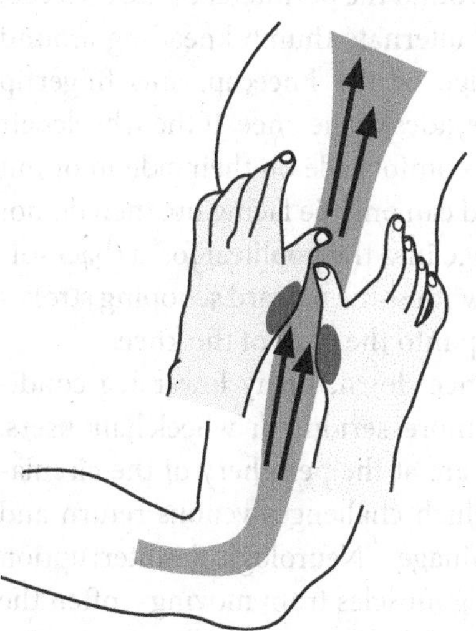

Long strokes with the heel of the hand. Use one hand or both at the same time.

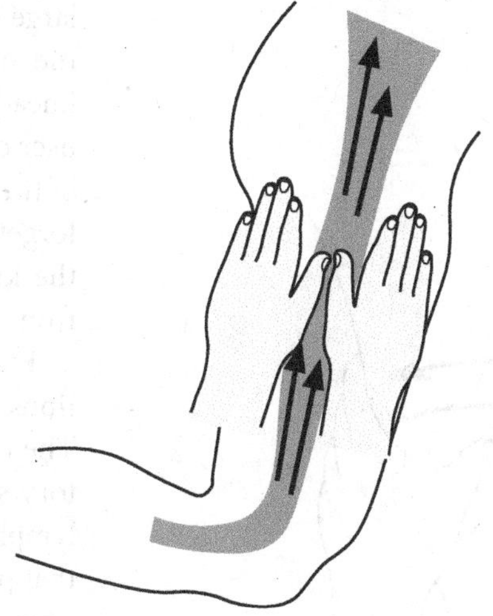

Long strokes with the thumbs.

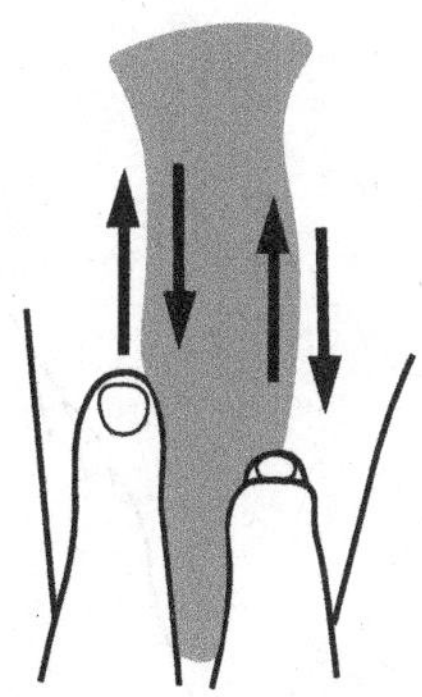

Short strokes with the thumbs.

FIGURE 4.28. Iliotibial Band: Transverse Skin Rolling

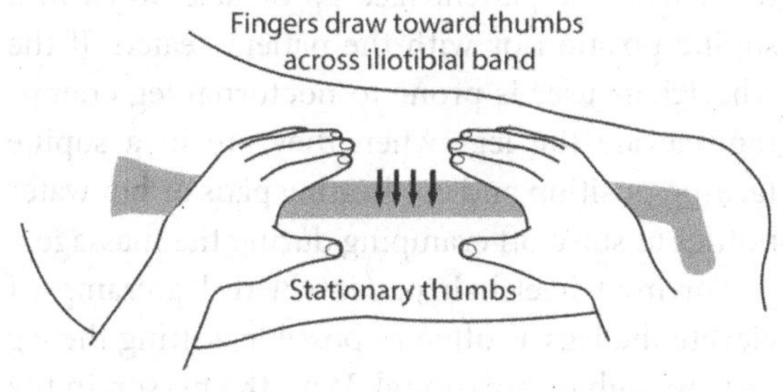

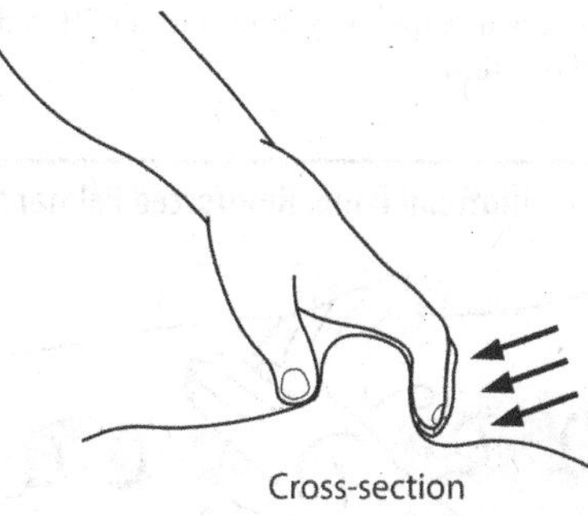

FIGURE 4.29. Iliotibial Band: Transverse Stroking: Heel of Hand

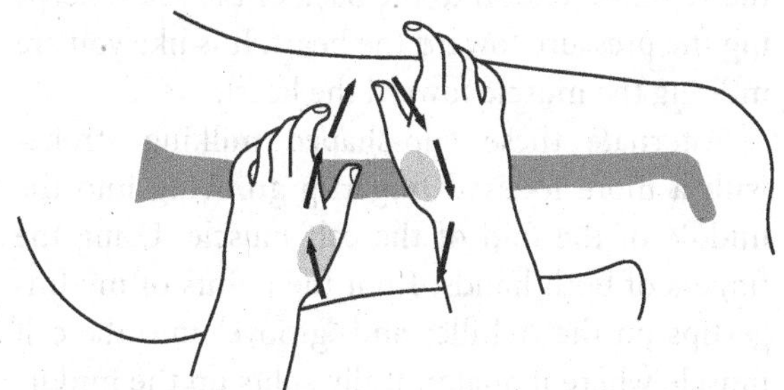

Stroke across the iliotibial band with the thenar eminence and palms.

At both attachments (hip and knee), but especially at and below the knee, use frictioning with ice or fingertips or a fisted knuckle. This back-and-forth movement helps break down adhesions. You can alternate kneading or wringing with frictioning to make the frictions more tolerable. This is an important structure, whether it has a problem or not, to keep as flexible as possible in order to guarantee mobility in the knee and hip joints.

Knee Problems

Bridging the top of the lower leg is the almighty knee, including the patella (kneecap). The knee is the largest joint in the body. Swimming (for

FIGURE 4.30. Iliotibial Band: Transverse Stroking with the Thumbs

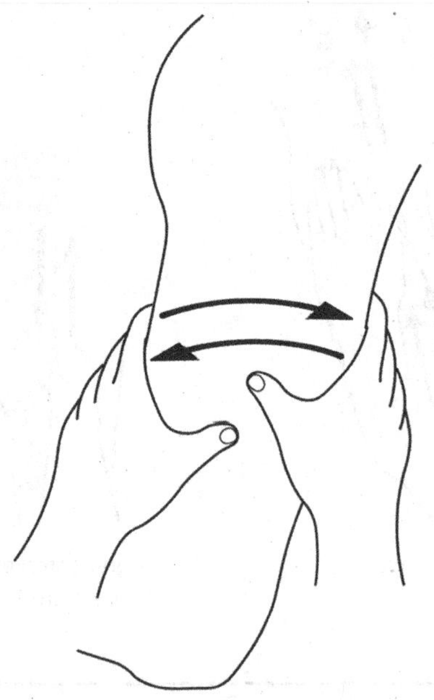

Position your thumbs slightly offet from one another and press them toward, then past one another. Then draw back to original position.

FIGURE 4.31. Iliotibial Band: Reinforced Palmar Kneading

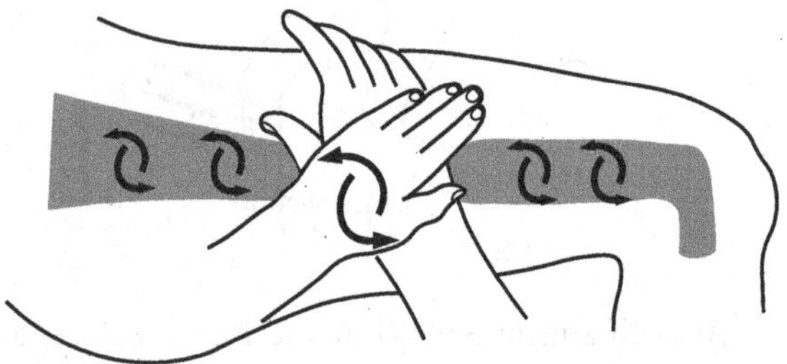

Reinforced palmar kneading.

wheelchair users who are able) is excellent to exercise and strengthen this joint.

Massage for the knee joint is an important focus in your overall massage routine, as this joint can so quickly contract and shorten, becoming fixed. A combination of massage and leg pumping is essential and should be done at least daily—even better, twice a day (morning and evening).

The most relieving stroke for any problems of the knee is wringing. I "slice" across the patellar tendon at the bottom of the kneecap. I also do a lot of frictioning around the perimeter of the kneecap, large oversized alternate thumb kneading around the outside edge of the kneecap, and fingertip kneading to the sides of the knee. If the wheelchair user cannot be comfortable on their side in or out of the chair, and can only lie facing up, then do not forget to massage into the popliteal fossa (back-of-the-knee area) with some upward scooping strokes from the calf up into the back of the knee.

From the knee down, many lower leg conditions become more serious in wheelchair users. The lower legs are at the periphery of the circulatory system, which challenges venous return and lymphatic drainage. Neurological interruption that prevents leg muscles from moving—often the situation for wheelchair users—challenges circulation even more.

Leg Cramping

Massage to alleviate leg cramps can be administered with the patient face-up or face-down in a supine position or with the patient seated. If the wheelchair user is prone to nocturnal leg cramping, elevate the legs when they are in a supine face-up position and use heating pads or hot water bottles to stave off cramping during the massage.

For my wheelchair patients with leg cramps, I elevate the legs as often as possible, setting the leg rests to high or horizontal. With the person in the chair or on their back, dorsiflex a leg, pulling the toes toward their head, stretching out the calf muscle (the gastrocnemius, a common location for leg cramping).

Alternating your hands, scoop up the leg from the Achilles tendon to the back of the knee, keeping the pressure toward the heart. It is like you are milking the muscle toward the heart.

Alternate these cup-shaped milking strokes with a more focused fingertip grooving into the middle of the fold of the calf muscle. Using the fingers of both hands, I put the points of my fingertips on the Achilles and "groove" into the calf muscle where it anatomically splits up the middle to the back of the knee. This divides the calf muscle in half, so I call this long stroke "splitting the

FIGURE 4.32. Knee Massage

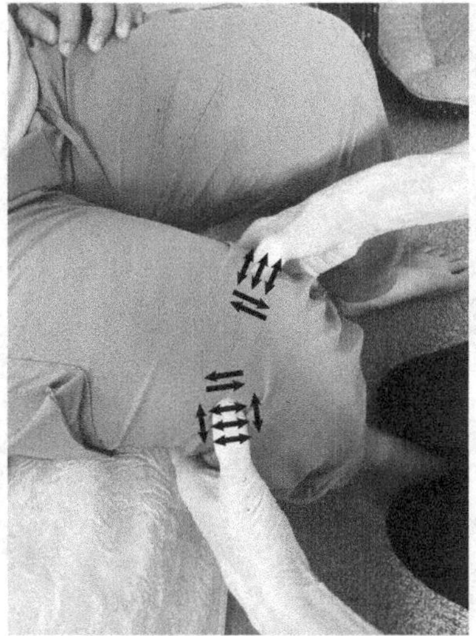

Thumb fricitoning.

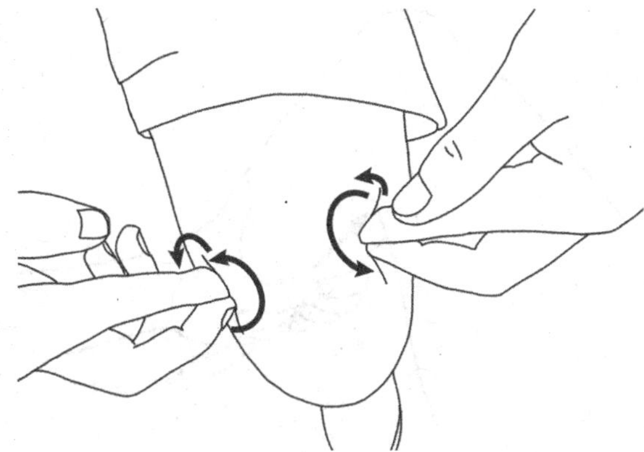

Reinforced fingertip frictioning.

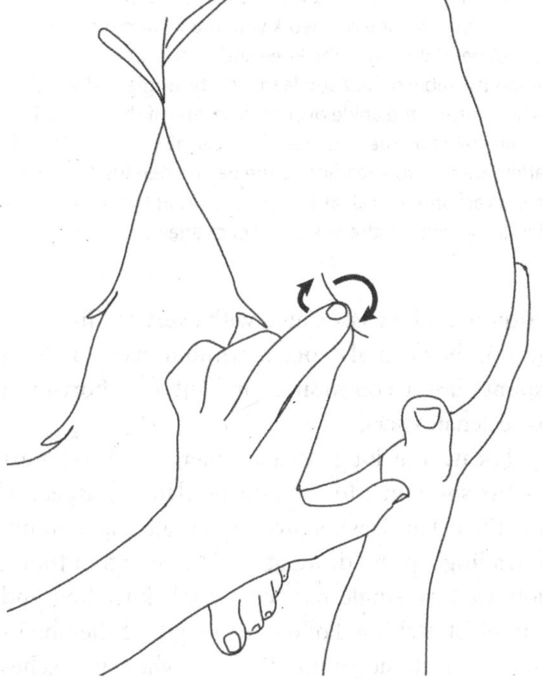

Single-handed reinforced fingertip frictioning.

FIGURE 4.33. Lower Leg Anatomy

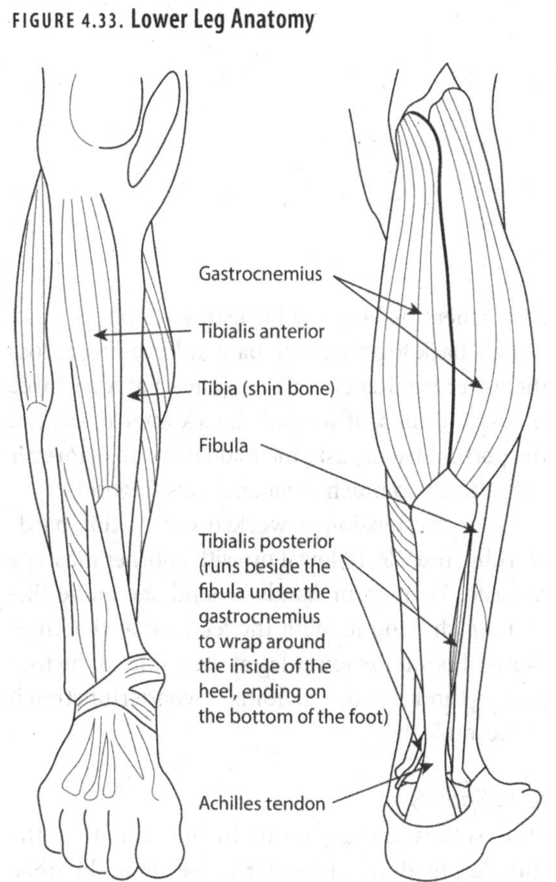

FIGURE 4.34. **Lower Leg Massage**

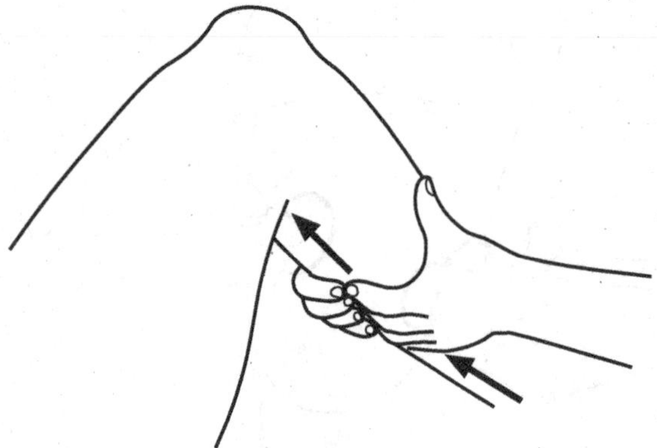

Splitting the gastrocnemius.

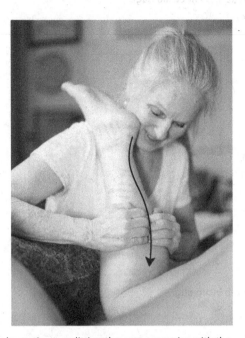

An alternative to splitting the gastrocnemius with the person lying supine is to work with them lying prone. I like to bend the leg at the knee and lift the ankle up. I sit on the table or bed and lean into the angle of the leg while putting the ankle over my shoulder. If the person is comfortable on their stomach, you can also do some good alternate thumb kneading to the gastrocnemius. Wrap your hands around the calf as you work. Start at the popliteal fossa and work to the ankle and back again.

gastrocnemius." On the backstroke, I put the calf muscle back together with palmar kneading across the lower leg. Repeat this movement at least three times, and more if wanted. Check after three, but the person usually asks me to do this stroke forever as it affords so much relief and feels so good.

Once the tension is worked out of this hard-working muscle, follow it up with another massage favorite. Wrap your hands around the ankle like you are choking it. With the leg bent at the knee, flex and point the lower leg at the ankle so the foot goes up and down, providing a wonderful stretch at the ankle.

Shin Splints

Shin splints are a painful inflammation of the muscles, tendons, and other tissue along the tibia. Although often associated with exertion (like running), they can also occur without exertion. Shin splints are a common complaint for short-term wheelchair users.

Locate the long tibialis anterior muscle next to the shinbone, to the outside (lateral) aspect of the tibia. This is where to do your alternate thumb kneading, up and down at least three or four times, followed by single-handed thumb kneading and thumb stretching. Follow the length of the tibialis anterior right down into the foot, where it attaches along the instep below the big toe.

With this condition, massage is important for the whole leg, not just the lower leg. Shin splints are so difficult to get rid of quickly once they arrive, so do all you can to prevent the condition. This is very much like plantar fasciitis in that once

FIGURE 4.35. Massage for Shin Splints

SINGLE-HANDED THUMB STRETCHING: TIBIALIS ANTERIOR

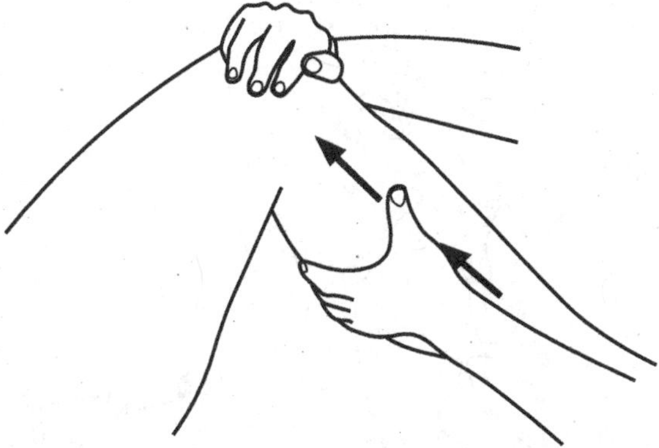

Supporting the leg with one hand, do some single-handed thumb stretching to the tibialis anterior.

THUMB STRETCHING AND KNEADING: TIBIALIS ANTERIOR

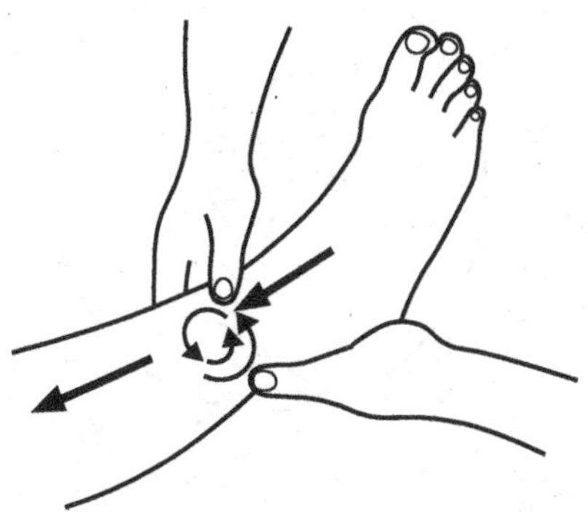

Cupping the heel with one hand, do some thumb stretching and thumb kneading to the tibialis anterior, with special attention to where it attaches to the tendon that connects the muscle to the inside of the foot.

OVERHANDED THUMB STRETCHING: TIBIALIS ANTERIOR

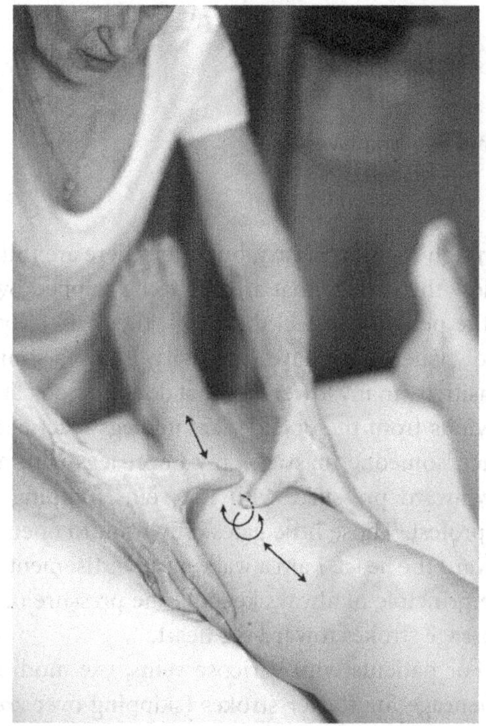

Overhanded thumb stretching is a series of short strokes about an inch or two long with a short, straight, stretching action and one thumb picking up where the other one left off. This is a good treatment for self-massage, at least if the person is able to reach their shins! They can work up and down the anterior tibialis with their fingertips, like playing a keyboard.

arrived, it is difficult to treat. Make prevention a priority: with any hint of shin splints, get massage and hydrotherapy and wheel to the pool for an antigravity workout!

Problems of the Calf Muscle

The muscle in the back of the leg goes from the knee to the heel of the foot, forming the Achilles tendon as it attaches to the calcaneus. Wheelchair users with chronic conditions such as MS, ALS, Parkinson's disease, and spinal cord injuries are all predisposed to a shortening of the calf muscle, resulting in a pointed foot. This results in the ankle joint also becoming fixed in a variety of deformities.

The gastrocnemius is a huge vascular system with lots of muscle, narrowing into a long line of inelastic tendinous attachments at the heel (Achilles tendon). It's really important to milk this muscle continuously to bring in fresh blood and counteract the natural slowdown at this distant circulatory turnaround. Milking the veins up toward the heart will at the same time encourage the elasticity of the tendinous, sinewy lower aspect of the muscle so it can't pull as hard to point the foot.

The strokes that I employ here are the splitting of the gastrocnemius from the heel to the back of the popliteal fossa (back of the knee). Do lots of

FIGURE 4.36. **Calf Muscle Massage**

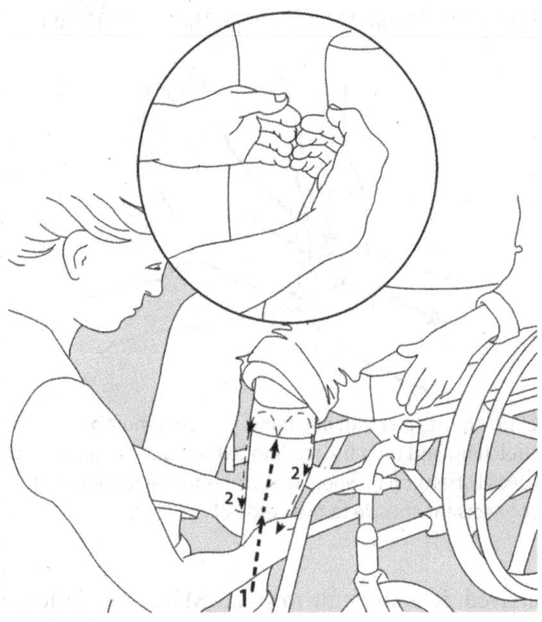

Splitting the gastrocnemius. Hold your hands in cupped positions and press the backs of your fingertips on either hand together. Use your fingertips to split the gastrocnemius.

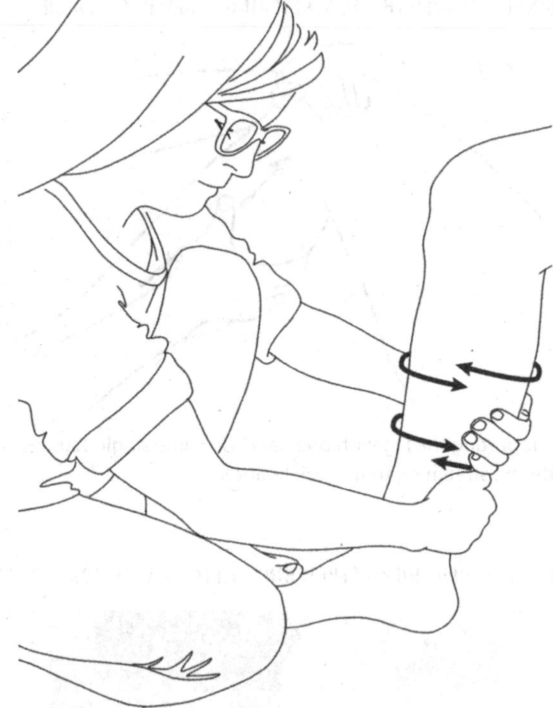

Palmar wringing, lower leg.

open C-wringing and fingertip kneading to the length of the gastrocnemius, always from the bottom to the top.

Varicose Veins

Varicose veins are lumpy, enlarged veins that usually appear in the legs. Spider veins, tiny blue or red veins on the surface of the skin, are a less severe form of this condition. This condition does not come from wheelchair use, but can be aggravated by wheelchair use. Varicose veins are challenged by gravity, weight gain, and immobility; they usually show signs of failure in the lower leg before the upper leg. Many long-term wheelchair users develop vascular lower leg problems simply from sitting in the chair with the lower legs unelevated.

I avoid massaging varicose veins entirely and only use hydrotherapy to help relieve the congestion. Avoiding obvious varicosity showing itself through the skin is easy, but often there are things below the surface that are still to be skipped over. If the person can feel their legs, they will let you know where they have sensitivity. I have a similar sensitivity in my lower legs that does not look at all obvious from the outside. Yet my legs react badly when someone massages my lower legs with any downward pressure, with my veins jumping up in protest. Those little gates only want to open up toward the heart. I am a walking advertisement for the principle of always keeping the pressure of all massage strokes toward the heart.

For patients with varicose veins, use modified effleurage for starter strokes (skipping over areas with obvious varicosity) and then do alternate thumb kneading and wringing, always dancing over the areas where you see varicose or spider veins. Wringing is perfect for adapting to different sensitivities as you can change the pressure in a split second when the massage recipient indicates a touchy or uncomfortable area. I always spend a lot of time on the feet of patients with varicose veins for a great relaxation response.

Cold, wet wraps on the legs can also relieve the congestion and pain. Those damaged, over-extended vein walls react well to the constriction prompted by cold water. Cold leg baths are also excellent remedies for poor circulation in the lower legs. You can apply a cold leg wrap while you're massaging other parts of the body before and after your leg massage routine.

With any varicose veins, be sure to elevate the legs during a full body massage by setting the wheelchair footrests high or horizontal. Since you can't massage the varicose veins directly, a good place to focus your massage is the hips and upper legs, where no varicosity is present, but where you might be able to open up and improve the circulation.

COLD WRAPS FOR THE LEGS

Although the idea of wrapping your legs in cold, wet sheets might sound terrible, a cold wrap on the legs is heavenly.

An absorbent flannel sheet works best. You may want to have two pieces of sheeting so you can wrap the legs individually. You will also need some plastic wrap, an extra blanket for insulation, some pillows, and possibly a hot water bottle.

1. Soak the sheet in a cold bath or container of ice water.
2. Warm up the legs with massage.
3. Wring out the sheet just until it isn't dripping. You want it to hold as much cold water as possible.
4. Quickly wrap the sheet around each leg separately and then cover the legs as tightly as possible with plastic wrap. You want to prevent air from getting to the cold wrap, which will heat it up. Wrap the legs right up to the upper thigh.
5. Elevate the legs on pillows and cover both legs with another blanket for insulation. You don't want the person to heat up too fast.
6. If desired, keep the rest of the body warm with a hot water bottle under the neck. You can massage the rest of the body while the person relaxes in their wrap.
7. When the wrap has heated up naturally (through the body's heat), you can repeat the cold wrap or just wash off the legs with witch hazel.

Ankle and Foot Problems

Two reasons we massage the feet of wheelchair users are: 1) to keep the ankles and feet mobile in case of a cure for people with, for example, spinal cord injury; and 2) because the feet are so far from the main pumping station of the heart. The techniques are the same: we start with general strokes, then focus on specific strokes for contracted structures in the lower leg, ankle, long foot bones, and toes.

My ideal timing for foot massage is early morning before the person is out of bed, making it easier for them to put their feet on the ground and to bend that sleepy ankle, and then again at night, with a recovery focus, as the person retires.

The anatomical curvatures in the feet due to immobility and prolonged sitting are as varied as the individuals they are attached to. Most commonly, one foot is very different from the other. My patient, Freya, for example, who suffered for twenty years with Parkinson's disease, had one pointed foot with the toes completely flexible but the calf muscle contracted. She had no visible deformity on that side. Her other leg was twisted at the ankle, had an involvement of the anterior tibialis, plus a shortening of the calf muscle. The big toe was completely hooked, curved, and contracted. Her more affected leg was also completely different in its circulatory and neurological functioning, with spasms and movement in the leg itself and ulceration in the heel. The other leg was completely flaccid yet flexible. I've also found this same differential with my spinal cord injury patients. You can never treat both legs the same, so the massager needs to be adaptable and creative with their massage strokes.

Any swelling in the lower extremities usually starts or shows itself in the toes, foot, and ankle first before extending further up the leg. Part of your foot massage will involve "reducing the ankle," which is a technique used to open the circulation

FIGURE 4.37. **Referred Pain in Foot Problems**

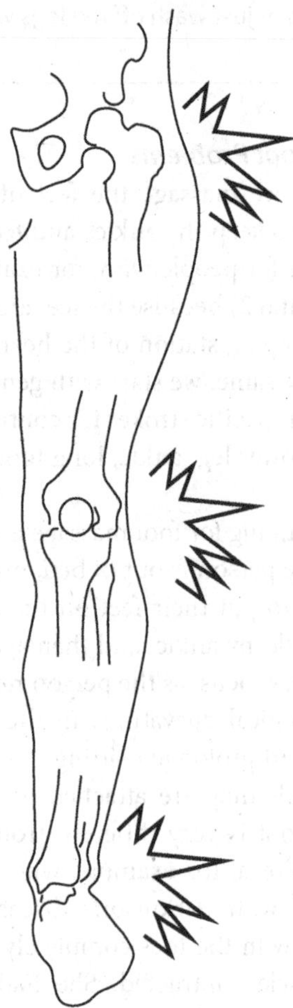

Pain caused by flat feet can be referred into the knee and hip, and are commonly experienced by short-term wheelchair users.

FIGURE 4.38. **Arches of the Foot**

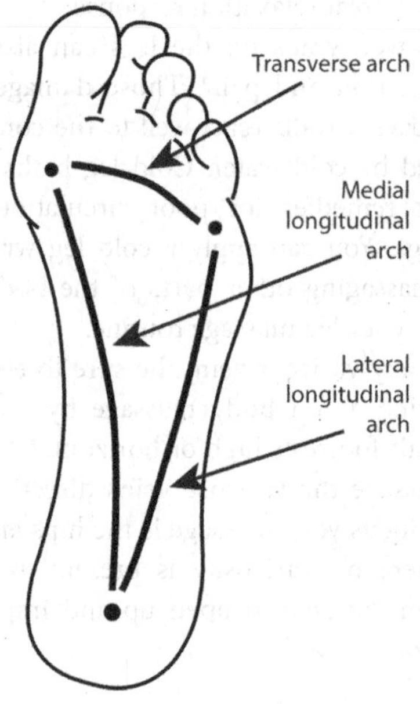

to the foot by reducing the congestion in the ankle and moving it further up the leg to be remedied in the trunk of the body.

The position of the wheelchair recipient for this foot massage can be seated, side-lying, or supine.

The basic massage strokes of effleurage and wringing break up the surface tension of the swollen lower leg and start to establish a better flow of lymphatics and blood. I use the knee as the starting place for this routine and work around that area first to open up the circulation to the lower leg and foot.

Begin by splitting the gastrocnemius and then focus your massage on the tibialis anterior, the muscle that runs down the front of the lower leg. You should be about one to two inches to the outer side of the ridge of the tibia. Follow that long muscle to its attachment at the inside edge of the top of the foot, crossing over at the level of the ankle. Use small, slow, firm strokes of alternate thumb kneading, fingertip kneading, and single-handed thumb kneading.

Move to open-handed wringing, alternating with long thumb stretching. This deep thumb stretching is the same stroke you use between the erector spinae muscles and the spine while massaging the back. Use it now between the tibialis anterior and the ridge of the tibia. Move very slowly and be sure to be right on the tips of your thumbs for the greatest depth and accuracy.

After massaging the lower leg, continue on with the foot and ankles. A thorough foot massage begins with thumb kneading to the anklebones and fingertip kneading to the attachments of the Achilles tendon to relieve any local discomfort.

Then you can begin some nitty-gritty strokes along the inner longitudinal arch that runs up the instep of the foot. First apply a mini-effleurage to the sole of the foot with your thumbs. Then move to thumb wringing across the longitudinal arch, alternating with thumb compression (just press each thumb in and hold for moment), alternate thumb kneading, and deep thumb stroking. With a firm touch, these strokes will give relief to this long arch. Encourage your patients to breathe deeply into each stroke.

The same sequence of strokes can also be done on the transverse arch at the base of the toes. This massage can be uncomfortable at first, but after about five minutes, most of this discomfort subsides.

The more foot massage the better, combined with cold footbaths and other cold applications. Epsom salt footbaths are a must!

FOOT MASSAGE MENU

Use these strokes for hooked and contracted toes, and ankle and foot spasticity or flaccidity.

1. **Gastrocnemius massage:** Split the gastrocnemius, using both hands in an upward direction from the Achilles tendon to the back of the knee.
2. **Thumb stretching and thumb kneading to the tibialis anterior:** Use a single-handed stroke.
3. **Thumb stretching to the tibialis posterior.**
4. **Kneading to the malleoli (anklebones).**
5. **Thumb stretching to the top of the foot.**
6. **Thumb stretching to the medial longitudinal arch.**
7. **Static frictioning to the medial longitudinal arch.**
8. **Thumb stretching to the upper side of the foot:** Stretch in the groove between the long bones.
9. **Thumb wringing to the sole of the foot.**
10. **Transverse arch mobilization:** With both hands, hold a foot at the base of the toes where the toes join the foot. Put your thumbs on the bottom of the foot and your fingers on top. Working from toe joint to toe joint along the transverse arch, move one hand up and one hand down to mobilize each joint.
11. **Digital compression:** Alternate left and right thumb tips to apply pressure slowly and firmly all over the sole of the foot. Treat the sole of the foot like a series of trigger points, with the patient breathing into the steady pressure of each thumb. Digital compression is always the favorite stroke in this routine, but ask for lots of feedback to be sure your pressure is right.
12. **Frictioning to the medial longitudinal arch.**
13. **Frictioning to the joint at the base of the big toe.**
14. **Eversion/inversion:** Twist the foot toward the inside and then the outside, holding the foot with one hand and the ankle with the other hand.
15. **Transverse arch stretching:** Slide your hands from the ankle to the toes like you are squeezing the foot to make it longer. When you get to the base of the toes, bend the toes downward. Your thumbs are on the top of the foot, fingers on the bottom. Then reverse your direction up to the ankle.
16. **Transverse arch mobilization with thumbs on top.**
17. **Toe flexing:** Use your palm to flex the toes at the transverse arch. Then bend each toe up and down individually. Massage according to the contracted or flaccid condition. With spasticity, I spend more individualized time on those curled toes and use ice massage on the individual joints.
18. **Alternate thumb kneading and wringing:** Wind down the massage with alternate thumb kneading to the entire foot, a mini-effleurage up the leg to the knee and tibialis anterior, and wringing to the whole leg, especially the lower leg right out to the toes.
19. **Effleurage to the entire leg, three times:** Adjust by leg, as appropriate: you might be focusing significantly more massage time on the deteriorated leg.
20. **Light reflex stroking to finish.**

FIGURE 4.39. Strokes in Foot Massage

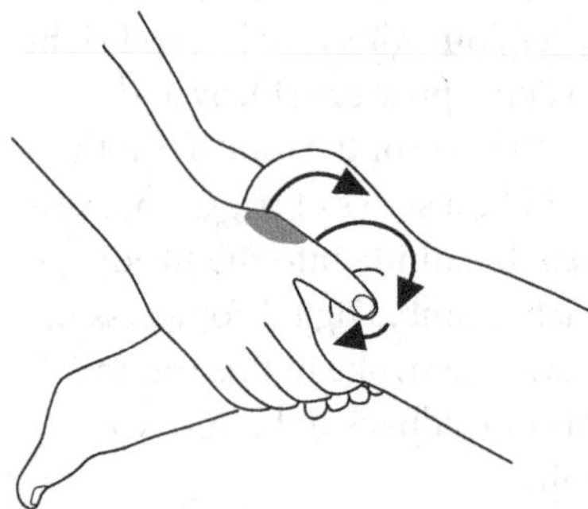

a. Kneading to the anklebones (with the heel of the hand).

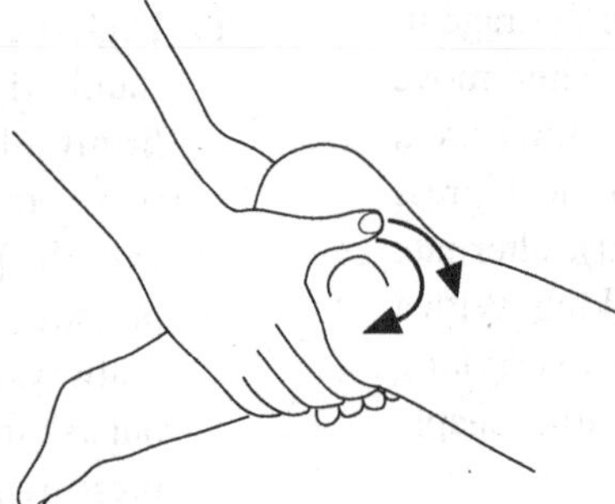

b. Kneading to the anklebones (with the thumbs).

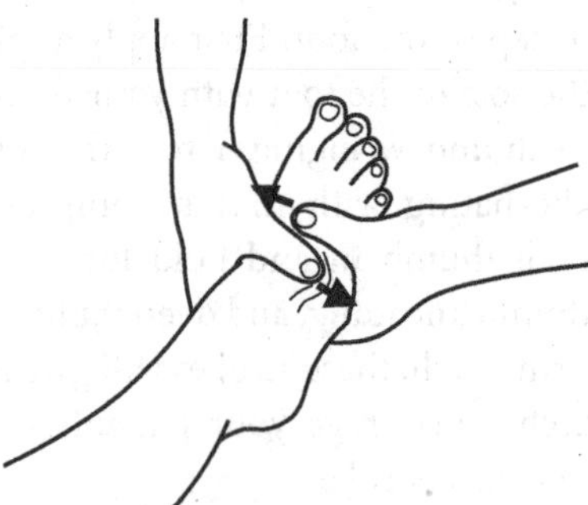

c. Dorsal thumb stretching.

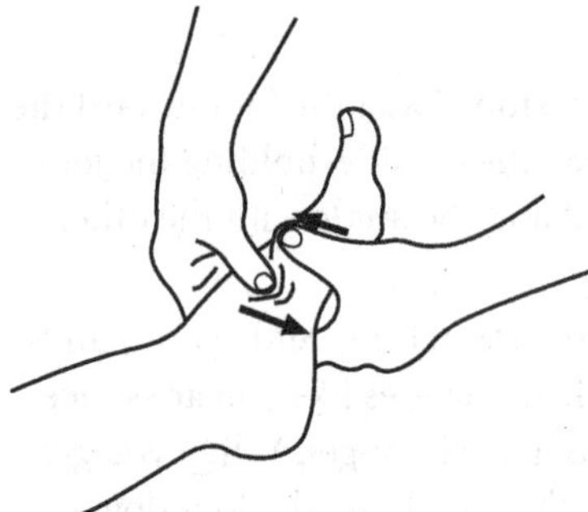

d. Medial thumb stretching.

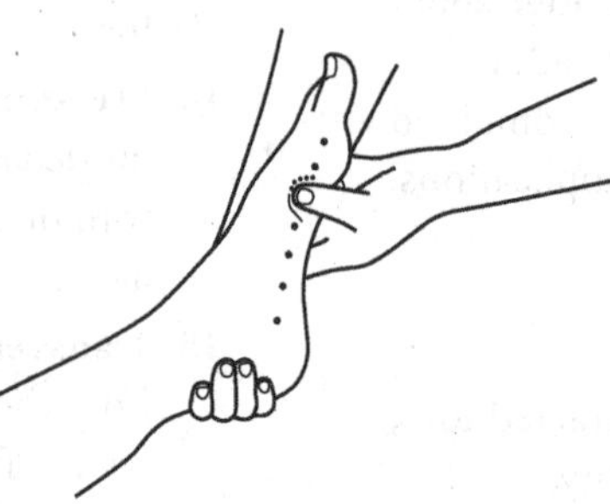

e. Frictions on the medial longitudinal arch.

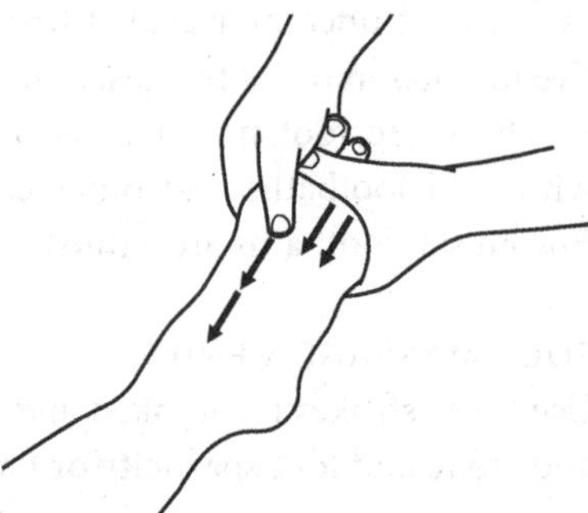

f. Thumb stretching.

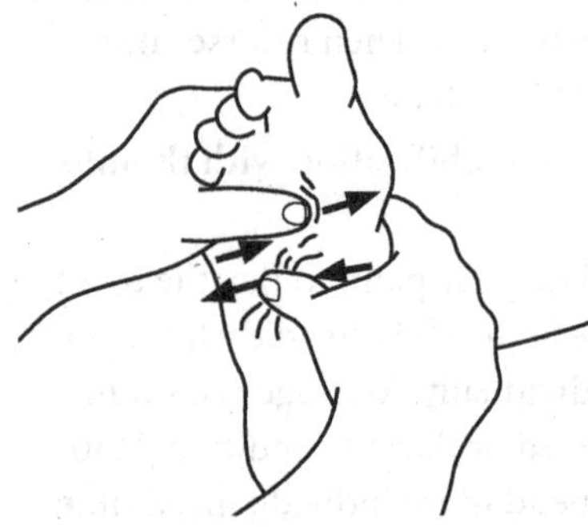

g. Thumb wringing.

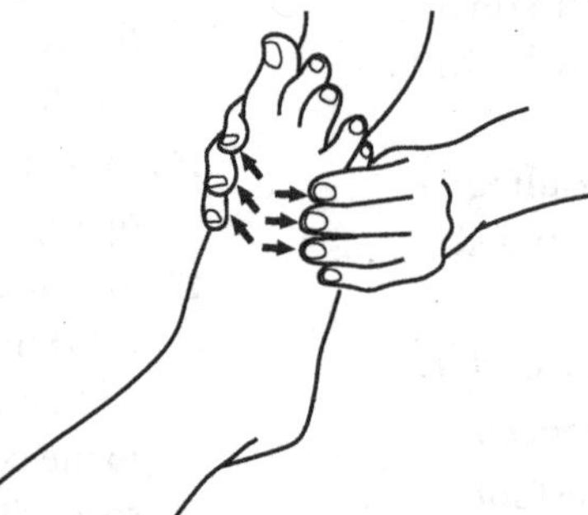

h. Transverse arch mobilization (dorsal view).

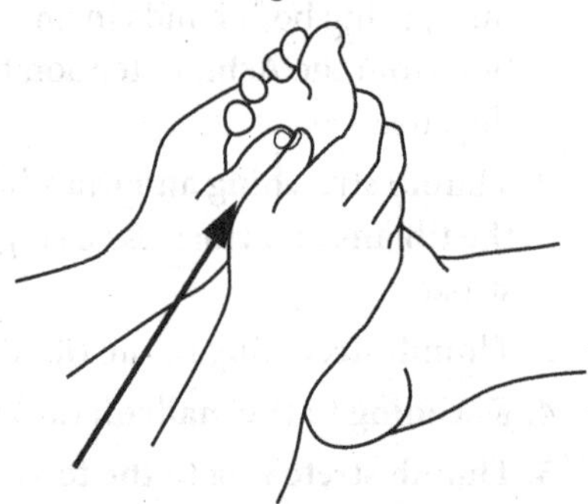

i. Transverse arch mobilization (plantar view).

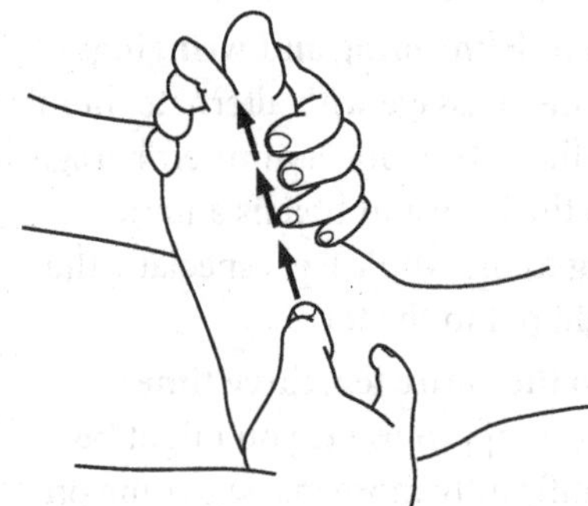

j. Frictions to the medial longitudinal arch.

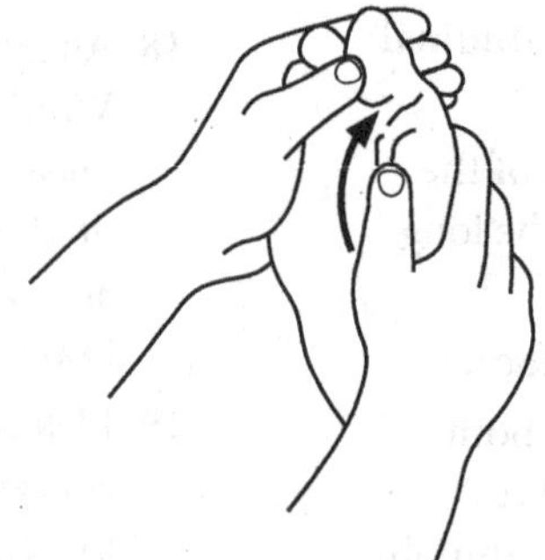

k. Frictions to the base of the big toe.

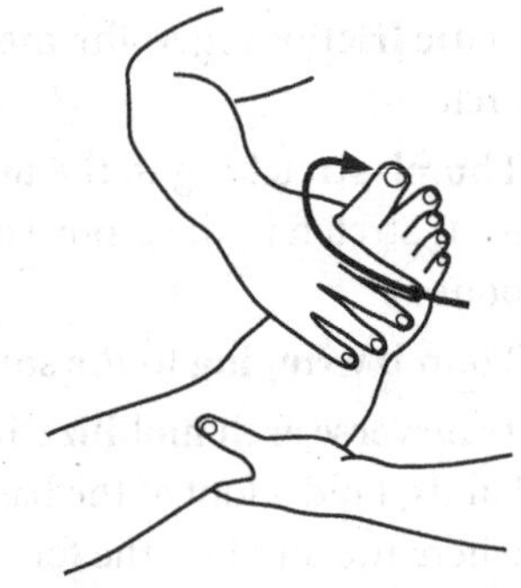

l. Eversion.

FIGURE 4.39. CONTINUED

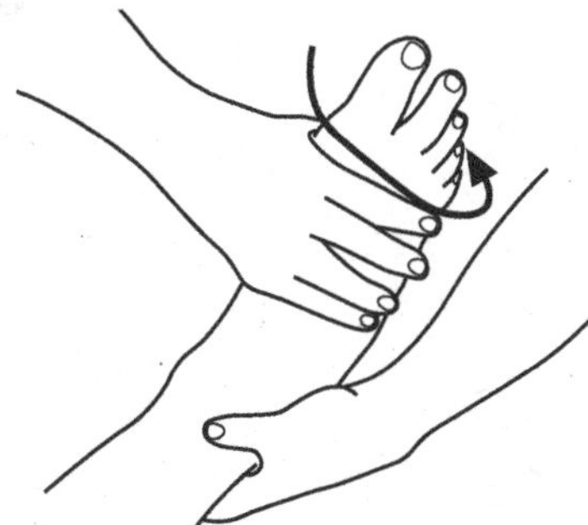

m. Inversion.

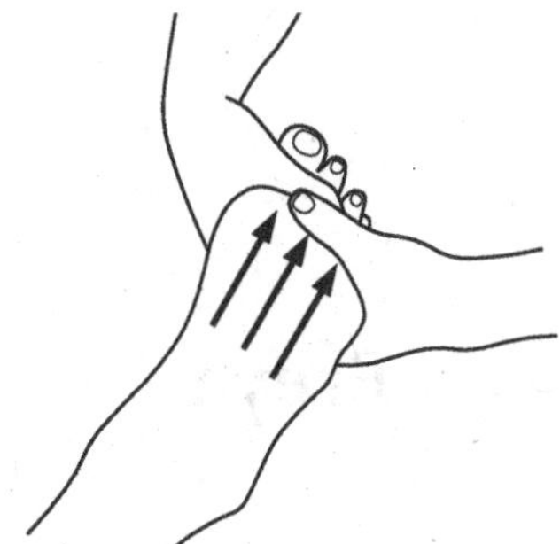

n. Transverse arch stretching.

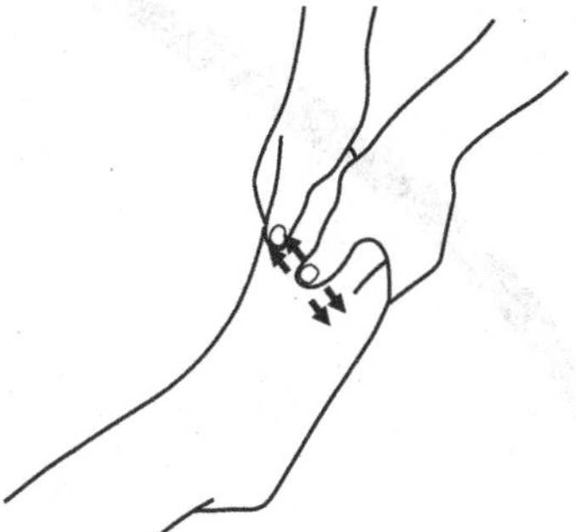

o. Mobilizing the transverse arch thumbs on top.

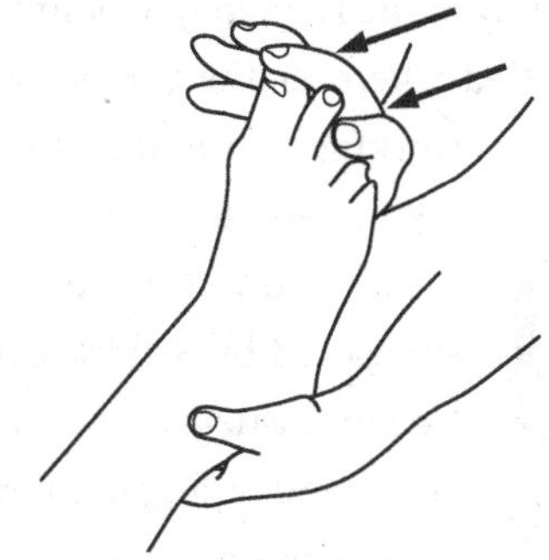

p. Flexion.

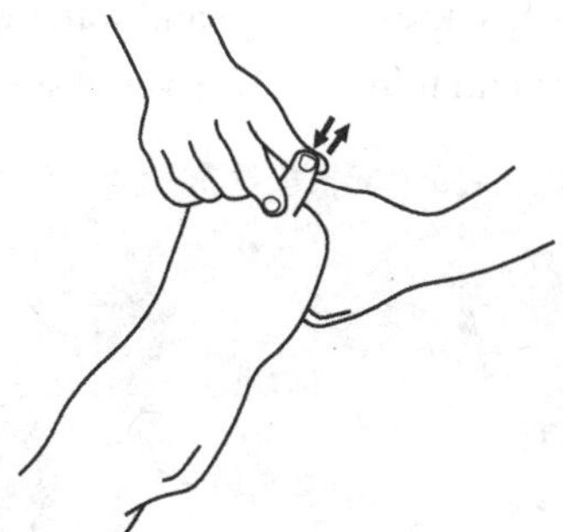

q. Toe mobilization.

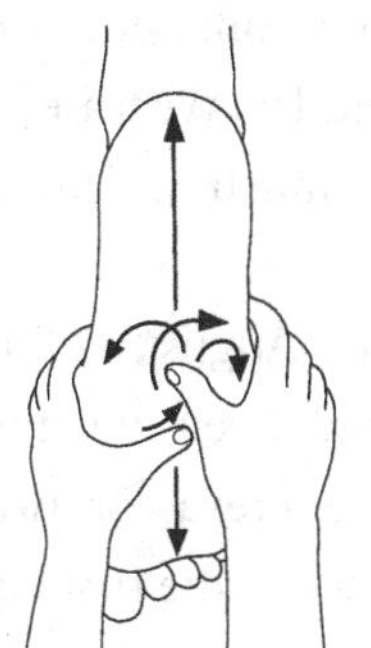

r. Alternate thumb kneading to the sole of the foot.

VIDEO LIBRARY

Visit brusheducation.ca/wheeling-in-good-hands to watch these videos:

- **Wheelchair transfer technique:** Wheelchair to bed
- **Wheelchair transfer technique:** Wheelchair to table – modification for leg injury
- **Wheelchair transfer technique:** Wheelchair to car – modification for leg injury
- **Wheelchair transfer technique:** Wheelchair to car with transfer board – modification for leg injury
- **Wheelchair transfer technique:** Wheelchair to car – 24-hour wheelchair experience
- **Specific massage treatments:** Headaches – head tilts and rotations
- **Respiratory massage:** Rib raking with chest compression and suctioning – acute hospital care
- **Respiratory massage:** Cupping – supine – teaching friends and family
- **Respiratory massage:** Compression and percussive tapotement
- **Hip mobilization:** Supine – out of the chair with Ed
- **Hip mobilization:** Supine – out of the chair with Mary-Jo
- **Leg cramping:** Splitting the gastrocnemius – in the classroom

Freya

I can still feel the sensation of connecting with Freya on a conference call with two of her kids, Ailsha and Jay. We teased her, sang to her, and told her how much we loved her.

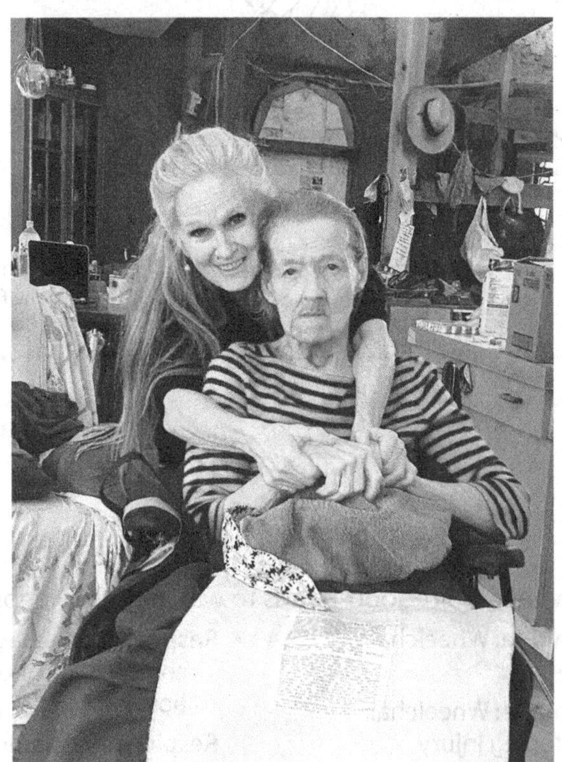
Freya Gray and me.

It was August, 2021, and I had been missing massaging Freya for two months now—the first big gap in a couple of years where it had been easy to get my hands on her. We were now separated by distance (she was in the Slocan Valley in the south of British Columbia, and I was in Fort St. John in the north), forest fires, and Covid.

Over the past two years, I had been paying back Freya, with massages, for her huge influence on my young life, my middle life, and now my life as a senior over seventy. Freya taught me many practicalities about animal husbandry, rural architecture, and raising kids the right way.

When I met Freya, she was married to her first husband, Tony, and they had six children.

I was working on a documentary crew for an air and water quality study of the Kootenay-Columbia river system. I traveled wherever the teams were working, filming them taking samples and testing the air and water. We were sponsored by Selkirk College in Castlegar. I became very good at lugging huge video equipment. In those days, reel-to-reel recording machines were like packing a dozen beer on your hip up and down country roads. We were young and we were enthusiastic about preserving our natural environment.

I was looking to live closer to the college. I saw an ad from one of the professors, which turned out to be Freya's husband, to housesit while his family was building in the Slocan Valley. When I visited their home in Blueberry Creek, they had a couple of goats in the backyard, which they milked to feed their youngest kids, Catlin and Jay, who were barely toddlers, still in diapers. I was able to stay at their place and started to help them build the foundations for their new dream home on the river in Vallican.

Freya and I became instant friends. She taught me how to dance free form in some new age, contemporary, flowing type of swirling and twirling. The kids were used to this type of interpretive dance, but it was new territory for me. I was still in the land of rock and roll.

That summer was a turning point in my life. I became committed to living an ecologically sound lifestyle, and in the years that followed, I got my own goats. I also expanded my dance repertoire!

I had a volunteer job at the local crisis center in Castlegar, and I introduced Freya to the staff. They also began to help with the construction of the new house, which would accommodate six kids (then), two parents, and a community of friends and relatives. Freya's second marriage to my friend Dan resulted in her seventh child, my godson Shamus. But Freya was saving the best for last.

Freya's teams of helpers were evident in the house-building project, and later in her palliative care. The partner of her last thirty-seven years, Stan, was the center of her palliative care team and loving universe. He became her most supportive and collaborative lifelong partner. He respected her manifested desires to the best of his ability until her peaceful parting.

Stan was able to set up a palliative program through Choice in Supports for Independent Living, a government program in British Columbia, with the help of Freya's daughter Ailsha, a licensed practical nurse working at the regional hospital.

Freya taught me, especially in her last couple of years living with Parkinson's disease, about life's principles of giving and receiving. My hands-on help went beyond my professionalism into our girlfriendism! Now I could get Freya the clothes that made her look great and the hairdos that only girlfriends can organize. Freya was my "die good-looking" project! She was always a beautiful blond.

We did her wheelchair outdoor walks underneath her cathedral of cedars as she bathed in their colors of grey and brown, rich green with tones of yellow and gold. Ailsha, had inherited Freya's artistic talent, so we enlarged Ailsha's painting of sunflowers and "planted" them on the newly painted wall that Freya gazed at every day. Her legacy of talent is carried on today with the art of her children!

In the last year of Freya's life, we had great house-finishing projects, clearing-the-car-wrecks projects, and a general back-to-the-beginning project to return her land to its rural roots of A-frame barns and basement foundations!

But Freya's greatest love was Stan. He had a warmth and talent with people that was never experienced on that land before. He was focused on Freya's care and still allowed us to care for him. Massaging Stan after massaging Freya was a classic palliative massage dream come true for me. Years earlier, the massage that I had received from Joe Fedoruk on Freya's dining table after a rambunctious Gestalt therapy weekend forever changed the direction of my life from filmmaking to massage therapist, from back-to-the-land farmer to downtown Toronto student.

The community that Stan created around Freya of love, affection, caring, and admiration was a loving circle of talent.

Now it was fifty years later, massaging Freya's care team around that same dining table, helping to show the love that we had for them all.

Freya outlived her prognosis. Her palliative care physician, Dr. Trevor Janz, said her situation was as good as it could possibly be, and he reinforced the feedback that I constantly gave Stan, Liz, Janet, Kate, and Peggy: Freya had the best team ever!

As her team massaged her, they hoped maybe she would make it to Christmas, then maybe New Year's Eve. But she continued past all expectations, still able to lift that one arm toward the ceiling and spend hours looking up. I think we were all blessed by such a gentle departure. She seemed to elegantly glide over the edge and come back again, never wanting to discuss how she wanted to die. As the mystery of her departure date and flight pattern swirled around us, we all learned to practice that eternal principle of one day at a time.

In her last years, for every day she lived, Freya was massaged, touched, cuddled, and kissed. She starred in my palliative underwater massage movies in Ainsworth Hot Springs and then at home in her own elegant bathtub, complete with wheelchairs and rolling mechanical lifts and hoists. She helped me teach palliative massage via Zoom across the country with the Institute of Traditional Medicine in Toronto and the gerontology nursing program at Selkirk College in Castlegar. Her Zoom presence, willingness, and support for my work will always be a blessing. Freya continues to influence me today, more than fifty years from our first meeting. I still watch Freya wheeling under her canopy of giant old-growth cedars, soaking up their healing touch from here to heaven (complete with harp music!).

At the clinic where I work in Fort St. John, I tell mothers-to-be about Freya. I tell them about Freya raising all her kids on goat's milk, and about my husband using goat's milk to share the feeding of our baby daughter. He became a goat milk fanatic, tracing Crystal's strong bones back to Freya's influence.

In August, 2021, seeing Freya's number come up on my cell phone, I instantly panicked. As soon as I heard Jay's voice, I knew it was a happy call from Vallican. Jay's voice put me right there beside Freya. Jay had been my substitute massage person for Freya as he worked in the north every month during the time of Covid, when I had been unable to travel to Nelson to massage her. Now I had them together on the phone! I requested Jay to hug and kiss his mom, massage her feet, and bring back to me Freya's touch. With Ailsha on the line, we sang to Freya and caressed her with our words.

Now Freya has glided to the other side. I will always feel her as she held onto my hand as I massaged her. I can still feel her hands on me as her loving touch continues to color my life.

Thank you, Freya for your rainbow of blessings. I love you.

5

Underwater Massage for Wheelchair Users

Underwater massage can be done in a bathtub, hot tub, or public pool. The water gives buoyancy and ease of movement for people who are stiff and immobilized. It also allows additional mobility therapy for hard-to-move hips, shoulders, heads, and necks.

Two of my favorite underwater massage recipients, my mom and my friend Freya, loved Ainsworth Hot Springs on Kootenay Lake in British Columbia. For them, the drive to the hot springs was relaxing in itself, and getting in the pool even more so.

Simply floating a person in warm water is therapy. It triggers a strong relaxation response in the body, marked by increased serotonin production and endorphin activity—which is no doubt why naturally occurring hot springs from Alaska to Asia have long been locations of health-giving institutions. A 2019 study[2] documented the effects of warm water on fibromyalgia patients: increased relaxation, reduced anxiety, enhanced overall well-being, and reduced pain, reduced fatigue, and improved quality of life.

First Steps in Underwater Massage

The Three Nos

Underwater massage has three special requirements to keep in mind:

- **No oils:** The water provides lubrication.
- **No effleurage:** The water already provides a kind of gentle massage.
- **No pressure without counterpressure:** This is because your patient is buoyant. You need to provide opposing support for each stroke, as the pressure of the massage stroke will cause the patient to be pushed away from you.

Considerations about Bowel Evacuations

Bowel evacuation can be a big topic for people living in wheelchairs and needs to be considered as part of your underwater massage preparations. Underwater massage, like all massage, works to stimulate the three major systems of the body: digestive, respiratory, and circulatory. Stimulating the digestive system can result in bowel movements, which presents a problem in a hot tub or public pool.

With some patients, simply spending twenty minutes suspended over their bed in a sling will stimulate their bowel and completely empty it. So this might be a good step before a pool massage. You can also perform abdominal massage with leg pumping while the patient is still in bed to help evacuate the bowel. Talk it over with your patient and choose a strategy that suits them best.

For tub massages, remember that you can always empty the tub if the person has a bowel movement (it's a positive problem). You don't have to transfer them in and out of the tub to do this: you can just fill tub again. I like to add Epsom salts!

Pool Massage

Pool Transfers

Some pools have ramps that let you wheel right into the pool. If your pool does not have a ramp, though, you'll have to transfer the wheelchair user to the pool. Transferring to a pool from a wheelchair requires several helpers or a mechanical hoist or lift. Hoists and lifts are easy to rent from Red Cross outlets. Robotics may deliver other solutions soon: engineers are now designing and building robots for exactly this purpose!

If you are working with human helpers, you need three: two to lift, and one to secure the wheelchair user from tipping backward (since a bathing suit has no waistband to grasp during the lift). The process is similar to the tandem transfer from a wheelchair to a car. Two people position themselves on either side of the wheelchair user and lift together. They can use their hands and arms to lift, or they can seat the person on a sling adapter and lift with that. The third person takes a position behind the wheelchair user.

Patient Positions for Pool Massage

Positions include:

- Seated on an underwater bench or step with back support.
- Seated on your knees or the knees of a helper—for example, a friend or family member.
- Floating with support. The support can be provided by pool noodles.

Getting to the Pool Bench for Seated Pool Massage

Think through the procedure for getting to the pool bench before you transfer your patient to the water.

1. Identify the pool bench you will use for the massage.

FIGURE 5.1. Pool Transfers

DECK TO POOL WITH THREE HELPERS

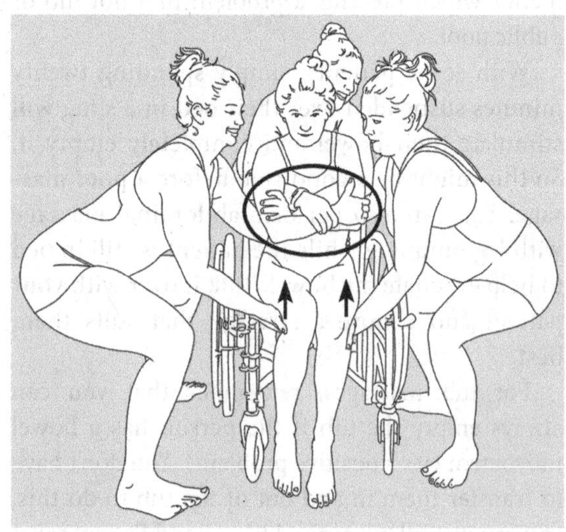

Lifting.

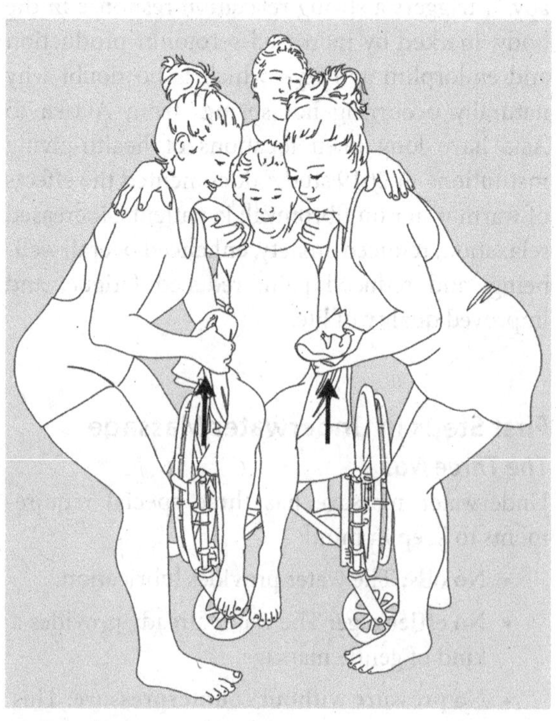

Lifting with a sling adapter.

FIGURE 5.1. CONTINUED

DECK TO POOL WITH THREE HELPERS

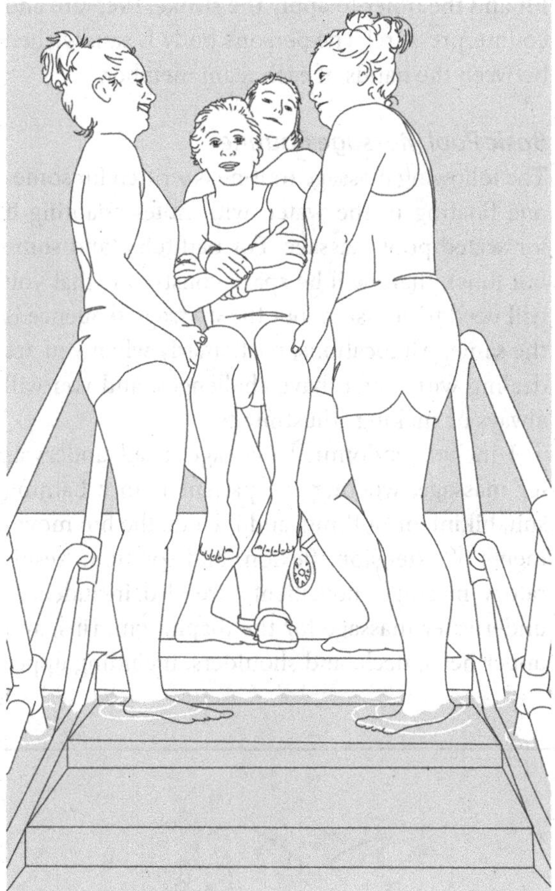

Stepping into the pool.

2. Support the patient in the water with either of these shoulder techniques:
   - Rest the patient's head on your shoulder. Hold the back of their neck with one hand and support their hip or sacrum with your other hand.
   - Rest the patient's head on your shoulder. Put your hands on either side of the patient's hips or under the hips, or put one hand on a hip and one under the sacrum.
3. Walk backward to the pool bench. Walking backward always gives you the best control. Be sure to do shoulder checks as you move through the water.

FIGURE 5.2. Walking to the Pool Bench

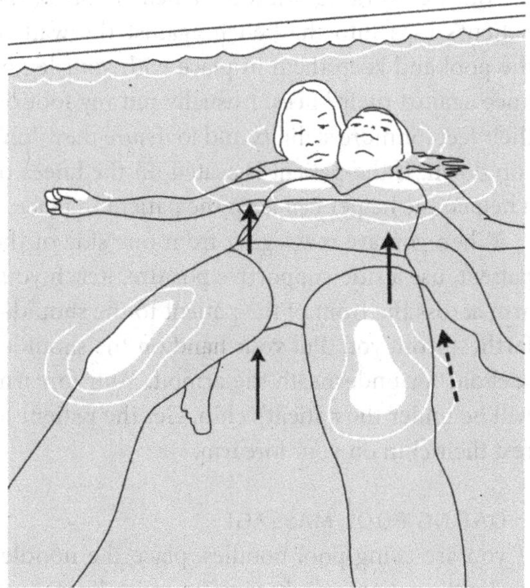

Walking backward with the patient's head on your shoulder and hands gently supporting the patient under their hips.

FIGURE 5.3. Supporting the Patient in the Pool

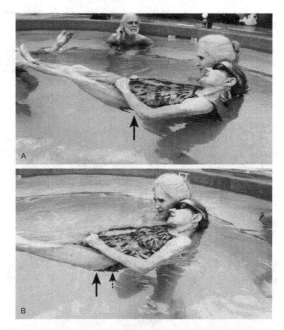

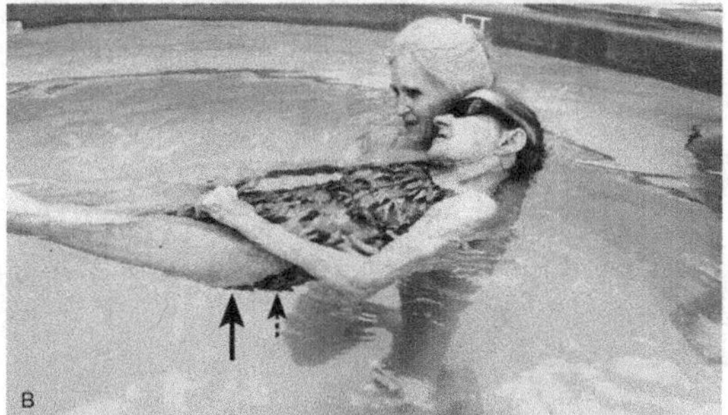

Freya and I demonstrate two positions: (A) Freya's head on my shoulder, with my left hand holding her neck and my right hand supporting her sacrum; (B) Freya's head on my shoulder, with my hands supporting one hip and her sacrum.

Therapist Stances in Pool Massage

SEATED POOL MASSAGE

If you are working without a helper, press the patient's hips into the bench against the wall of the pool and keep them in place with your leg or knee against their knees. I usually put my foot on their feet for more stability and to insure they don't slip down. If the patient is seated on the knees of a helper, the helper can keep the patient in place.

When you are massaging from one side of the patient, use a side-supportive posture. Reach your arm across the front of the patient to the shoulder farthest from you. Put your hand on the shoulder (deltoid) or underneath the armpit. Your forearm will be under the patient's chin. Get the patient to rest their chin on your forearm.

FLOATING POOL MASSAGE

If you are using pool noodles, place the noodles under the patient's neck, armpits, waist, knees, and ankles. You can do a full massage with your patient in this floating position while you are seated or squatting in the pool. I recommend, however, a tandem massage team for stability. Each team member adopts a stride stance on opposite sides of the patient. They each use one hand to control the lift and the other to apply the stroke. Pressure and counterpressure! The person's body is sandwiched between the hands of each team member.

Basic Pool Massage Routine

The following massage routine is written for someone floating in the water, with notes adapting it for seated pool massage. For bathtubs (and some hot tubs), there will be space constraints that you will need to adjust to, but the massage sequence is the same. All locations, particularly when you are dealing with water, have challenges, and you will always be making adjustments.

I include abdominal massage in all underwater massage, whether the patient is in a bathing suit, bikini, or nothing, and include the hip movements of extension, flexion, and rotation. Respiratory massage movements are also included in underwater massage for the diaphragm, ribs, and upper head, neck, and shoulders, including upper

FIGURE 5.4. Position for Seated Pool Massage

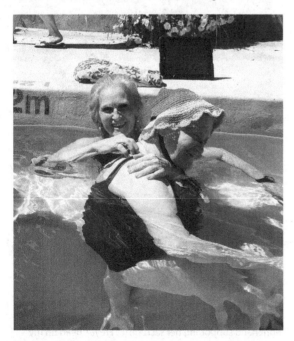

You can sit the patient on your knee.

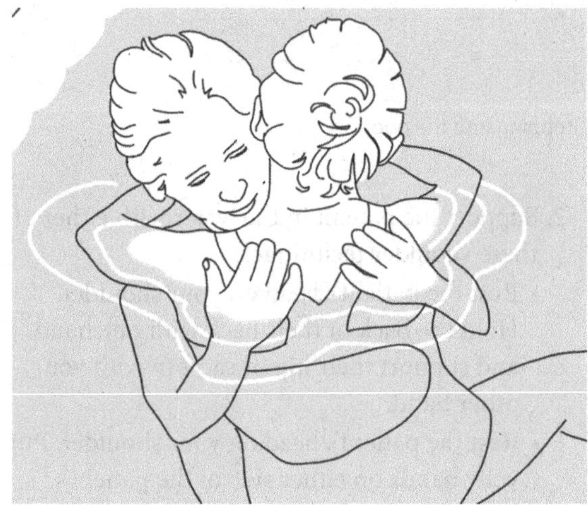

Or you can face the patient towards you in a hug position.

FIGURE 5.5. Position for Floating Pool Massage

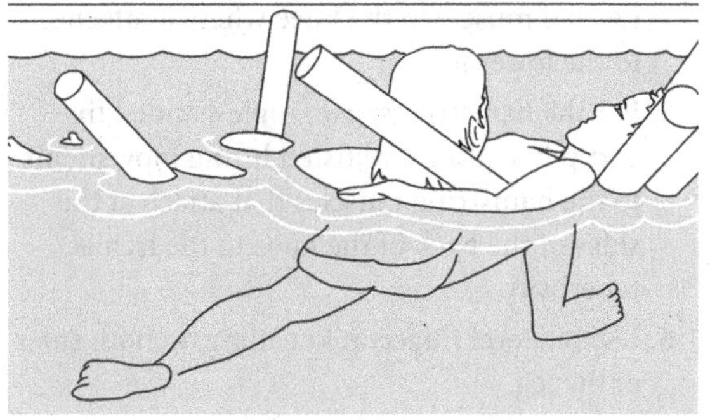

Every pool has noodles useful for floating pool massage.

respiratory facial massage. From the person's air intake at the nose, all the way down to the diaphragm, a person can be massaged in a pool or tub.

The routine outlined here starts with the back, but you can also start at the hands or feet. Many people shake hands as a greeting, and I often employ this idea as a starting point. Although I always teach the principle of opening up the circulation to an extremity by starting at the shoulder or the hip, sometimes I find it better to start at the hands or the feet to get the quickest relaxation effect without disturbing the patient. It also gets the person used to my touch and used to having a massage under the water. If I am doing the hands or feet first, I am careful to reach into the water, not lifting the hand or foot out of the water, in order to keep the extremity warm.

BACK MASSAGE

1. Place one hand on the abdomen to counteract the upward direction of pressure as you massage the back. I use shallow water so I can stand above my patient and be able to do the lifting strokes from above them.
2. Slowly work from the lower back up to the shoulders with pressure indicated by the patient.

For a seated patient: Stand to one side of the patient. Using a side-supportive posture, massage the patient's back with fingertip kneading levered against the wall of the pool.

NECK AND SHOULDER MASSAGE

1. Support the patient's forehead with one hand and use single-handed fingertip kneading to the neck muscles up to the occipital ridge attachments of the trapezius and erector spinae muscles.
2. With one hand on the patient's chest, use single-handed fingertip kneading to the rhomboid muscles between the shoulder blades.

For a seated patient: With the patient resting their chin on your supporting arm, massage with single-handed scooping strokes to the entire neck, then massage the rhomboid muscles.

ARM AND HAND MASSAGE

1. Reach around the shoulder girdle and massage the back of the deltoid using single-handed palmar kneading, single-handed thumb kneading, and single-handed fingertip kneading.
2. Use alternate thumb kneading and single-handed thumb kneading to the biceps and triceps of the upper arm, especially the attachments on either side of the elbow to increase flexibility.
3. Massage the inner elbow using alternate thumb kneading with the elbow bent, and cupping and palmar kneading to the olecranon process of the outer elbow.
4. Use alternate thumb kneading and single-handed thumb kneading to the forearm flexors.
5. Use alternate thumb kneading and single-handed thumb kneading to the extensors all the way to the dorsum of the hand.
6. Massage the wrist with tiny alternate thumb kneading strokes.
7. Massage the hand with alternate thumb kneading to the dorsum and the palm aspects. Also flip the hand at the wrist to alternate thumb kneading from the heel of the hand to the base of the fingertips.

8. Massage each finger with rotational movements (corkscrewing) three times per finger.
9. Wring the entire arm (can be done at any time throughout the arm routine).

For a seated patient: Move to the front of the patient to massage the arms.

LEG MASSAGE

With a floating patient, we can bend the leg at the knee and lean it over to the opposite side and stretch those hip muscles, all the while massaging with fingertip and thumb kneading.

1. Use single-handed fingertip kneading to the entire hip with a focus on the ischial tuberosity and the head of the femur.
2. Wring the entire upper leg. Wrap one hand way around to the back of the thigh, pulling up and across the thigh and passing the other hand, which is bent down as far as possible.
3. Do bilateral wringing at this point, and at the end of the upper leg session, and also at the very end of the leg massage routine. Wring up the whole leg from top to bottom or bottom to top three times.
4. Use alternate thumb kneading on the quadriceps up and down the length of the four-headed muscle to the knee where it attaches to the lower leg.
5. For the hamstrings, use single-handed fingertip kneading and fisted lifting movements to the hamstring muscles that attach at the sides of the back of the knee to the ischial tuberosity.
6. Use bilateral fingertip kneading on both sides of the leg.
7. Massage under the leg with sweeping strokes of fingertip pressure starting at the top at the ischial tuberosity and working your way down to the posterior attachment on either side of the knee itself. I use an alternating fingertip stroking with both hands or one hand.

For a seated patient: Stand facing the patient, and either 1) straddle each leg, controlling it between your knees, or 2) stand at the knee. Use levered single-handed fingertip kneading and fisted lifting movements to massage under the patient.

FIGURE 5.6. **Underwater Alternate Thumb Kneading**

BACK OF HAND

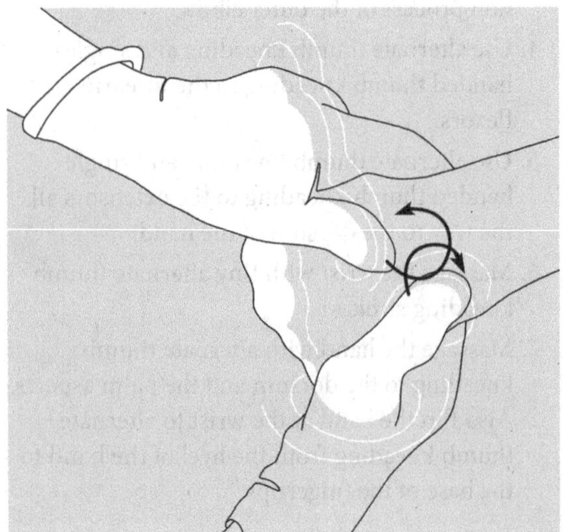

PALMS

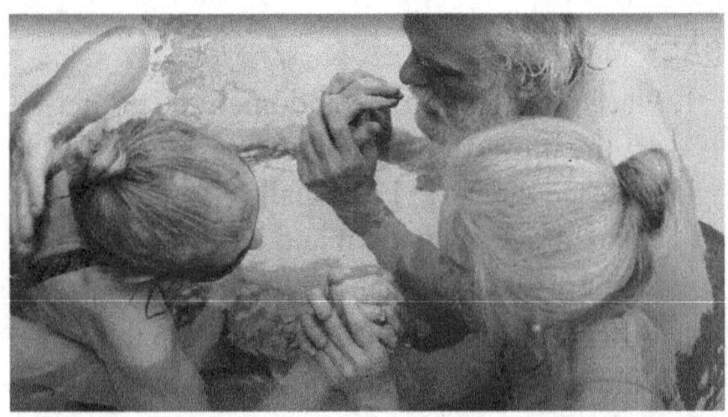

KNEE MASSAGE

1. Use a modified wringing to the entire knee, wedging the patella with one hand above and one below the kneecap. Again, wrap your hand completely around the knee itself.
2. Hold the lower leg with both hands as you massage.
3. Use fingertip kneading bilaterally up and down the sides of the knee.
4. Use fingertip kneading in the posterior aspect of the knee, maintaining upward pressure in a lifting motion while using alternating and simultaneous strokes.
5. Passively move the patella back and forth to maintain its mobility.

For a seated patient: Move to the front of the patient to massage the knees, using alternate thumb kneading around the patellar perimeter with a huge singular alternate thumb kneading tracing around the patellar edge.

LOWER LEG MASSAGE

1. Wring from the side of the patient.
2. Use alternate thumb kneading to the tibialis anterior into the foot attachments.
3. Use single-handed fingertip kneading to the calf muscle (gastrocnemius).
4. Use bilateral splitting of the calf muscle from the Achilles to the back of the knee.
5. Use open *C*-wringing to the lower leg.

For a seated patient: Stand in front of the patient to perform wringing.

HIP ROTATIONS

These can be done now or at the end of the leg massage.

ANKLE MASSAGE

Holding the leg outstretched and straight, massage the anklebones with alternate and simultaneous thumb kneading around the malleoli.

FOOT MASSAGE

1. Use thumb wringing to the top and bottom of the foot.
2. Use finger-wrap wringing to the whole foot with a focus on the bottom of the foot.
3. Use alternate thumb kneading to the top of the foot.
4. Apply digital thumb compression to the sole of the foot, especially the transverse arch at the base of the toes.
5. Wring each toe slowly and thoroughly.
6. Use a passive ankle rotation three times in each direction stabilizing at the ankle joint.
7. Do flexion and extension at the ankle joint fixing the joint with one hand and mobilizing it with the other hand.

For a seated patient: You can massage the foot facing toward or away from the patient.

LEG PUMPING

In the water, leg pumping works best with two people for balance. This stroke mobilizes the hips and aids digestion. Use all three basic strokes, preferably with a helper so there is one person on each leg: alternate pumping; simultaneous pumping, bending both knees to the chest; and rotational pumping, three times in each direction.

FIGURE 5.7. Underwater Foot Massage

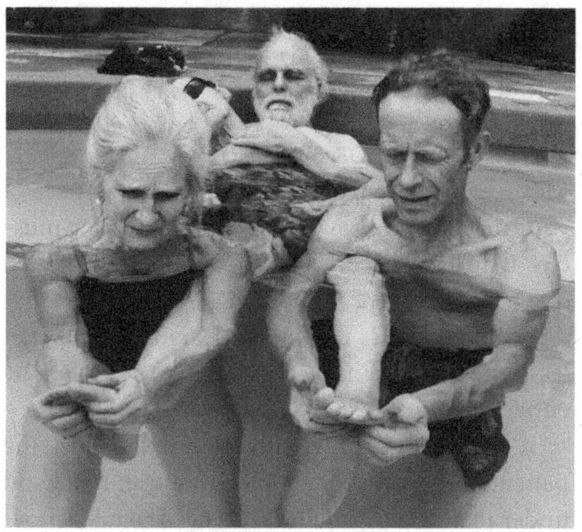

Freya sits on her husband Stan's lap while her son Finn and I massage her feet.

ABDOMINAL MASSAGE

1. Start with palmar kneading to the anterior (front) of the abdomen.
2. Sandwich the abdomen, with one hand on top and one on the lower back. Move both hands in circles at the same speed and in the same direction. Then move them in alternating directions. Do this at least three times slowly and firmly.
3. Single-handed fingertip kneading is performed in the same direction, lingering in each of the four corners of the abdomen.
4. Continue with a palmar vibration on the abdomen. Working in tandem, one team member puts their hands under the patient and the other team member puts their palms, one on top of the other or side by side, on the tummy. If you are working alone, you can put one hand under the person and use the other hand to do a single-handed vibration.
5. Finish with light reflex stroking in the same direction of digestive movement using a very light touch and a continuous momentum.

For a seated patient: Massage the abdomen as you would if the patient were seated in a wheelchair. Remember the "sandwiching"!

FACE AND SCALP MASSAGE

Hold the head firmly with one hand and use the other hand to massage the opposite side of the face and scalp. Change hands and massage the other side of the head and scalp.

WATER MOVES FOR MASSAGE

Move your patient through the water as part of your massage to provide a lateral stretch for muscles that have become contracted and shortened due to immobility.

If the patient is floating with noodles, you can leave the noodles in place, and move the patient by either walking backward or forward.

If you are working without noodles, rest the patient's head on your shoulder and put one hand under their hip or sacrum. You need to keep moving, walking backward constantly so the patient doesn't sink. This requires that you find a comfortable gait and posture that works for you and your patient. The right gait and posture for me is with bent legs so my shoulders are at water level, but a taller person might need to do a squatting-walk backward.

Without noodles, you can use the shoulder technique you used to move the patient through the pool at the start of the session, walking backward.

As you push or pull the patient through the water:

- Make circles in one direction and then the other.
- Make wave-like motions, up and down.

Tub Massage

Tub Transfers

I use the classic transfer procedure for putting a patient in a tub for bathing. I push the patient's wheelchair to the side of the tub, put the brakes on and footrests down, and transfer the patient to a sitting position on the edge of the tub. Then I swing their legs into the tub and ease them into the water.

Remember that people getting out of the water will be relaxed and weak. Before they get out, I drain the water from the bath then put a towel over their shoulders and get in behind them, assisting with an armpit lift to the edge of the bathtub. I have them just sit for a while before we transfer to the wheelchair. I have the wheelchair beside the bathtub, right up against it, ready to wheel them back to their bed.

You can also use a mechanical lift for tub transfers. I recommend this for patients who are frail or who have limited or no use of their arms, such as people with high spinal cord injuries.

Important Features of Tub Massage

For your patient, the big difference between a normal bath and an underwater massage is the level of the water and the time spent in the tub.

- **Level of water:** If possible, the water should completely cover the person, including, their shoulders (the deeper the water, the better).

In practical terms, this often means pouring water over them as the person relaxes and their knees bend upward. You may need to increase the water level in the tub or simply use a hose to keep any body parts sticking out of the water warm and relaxed.

- **Time in the tub:** A tub massage usually takes twenty minutes to a half hour. Keep the temperature of the water consistent over the time spent in the tub. After you've done the massage, allow another fifteen minutes to half hour to simply let the person rest, listen to music, watch a nice view, or snooze on a supportive neck rest or pillow. I often use the airplane inflatables for neck support, and this allows the person to have a post-massage sleep in the hot water.

Patient Positions for Tub Massage

Positions include:

- **Seated or reclining:** A tub pillow for the patient's neck will make them more comfortable.
- **Supine, face-up:** When I'm massaging under a person in this position, I place one hand on top of the person to keep their body submerged in the warm water.
- **Side-lying:** Working from one side of the tub, you can roll a person toward you into a side-lying position to get better access to their back, in particular. Ideally, you should duplicate what you do on one side by going around the tub and rolling them the other direction.

Therapist Stances in Tub Massage

The side-supportive posture is important for patients who are seated or reclining. This is the same posture as for a patient seated in a pool, where you reach across the patient and rest their chin on your forearm.

You can use a supported stride stance or a half-kneel stance (one knee down, one knee up) with your tummy leaning on the edge of the tub.

Alternatively, you can use a stride stance with the forward knee bent and positioned on the edge of the tub, or with the forward foot in the tub.

Some strokes are best accomplished facing the patient. For these, I often climb right into the tub.

Routine for Massaging In and Out of the Tub

1. From outside the tub, massage with levered fingertip kneading, up and down the back close to the spine along the erector spinae muscles, working your way to the outside aspect of the submerged person's trunk. If the patient is in a sling, pull the sling to help maneuver your hand between the sling and the bathtub itself. The bathtub surface will provide resistance and power to the levered fingertip kneading.
2. From the outside the tub, massage the extremities, keeping the limbs underwater wherever possible. In a stride stance or half-kneeling stance, lever your body by leaning your tummy onto the edge of the tub. Use the basics of palmar kneading and fingertip kneading to open up the circulation to the extremities by working the shoulders and the hips first. Continue your massage down the arms and legs with alternate thumb kneading and wringing to all the upper surfaces, quadriceps, tibialis anterior, biceps, triceps, and forearm extensors and flexors.
3. To massage underneath the leg, use bilateral fingertip kneading from the hip and ischial tuberosity to the popliteal fossa at the back of the knee.
4. Stepping into the tub to massage the hips and legs is my best underwater massage technique. I step one leg in and lean diagonally toward the far-side hip, lifting the leg toward me at the back of the knee while using my extending hand to massage the gluteal muscles. I also sometimes fully enter the tub, with both feet in and knees bent, to provide bilateral levered fingertip kneading, starting at the ischial tuberosity where the person is making contact with the bottom of the tub.

5. To massage the hips, I like to be fully in the tub, in a kneeling position between the patient's knees. This allows access with both hands—one hand on either side of the hips—for levered fingertip kneading. I can massage the hips bilaterally (both hips at the same time) or unilaterally (one hip at a time). When I do one hip at a time, I bend the patient's knee slightly, holding one hand under the knee, diagonally positioning it so I have better access to the lower back and hip.
6. Still positioned between the knees, I work my way up the back to the shoulders and massage in the armpits. I massage up and down the erector spinae muscles, reaching as far as I can at the top and finishing at the sacrum.
7. To massage the legs, I turn myself around between the patient's knees to face their feet. I continue the principle of upward pressure toward the heart with long strokes up the back of the calf from the Achilles tendon to the popliteal fossa. This rhythmic stroking is

FIGURE 5.8. Massaging the Extremities

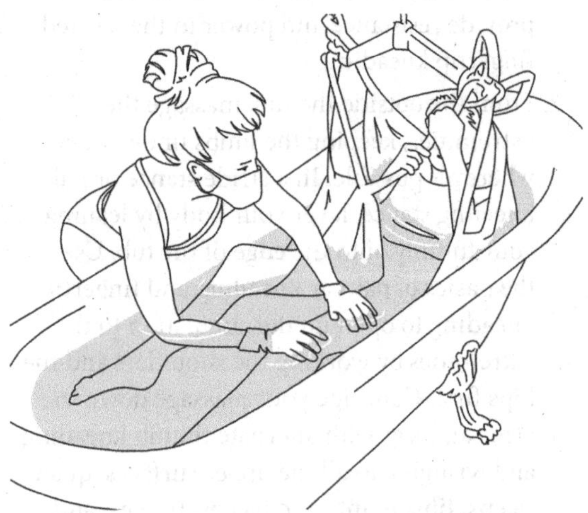

The therapist can lean on the edge of the tub for back support.

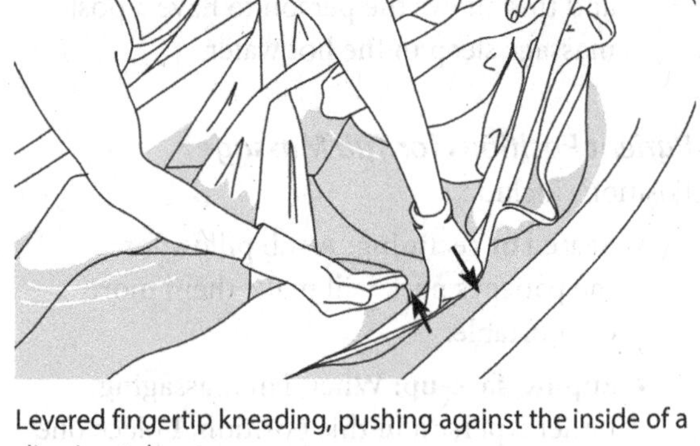

Levered fingertip kneading, pushing against the inside of a sling in a tub.

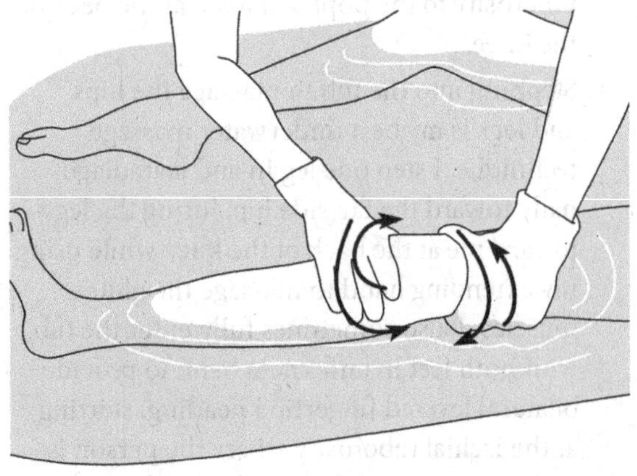

Wringing above and below the knee from outside the tub.

FIGURE 5.9. Leg Massage from Outside the Tub

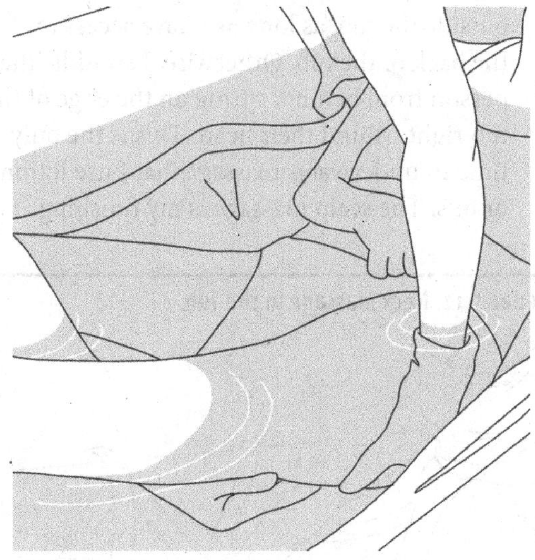

Reaching across the patient from outside the tub to massage under the leg.

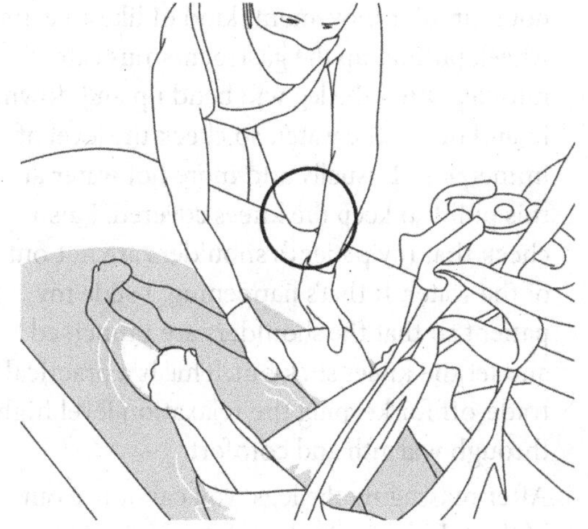

Bilateral fingertip kneading of the leg, one knee positioned on the edge of the tub.

FIGURE 5.10. Hip Massage Partly in the Tub

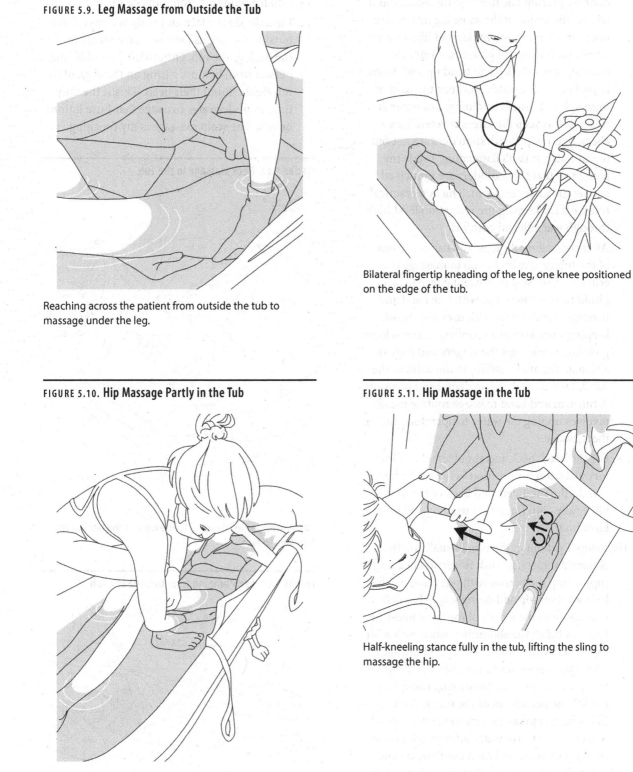

Stride stance with forward foot in the tub for hip massage. Here, my forward leg is between the patient's legs.

FIGURE 5.11. Hip Massage in the Tub

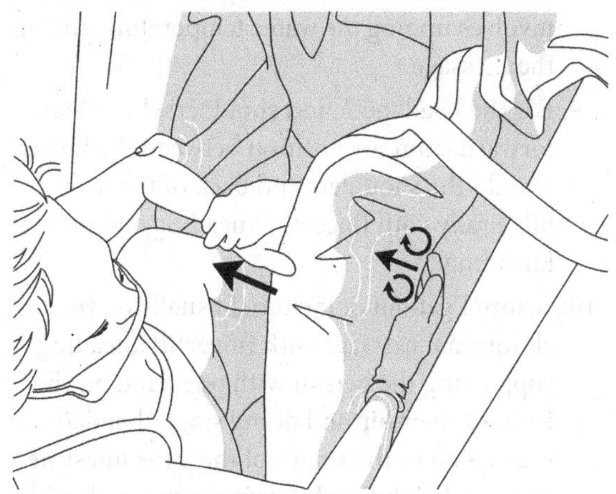

Half-kneeling stance fully in the tub, lifting the sling to massage the hip.

done by placing one hand on the outside and one on the inside of the same leg in a continuous circular movement, kind of like a Ferris wheel, pulling up the gastrocnemius calf muscle. Often the leg will bend up and down, in and out of the water, so check the level of immersion. I usually add more hot water at this point to keep the knees covered. I also check that my patient's shoulders are not out of the water. If that's happening, I slide my patient so that the shoulders are immersed and let the knees stick out. This is a practical trade-off for keeping the relaxation level high through warmth and comfort.

8. After massaging the legs, you can move out of the tub or stay in the tub to massage the arms. I like to stay in. Kneeling face to face, I hold the person's wrist with one hand and massage the shoulder with my other hand, keeping their arm in a semiflexed, bent-elbow position. Corkscrew the fingers and provide alternate thumb kneading to the palm of the hand, including alternate digital compression. A full arm and hand massage routine usually involves upping the water temperature during the massage.
9. For the head, neck and shoulders, I can lean forward from my position between the knees and do the shoulders and back of the neck bilaterally with fingertip kneading and palmar kneading.
10. Before I get out of the tub, I usually do the abdominal massage with fingertip kneading, supporting the person with one hand on the front of their hip and doing single-handed massaging to the length of the large intestine. I always finish the abdominal work with a lifting stroke with both hands around the back where the nerves for the digestive system exit the spine, at the same time being careful to not lift the person out of the water. A nice finish here is to take a handheld showerhead and circulate warm water around and around on the abdomen, and then continue up and down the legs and back before getting out of the tub to do the face and scalp.
11. I do leg pumping from outside the tub.
12. I usually do the face and scalp massage from outside the tub, as long as I have access to the back of the tub. Otherwise, I straddle the person from behind, sitting on the edge of the tub right behind their head. This is the only time in underwater massage that I use lotions or oils. The scalp massage is my finishing

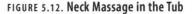

FIGURE 5.12. Neck Massage in the Tub

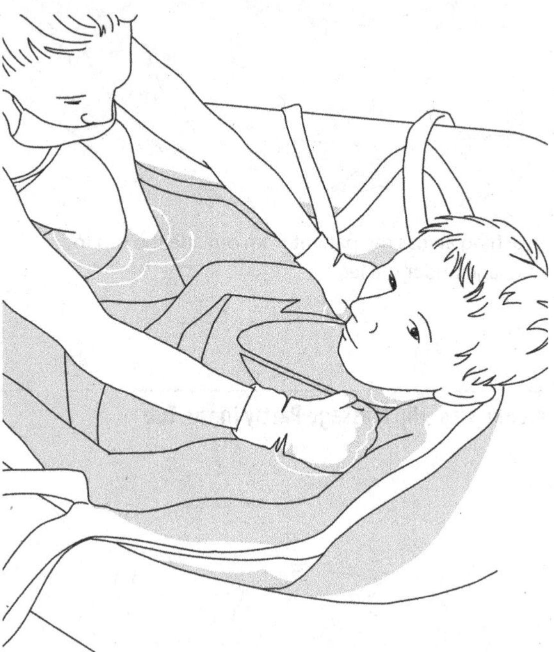

Bilateral fingertip kneading to the back of the neck in the tub, face to face.

FIGURE 5.13. Leg Pumping from Outside the Tub

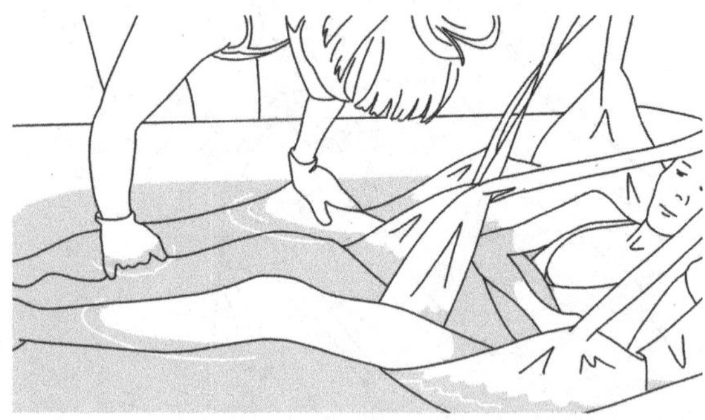

Leg pumping from outside the tub, with the sling lifting the patient slightly.

touch, reaching down if I am above them or reaching around at whatever angle is possible.

THE POLITICS OF WATER LEVELS

When you get out of the tub to massage the face and scalp, the water level will drop. This will not be popular with your patient!

Before I start the face and scalp massage, I increase the temperature and level of the water. This provides the perfect opportunity to use a handheld showerhead for a European-style underwater massage (which uses hoses instead of hands).

I once took some Canadians to Bad Wörishofen, a spa town in Bavaria, Germany, for Kneipp hydrotherapy, where I was introduced to hoses as a way to apply variable force to the body. My first experience of this massage created such a powerful reaction that I slept for three hours, so deeply that it was difficult to wake me up.

Using a handheld showerhead as a tool for applying pressure to stimulate the circulation is a matter of adjusting the strength of the flow of water. I grip the showerhead in one hand at the point where it sprays, which allows me to control the force and monitor the temperature.

VIDEO LIBRARY

Visit brusheducation.ca/wheeling-in-good-hands to watch these videos:

- **Patient positions for pool massage:** Seated bench locked-in position with Freya
- **Patient positions for pool massage:** Seated on massager's knees with Freya
- **Patient positions for pool massage:** Seated on massager's knees with bounce with Freya
- **Patient positions for pool massage:** Seated on massager's knees with stride positioning
- **Patient positions for pool massage:** Floating with support with Freya
- **Patient positions for pool massage:** Hugging position for back massage with Freya
- **Patient positions for pool massage:** Hug position back to front – securing at the waist
- **Tandem positioning for arm massage routine for underwater massage**
- **Tandem positioning for foot and ankle massage routine with massagers' backs to the patient** – underwater massage
- **Back massage:** Levering to the back using the wall of the pool – underwater massage
- **Neck and shoulder massage:** Adapting for a 3-on-1 – underwater massage
- **Arm massage:** Underwater pool massage
- **Leg massage:** Underwater pool massage
- **Leg massage:** Alternating fingertip kneading to the hamstring
- **Leg pumping:** Alternating, simultaneous, and rotational
- **Leg massage:** Adapting for 3-on-1 – underwater massage
- **Tub massage:** Tub transfer and therapist positioning

Bo

Through Brad Jacobsen, the creator of Peer BC, and Lori Slater, who was head of the Peer BC support group in Fort St. John, I discovered the wheelchair community of Northern British Columbia. Lori told me about Bo Hedges when she learned I was writing a book about wheelchair massage. Bo is a low-level (T12–L1) paraplegic. He grew up north of Fort St. John in a village called Wonowon on the Alaska Highway. He is also the captain of the Canadian men's national wheelchair basketball team.

Bo played for the 2012 team that won gold at the London Paralympics. When I met him, the team was training for the 2020 Paralympics in Tokyo (which Covid delayed until September, 2021).

The first time I met Bo was at his brother Bill's place in Fort St. John. My daughter Crystal filmed us as I gave Bo a wheelchair massage. During the massage, Bo let me know that he used all the practical applications of massage in his daily routines and in his basketball career.

I immediately liked everything about Bo. He was handsome and eloquent, with a voice made for radio and of course an athletic physique. But beyond his strong exterior, there was something special about his outlook on the world. He was a person helping others to dream bigger than their circumstances in life.

Over the next four years, Bo and I worked on a documentary called *Dream Big: Fort Saint John to Tokyo* with Ben Haab of Eagle Vision Video Productions as my executive producer. This film shows the enormous community support behind Bo, from the beginnings of his epic journey to the present day.

The title of the film changed four times over the years. First it was *Dream Big: Wonowon to Tokyo*, then it was *Dream Big: Dead Horse Creek Ranch to Tokyo*, then *Dream Big: Fort Saint John to Tokyo*, and finally *Dream Big: Fort Saint John and Beyond.*

"Dream Big" was the easy part of the title: those words were the backdrop for our Toronto footage in the Scarborough sports center, written large on the wall of the basketball court. We decided to drop "Dead Horse"—the name of Bo's family's ranch—because it was such a strong image that distracted from the theme of Fort St. John as a prime example of a supportive community, global and local.

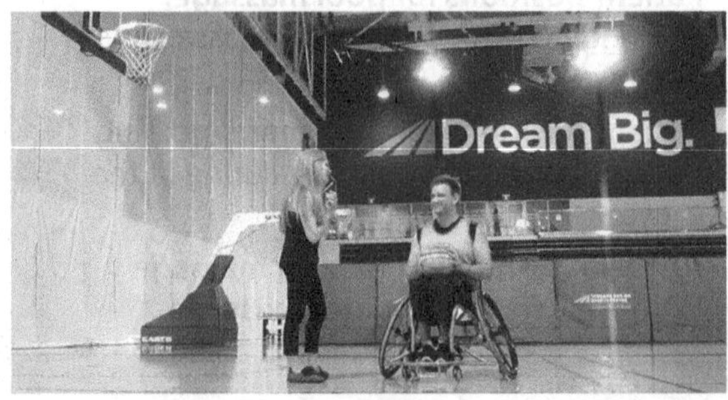

Bo Hedges and me in the basketball court at the Toronto Pan Am Sports Centre in Scarborough, Ontario, which is the national training center for Wheelchair Basketball Canada.

Fort St. John is a community with Bo's name all over it. In the city's million-dollar sports complex, I discovered Bo's winning wheelchair, his medals, and his history proudly on display. I knew that I was onto a good story! But again, most importantly, I was onto a huge swell of community support for Bo and for his story to be told in our film!

Bo was twelve years old when he broke his back. He was already a basketball player before the accident, and once he landed in the chair, his family and friends started playing basketball in wheelchairs to support him. He always wanted to be active, so being in a wheelchair was not going to stop him. Bo achieved his goals because of the support of his family and friends, and because of support that went beyond his family and friends: from Fort St. John, northern British Columbia, his home town, and the entire community. In making the documentary, I realized that the film was solidly about community rising to the occasion—in this instance, getting twenty to thirty wheelchairs in this northern community for the formation of a local basketball team.

In making the film, we were able to record Bo in numerous contexts—from his work on the family ranch raising cattle in British Columbia, to the intimacy of his home with his partner Weibke in Toronto, to Wheelchair Basketball Canada's National Training Centre in Scarborough.

I visited the family ranch, just off the Alaska Highway, and fell in love with the Simmental cows that the Hedges are known for breeding. I left there knowing why Bo is the way he is. I met his mother, Marilyn. She is a female version of Bo—thoughtful, smart, very observant, and generous with her time and her steaks!

When I initially approached Bo, my interest was in wheelchair massage, but our connection grew beyond that when we started working on the film.

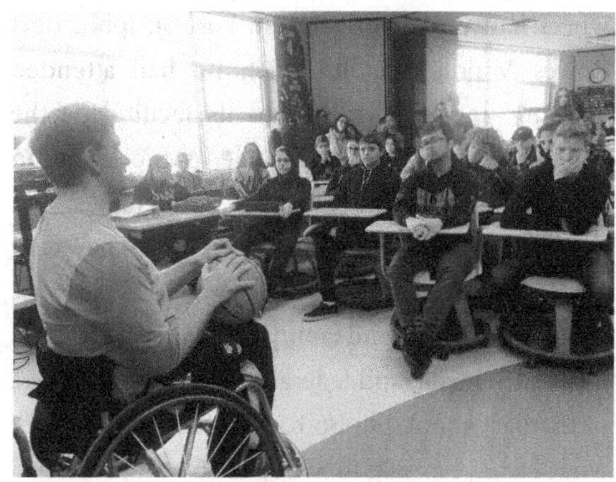

Bo has talked to many students about the life of a wheelchair athlete and how to play wheelchair basketball. Students learn to expand their imaginations about life's challenges.

Beginning with that first sports massage shoot at Bo's brother's place, and including Zoom sessions to teach Bo and Marilyn to massage each other's head, neck, shoulders, arms, and hands, I have appreciated the tactile, hands-on nature of this wonderful family. The hard work of cattle ranching informs their gifted hands. All the Hedges have drive, determination, and thoroughness. Bo started with solid work ethics, and he took them from the Alaska Highway to Tokyo, Japan.

In the summer of 2021—just before the Paralympics in Tokyo—I opened the local Alaska Highway newspaper and was surprised to see a lineup of wheelchair athletes. I recognized them from the winter games where I had taught wheelchair massage all day long! The article was announcing the launch of a new wheelchair basketball club, the Energizers. I wondered if the newspaper was doing this just for me to have the most perfect ending for the documentary about Bo!

I knew that Bo was planning to return to Fort St. John that September to help with the cattle roundup. I was planning to film a wheelchair basketball game with Bo and local people, including those that had started with him on the first wheelchair basketball team in Fort St. John. Bert Bowes Middle School, which Bo had attended growing up, had volunteered its facility for the game. I had planned the game as a celebration to welcome Bo home from the Paralympics, and as the final piece of the documentary. The event would include long-time supporters, players, sponsors, friends, and family, including politicians local, provincial, and federal. I had a strong image of that last shoot, but Bo had no idea the scope of what I was planning to honor him.

When I had told him about my idea for a local basketball game, Bo had commented that it would look pretty "sloppy." I didn't mind what it looked like because it was to be an event to honor him and show the community's appreciation for his dedication to the game.

The Paralympics went live in Tokyo on September 5, 2021. With rules about Covid restrictions, testing, and isolation, these games would be different than anything Bo had experienced in his other international competitions.

Unfortunately, because of Covid, we were not able to film in Tokyo. Now, it was my job to work the Fort St. John end of things. Interviewing Bo's family, his best friend, former players, and the mayor during the lead-up to the games was my daily documentation. I was counting on Bo and his teammates to give me clips from the games themselves for the climax of the sporting aspect of the film.

The term *para* in Paralympics comes from *parallel.* When listening to the CBC coverage of the games in 2021, I was struck anew by their meaning. For me, the Paralympics are the true essence of sport. They deliver on the true meaning of rising above physical circumstances and challenges. During the challenges we all faced with Covid, their message had deeper impact.

Every parathlete has achieved beyond their dreams just to compete in the Paralympics. Their courage, determination, and hard work deserve the same recognition as we give Olympic athletes, or maybe even more.

I filmed Bo's entire family, including cousins and more-distant relatives, during each of the international games leading up to Tokyo and each of the games in Tokyo. In the end, Canada finished out of the medals. But, the enthusiasm of the community of Fort St. John, from locally owned tiny companies like spas to the giant gas and oil companies, gave the conclusion of the project a fresh injection of the indomitable spirit of the north. For myself as the filmmaker, the overwhelming enthusiasm for Bo on his Tokyo adventure is inspiring. There's something about the north that breeds even more Canadian generosity of spirit.

Faced with the resurgence of Covid, the opening ceremony of the Tokyo Paralympics felt just short of a miracle. My footage captures the voice of Marilyn Hedges and the voices of Bo's brothers, Bill, Rod and Matt, and I'm re-reminded of the original team that helped Bo put Olympic wheels beneath him. I was refreshed by their willingness to be filmed again, to be interrogated by my constant phone calls, and yet remain supportive of this long-standing film project. I realized that they had been on this journey with Bo for over thirty years, so the four years of this film were no big deal to them.

Fort St. John is now the home of the Energizers, the local wheelchair basketball club created by Rob Stiles, the heartbeat of adaptive sports in the north. Bert Bowes Middle School is the central location of this fabulous club, which is now creating its first Wall Of Fame. This includes a dedication to Bo, and images of him showing his gold medal and reaching for the ball high in the air next to a Japanese player at the Tokyo Paralympics. Honoring Bo in the hallways of his school is a fitting finale.

From Bo, I learned about cattle ranching at its best! As a vegan vegetarian, I can now boast about the best red meat: Simmental from Wonowon!

Bo also helped me create wheelchair sports massage teaching films and added an all-important family element to them by including his mother, Marilyn, and his partner, Weibke. With this book, we will keep delivering these lessons for years to come, bridging the country with the power of touch. Thank you Bo and all the Hedges (Weibke and daughter, Matilda), and thank you to the power of Fort St. John.

6

Massaging Wheelchair Athletes

Sports massage was used in Europe years before we were using it in North America. The first use of sports massage was the Paris Olympics in 1924. These days, it is commonplace at all levels of professional and recreational sports. My former business partner, Grace Chan of the Sutherland-Chan School, was instrumental in organizing the first sports massage association for Canada and the United States back in the 1970s. In 1988, more than a hundred massage therapists, mostly American, paid their own way to Calgary, Alberta, to be part of our Calgary Winter Olympic massage team.

We had two sites for this international Olympic clinic, one in Canmore, Alberta, and one in Calgary at the Oval Dome, where I was a clinical supervisor. We organized the clinics to serve all athletes, and I loved the "internationalness" of the experience. I would be cheering for my Chinese speed skater and the therapist next to me would be rooting for her European athlete.

I have taught sports massage for more than twenty years. In 2013, I was thrilled to attend the international wheelchair rugby finals in Pretoria, South Africa, meeting the team therapists and members from all over the world. I was in heaven! My most instructive South African experience was a wheelchair athlete wanting to learn how to massage his partner. It reminded me of the important role families play in keeping wheelchair athletes at their best. This was the highlight of my teaching internationally.

But, of course, when you teach, you also learn. Zak Madell, an Albertan wheelchair sports athlete, and Bo Hedges, the captain of the Canadian men's wheelchair basketball team, have been instrumental teachers. Brad Jacobsen, who died in 2021, was another—Brad and I taught wheelchair massage at GF Strong Rehabilitation Centre in Vancouver, and he was my first wheelchair sports massage co-teacher. But I have learned the most from the friends and family of sports athletes who give massages on a regular basis.

The families of Zak Madell, Bo Hedges, and Brad Jacobson have all provided hands-on support. For Zak and Brad, their mothers were their massage mainstays throughout their early recovery.

The focus of family and friends on preventing pressure sores and overuse stress injuries makes a big difference to the success of wheelchair athletes.

The common denominator of all wheelchair sports is the extreme use of the hands and arms, so much of this chapter focuses on the upper body. Massaging the lower body is important for pressure sore prevention and continued security in the chair. To have the hips mobile and not locked up from being in a seated competitive position for long periods means massaging the entire gluteal area to open up the circulation to the lower extremity.

Five Categories of Wheelchair Sports Massage

My wheelchair athletes have shown me the importance of the following five distinct categories of wheelchair sports massage:

1. Conditioning and training massage
2. Pre-event warm-up massage
3. Intra-competition massage

4. Post-event massage
5. Recovery and maintenance massage

The most important aspect of wheelchair sports massage is family. I encourage all massage professionals to keep a hands-on partnership with the families of wheelchair athletes.

Conditioning and Training Massage for Wheelchair Athletes

Massage during training for an event is important. It can be a weekly massage when the event is still months away, or a daily massage when the event is a week away. Either way, the focus is relaxation. Relaxation is key as the event draws near. Total relaxation is the goal: it lets all the developing neurological pathways for winning (extreme exertion) be as responsive as possible. Relaxation and visualization exercises are part of the training formula employed by most top athletes. The ability to completely relax is an asset to every athlete. A full body wheelchair massage, from the toes to the nose, can achieve this. At the end, the athlete can lean forward onto pillows and deeply relax, or if the massage was on a massage table, the athlete should rest for at least twenty minutes.

In the days before an event, some modifications can be made to the full body massage. These changes might involve the duration of massage. Regular weekly or bi- or tri-weekly massages may have taken an hour each time, but now they might be shorter or longer. When I work with families that can reproduce my massages with exactness, they begin to know what modifications work best on arrival at an event destination. Massages might take on new goals, too, like getting over jet lag if the athlete has traveled across time zones, or compensating for confined spaces during travel or the stress of pregame preparations.

Twenty-Four Hours before Competition

When an athlete is focused on all the ingredients for winning, massages that are within twenty-four hours of an event are instrumental. Keep your focus on the needs of your athlete: the athlete is in a heightened state and therefore hypersensitive before competition. You want everything about your session to be relaxing, so avoid stimulating or superficial conversation, and avoid introducing new or unfamiliar ideas or treatment approaches. Do everything to accommodate the emotional, psychological, and physical needs of your athlete.

Ask your athlete what they would like in your sessions. Instruct them to soak in a warm bath or shower before and after each massage. This combination of hydrotherapy and conditioning massage will be familiar. It is mandatory for the athlete to have had this combination throughout their training.

The duration of the massage should fit the athlete's concerns or wishes. When they feel finished, your treatment should have produced a feeling of total relaxation.

Whether you are massaging through their clothing in their wheelchair or on a massage table with traditional draping, be sure to keep them warm. I use heating pads and wool blankets to conserve the heat produced by the massage treatment. I also use hot water bottles and ask all my athletes to travel with hot water bottles in their suitcases. Two bottles means that I can use contrasting temperatures, with one bottle hot and one cold. You can also use both hot and both cold.

Again, keep in mind that this important massage treatment should be familiar. This means that the hot and cold applications should already be commonplace for your athlete.

Using ice packs and other ice treatments is not recommended within the final twenty-four hours; however, if your athlete is coming into competition with an injury, that is going to be a familiar addition to the basic relaxation massage.

You can also provide a non-full-body massage with a focus on the back first, but keep most of the focus on the wheelchair athlete's arms. This may mean leaving out the anterior trunk, chest, and abdomen due to time constraints or the athlete's requests, but you can still easily achieve the goal of total relaxation.

Tandem Massage

With all my wheelchair athletes, I use tandem massage as way to teach family and friends, who might be replacing me at an event. Most families and friends will be happy to massage together.

PRINCIPLES OF TANDEM WHEELCHAIR SPORTS MASSAGE

1. Mirror each other's strokes: keep your strokes at the same place at the same time.
2. Trade sides so the athlete is balanced, as you and your tandem partner may not have identical pressure and touch.
3. Check in about pressure with your athlete often. Get them to direct you and your tandem partner to be similar in your touch. Keep asking.
4. Check in about your athlete's posture and pillow support.
5. Ask your athlete about where they would like more time or attention, and then divide up the chores between you and your tandem partner. Your athlete might say "my hands need a bit more," in which case both of you can work on the hands again. Your athlete might ask for more time on several places, like the neck and shoulders and one elbow; divide up the work between you.
6. Relaxation is the most important outcome, so a working tandem pair has to be quiet and coordinated with their hands and their voices.

Pre-Event Warm-Up Wheelchair Sports Massage

This short massage is given before the athlete starts their team or individual pre-competition warm-up routine. It invigorates and stimulates the muscles, which helps prevent injury and aids in peak performance. The physical benefits of warming up the muscles are as important as the psychological benefits. The nervousness of the athlete is a natural phenomenon before any type of performance.

When I worked with racehorses, it was obvious that these high-strung animals needed to race and compete; it was part of their nature, what they were bred for. With wheelchair athletes, it isn't any different. They are trained to compete and win.

Wheelchair athletes, whether in team sports (basketball, rugby) or individual sports (swimming, skiing), are revved up for racing against others. The warm-up massage can take the nervous edge off the individual and still leave them with the pent-up energy to push beyond their limits. The massage will often make the athlete more centered and grounded. That same nervousness that escalates blood pressure and heart rate can also steal the energy needed to excel.

The tension produced by anxiety and worry causes the muscles to tighten, draining oxygen and creating more lactic acid. Massaging the muscles helps them gain flexibility and responsiveness. The athlete should be prepared at a physical level to have their muscles react positively, not negatively, in their warm-up routine and their competition.

I use superficial strokes quickly and efficiently. I use different strokes compared to the massages that lead up to this pregame massage treatment. Be sure to use some of these pre-event massage strokes in the days leading up to the sports event so everything is familiar.

When everything else is different—the venue, putting on the uniform, the public gaze—the massage routine should be the same. Remember, positive talk if any talk. Get feedback about pressure and speed.

The massage sequences outlined below can be performed in five minutes, but could be extended to forty minutes, depending on how much time is available. Ideally the sequences could be done in tandem to cut the time and increase the thoroughness.

Short Warm-Up Massage Routines, Pre-Event

ARM MASSAGE: SHORT PRE-EVENT

Massage the arms at the beginning of the warm-up massage and again at the end.

1. Apply superficial effleurage up the arms (in tandem or solo), three times.
2. Apply palmar kneading to the deltoid muscle at the top of the arm, three times.
3. Use alternate thumb kneading on the biceps and triceps.

FIGURE 6.1. Short Pre-Event Arm Massage: Effleurage

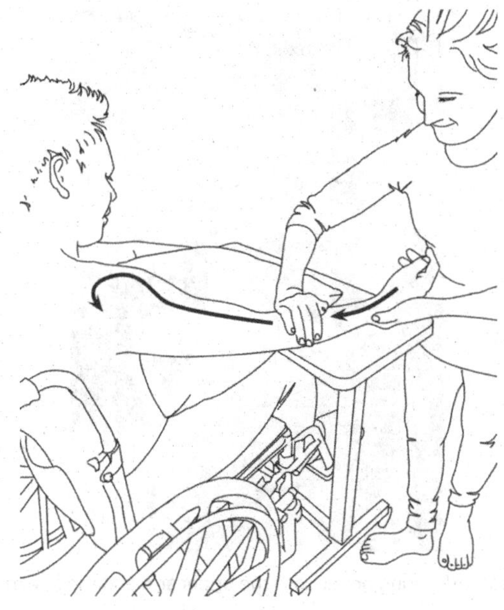

FIGURE 6.2. Short Pre-Event Arm Massage: Single-Handed Palmar Kneading to the Shoulder

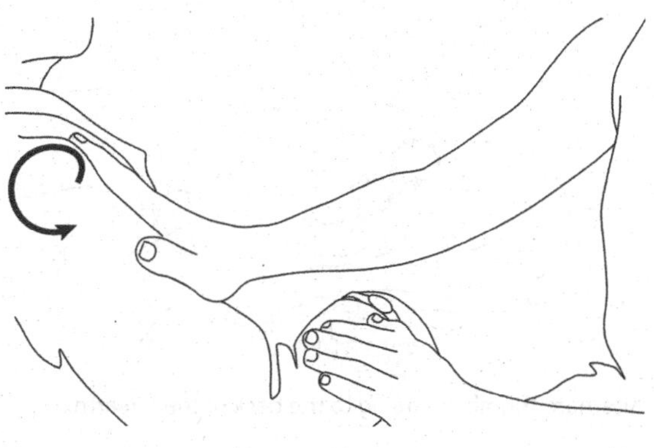

FIGURE 6.3. Short Pre-Event Arm Massage: Biceps

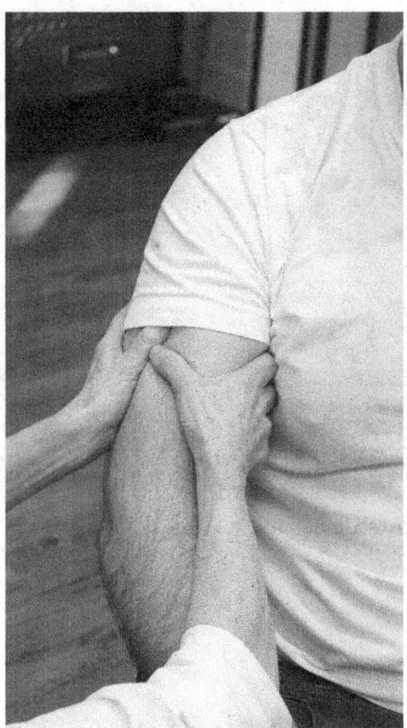

I am working on Bo Hedges here, who is featured throughout this chapter!

FIGURE 6.4. Short Pre-Event Arm Massage: Elbow

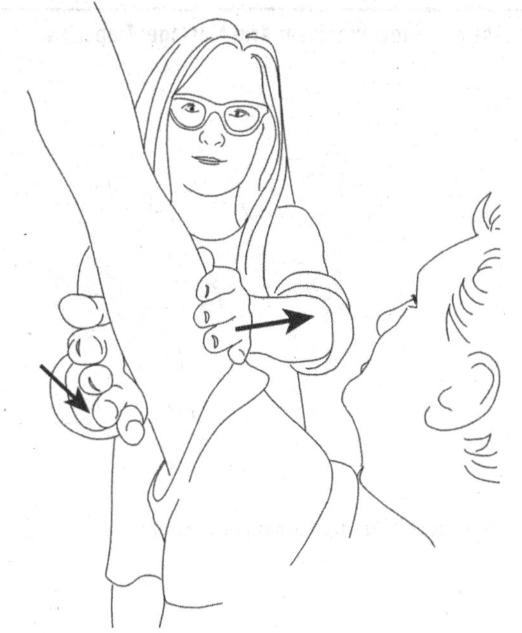

Brisk palmar rolling of the elbow.

FIGURE 6.5. **Short Pre-Event Arm Massage: Forearm**

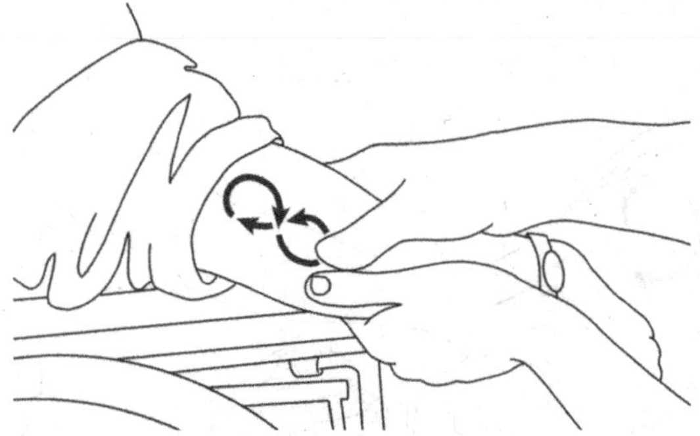

Alternate thumb kneading to the back of the forearm.

FIGURE 6.6. **Short Pre-Event Arm Massage: Wringing**

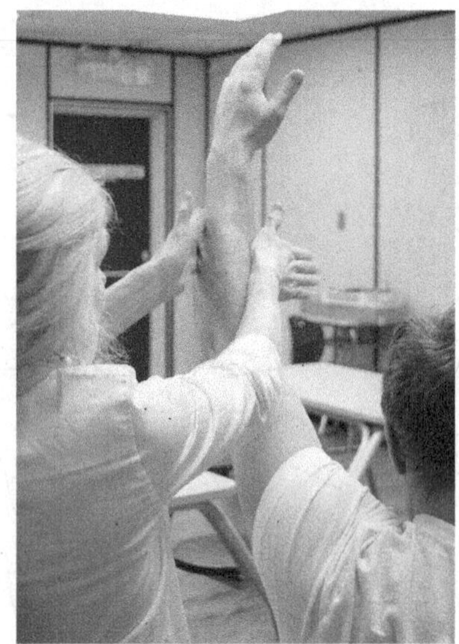

Vigorously wring or roll both the upper arm and the forearm.

FIGURE 6.7. **Short Pre-Event Arm Massage: Trapezius**

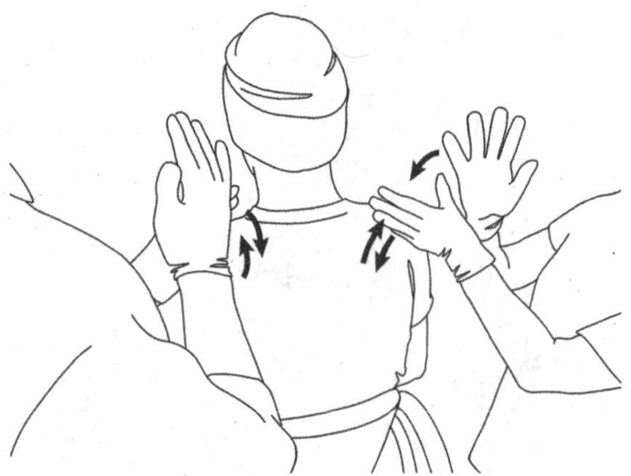

Tandem loose fingertip hacking to the trapezius.

FIGURE 6.8. **Short Pre-Event Back Massage: Rhomboids**

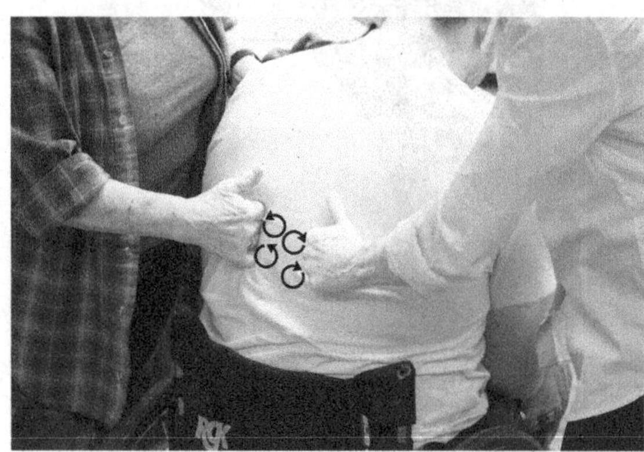

Tandem fisted kneading.

4. Do palmar rolling of the elbow between both hands, vigorously.
5. Use alternate thumb kneading on the forearm flexors and extensors.
6. Do palmar rolling of the forearm.
7. Squeeze the hand and wrist with a fingertip piano-playing movement, alternating digital compression.
8. Hold the arm straight up and roll the entire arm with vigorous back-and-forth movements between your two hands (palmar aspect), up and down. Don't forget the fingertips!
9. Use a percussion loose fingertip hacking to the trapezius as you cross over to the other arm. If working in tandem, you can do your tapotement up and down the arm.
10. Finish with light, fast fingertip stroking, three times.
11. I often repeat step 6 at this point, because the vigorous rolling gets the athlete revved up for competition.

BACK MASSAGE: SHORT PRE-EVENT

Have the wheelchair athlete lean forward and loosen their seatbelt.

1. Use tapotement down the erector spinae muscles from the occipital ridge to the sacrum.
2. Use a rolling fisted percussive stroke to the erector spinae muscles, spending extra focus at the sacrum.
3. Apply superficial fisted frictioning, vigorously and quickly, to the areas of significance for the sport. In swimming, this is the shoulder girdle. In hockey, rugby, and basketball, this is the shoulders.
4. The rhomboids underneath the trapezius deserve some vigorous kneading.
5. Apply loose fingertip hacking and other percussive strokes to the entire back.

HEAD, NECK, AND SHOULDER MASSAGE: SHORT PRE-EVENT

Stand behind or to the side of the athlete.

1. Use vigorous single-handed fingertip kneading on the neck if you are standing beside the athlete. Use both hands at the same speed if you are standing behind the chair.
2. It can be useful for the athlete to drop their head down, so the erector spinae stretches as you do the temporal kneading. I always include the strokes for the jaw and temples in this tense time.
3. Use all the percussive strokes on the shoulders and top of the trapezius.

FIGURE 6.9. Short Pre-Event Head Massage

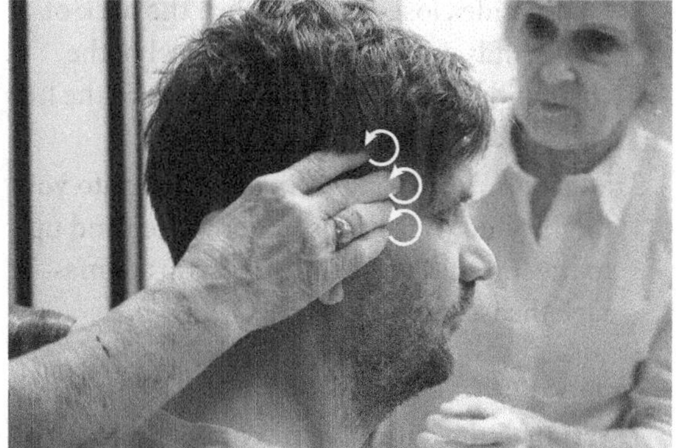

Temporal kneading.

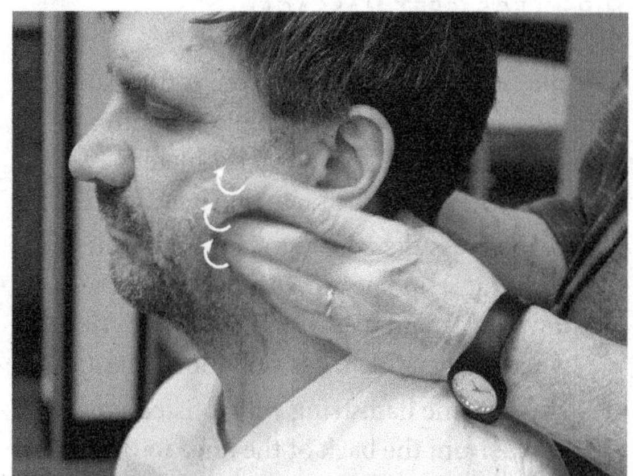

Jaw kneading.

FIGURE 6.10. Short Pre-Event Trapezius Massage

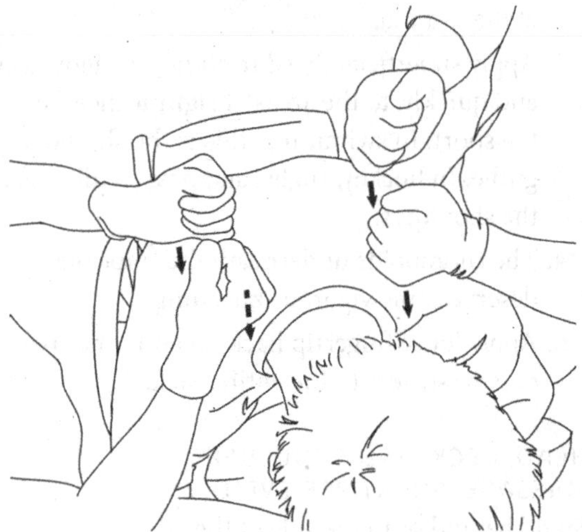

Tandem percussion on the trapezius.

FIGURE 6.11. Short Pre-Event Leg Massage: Quadriceps

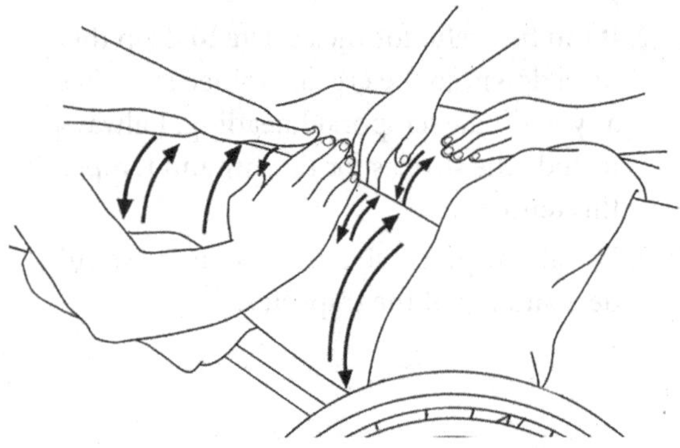

Tandem wringing to the quadriceps.

HIPS, LEGS, FEET MASSAGE: SHORT PRE-EVENT

The quick version of this massage is often done in a variety of stances—for example, standing to the side or crouching in front of the athlete.

Be sure to secure the seatbelt when finished.

1. Lean across the athlete to curl under the hip with fingertip kneading to loosen up the lower back and create stability in the chair, whether the athlete has sensation or not.
2. Massage the hamstring with a fisted upward stroke from the back of the knee to the ischial tuberosity.
3. Apply vigorous wringing to the quadriceps and hamstrings.
4. Do palmar rolling on the lower leg, as you did for the upper arm.
5. Squeeze the feet through the sports shoes, three times.

Longer Warm-Up Massage Routine, Pre-Event

Warm-up massage is important for the lower legs to keep the athlete comfortable in their chair.

Whether they can feel their feet or not, the importance of treating the entire person is neurological in nature. Often the people I have worked with who have a spinal cord injury report being able to feel sensation distant from the nerve interruption. I have always taken the attitude of working the entire length of that nerve route on both legs so there is a neurological balance and to promote connection up into the central nervous system by stimulating all the skin. I figure the cortex of the brain will like it!

I lift the foot onto my leg or elevate the foot in the leg rest to give some room under the thigh, which creates easier access for massaging. I also move the leg to whatever position will give me the best access to the back of it. Sometimes I even rest the athlete's ankle on my shoulder!

HIPS, MASSAGING THREE WAYS: LONGER PRE-EVENT

1. Reach across to the hip. Curl your hand under the hip and perform levered fingertip kneading to the gluteal muscles.
2. On the side closest to you, push the back of your hands down against the wheel of the chair and lever your fingertips up into the hip and gluteal muscles.
3. Squat down in front, lifting the foot onto your thigh. Slide your hands under the leg and up to the hip, and lever your fingertips to massage the ischial tuberosity.

LEG MASSAGE: LONGER PRE-EVENT

1. Wring to the entire thigh. Wrap around to the back of the thigh, engaging the hamstring with the quadriceps from back to front.

FIGURE 6.12. Short Pre-Event Feet Massage

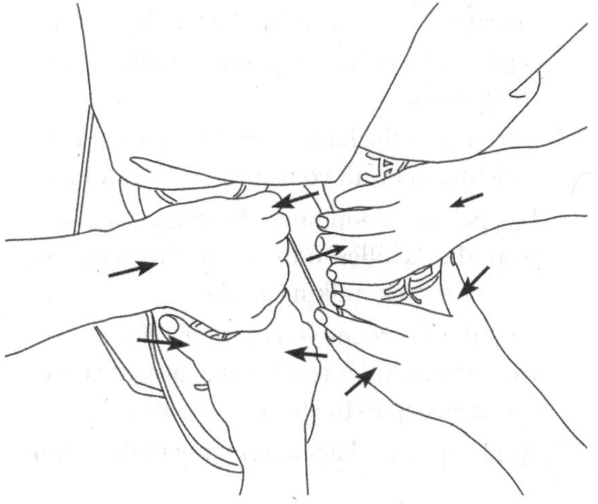

Tandem squeezing.

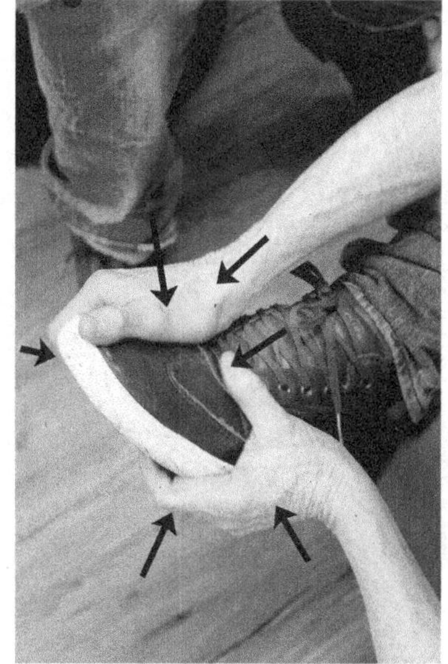

Feet squeezing on Bo.

FIGURE 6.13. Longer Pre-Event Hip Massage: Gluteal Muscles

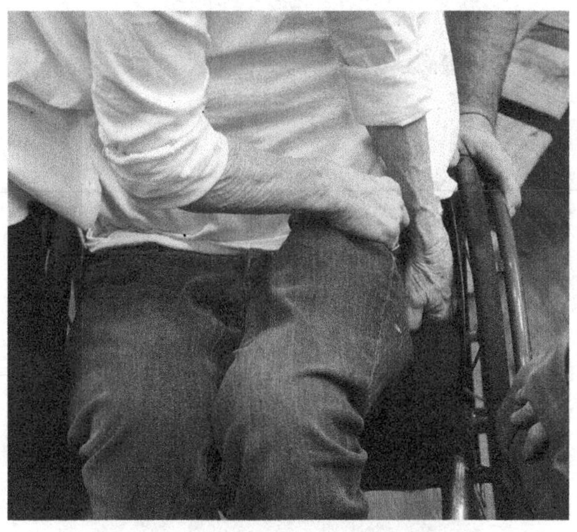

Levered fingertip kneading to the gluteal muscle.

FIGURE 6.14. Longer Pre-Event Hip Massage: Ischial Tuberosity

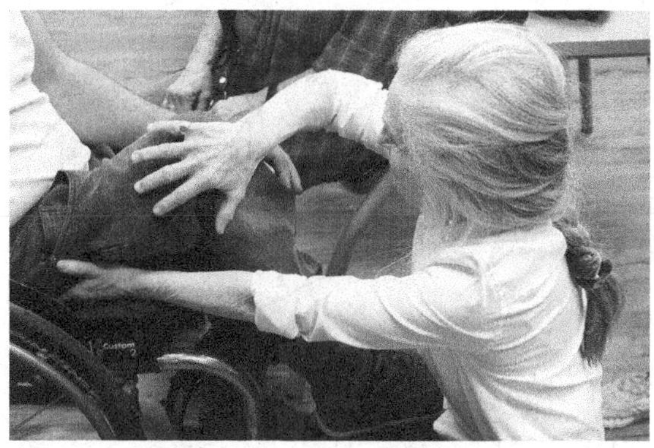

Squat in front of the athlete, put one of their feet on your thigh, and slide your hand under the lifted leg to the hip to provide levered fingertip kneading.

FIGURE 6.15. Longer Pre-Event Kneecap Massage

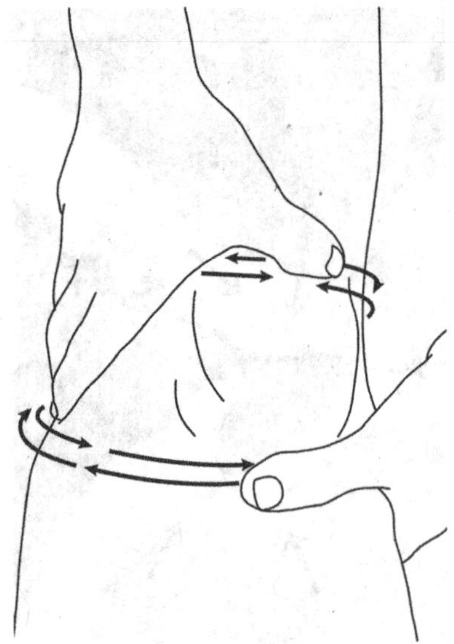

Kneecap massage.

2. Apply alternate thumb kneading to the quads.
3. Use modified wringing and alternate thumb kneading for the patella, then do leg pumping (three types: alternating, simultaneous, rotational).
4. Lifting into the back of the knee, work all the attachments with your fingertip kneading.
5. Use palmar scooping to the gastrocnemius from the Achilles to the back of the knee with an alternating milking stroke.
6. Split the gastrocnemius with the fingertips from the Achilles tendon attachment at the calcaneus up to the back of the knee.
7. Apply open *C*-shaped wringing to the lower leg.
8. Wring the ankle.
9. Apply fingertip kneading to the anklebones/malleoli.
10. Do a thorough foot massage with ankle rotations in both directions.

FIGURE 6.16. Longer Pre-Event Leg Massage

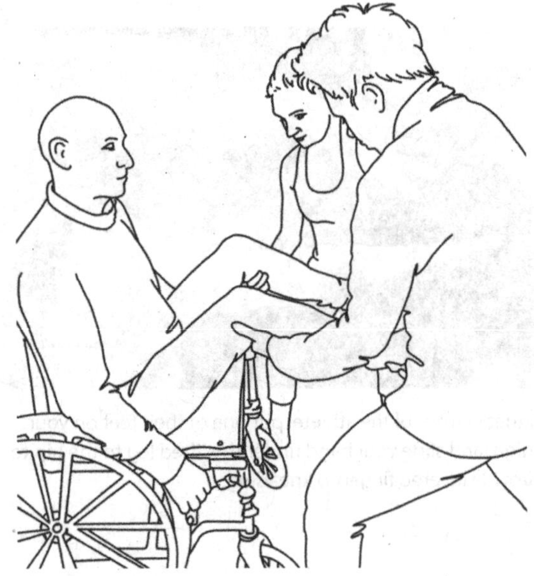

Simultaneous tandem leg pumping.

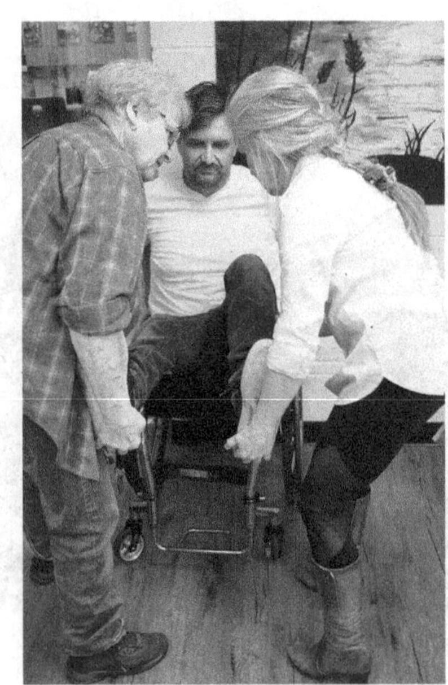

Alternate tandem leg pumping on Bo.

FIGURE 6.17. Longer Pre-Event Gastrocnemius Massage

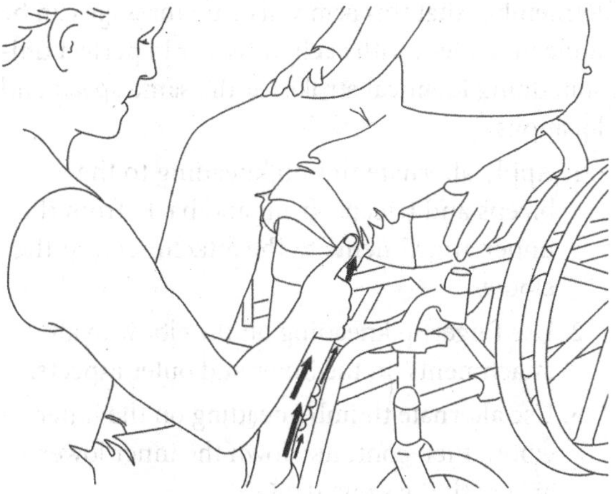

Upward palmar milking of the gastrocnemius.

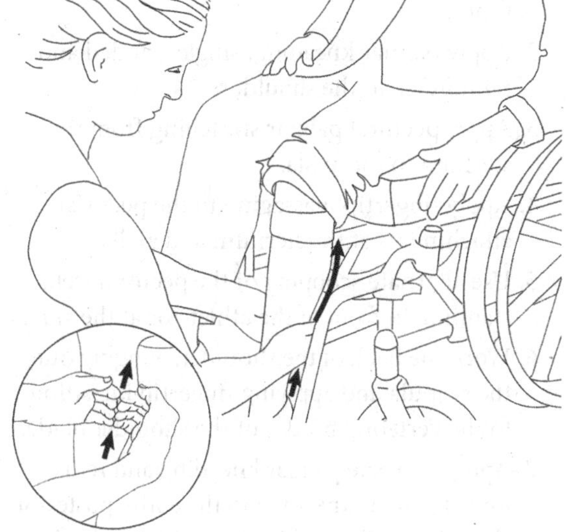

Splitting the gastrocnemius.

FIGURE 6.18. Longer Pre-Event Lower Leg Massage

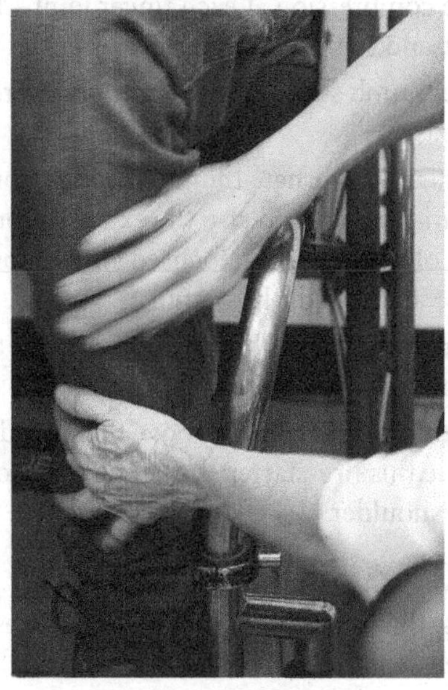

Wringing Bo's lower leg with his leg down.

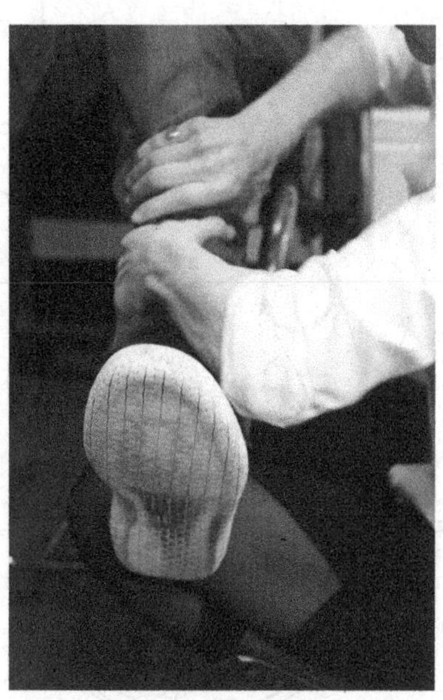

Wringing Bo's lower leg with his leg supported on my knee.

SHOULDER MASSAGE: LONGER PRE-EVENT

1. Use brisk effleurage on the entire arm, three times.
2. Apply palmar kneading, single-handed and reinforced, to the shoulder.
3. Apply pectoral palmar stretching from the sternum to the axilla.
4. Apply fingertip massaging to the pectoral attachments at the sternum and axilla.
5. Use alternate scooping of the pectoral web, standing in front of the athlete or at the side.
6. Work the back of the shoulder, winging out the scapula and applying fingertip kneading to the vertebral border of the shoulder blade.
7. Apply alternate palmar kneading and reinforced palmar kneading to the entire posterior shoulder girdle, pushing from front to back.
8. Have the athlete stretch their entire arm above their head and rub back and forth vigorously from the fingertips to the armpit (like you were starting a fire!).

FIGURE 6.19. **Longer Pre-Event Shoulder Massage**

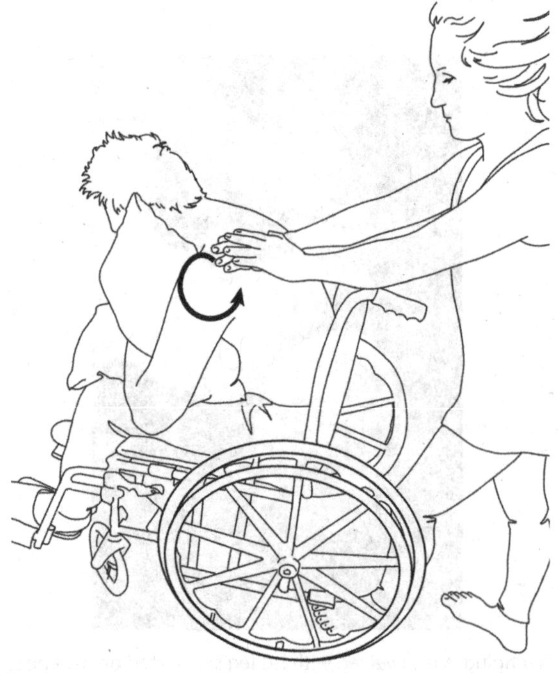

Palmar kneading.

UPPER AND LOWER ARM AND HAND MASSAGE: LONGER PRE-EVENT

Remember that this arm warm-up massage can be done in tandem with each massager in perfect unison, doing identical strokes at the same speed and locations.

1. Apply alternate thumb kneading to the biceps and triceps, front and back, from the upper attachments to the attachments at the elbow.
2. Use fingertip kneading on the elbow to all attachments on the inner and outer aspects.
3. Use alternate thumb kneading on the inner elbow, then continue down the inner lower arm with the same stroke.
4. Finish the forearm with alternate thumb kneading, focusing on the next joint of importance: the wrist. The speed of the arm massage slows down to be thorough for all attachments at the wrist and hand.
5. Apply digital compression to the hand with your thumbs all over the palmar aspect, focusing on the base of the fingers and base of the wrist.
6. Corkscrew each finger at the joints from the base of the finger to the tip.
7. Use compression at each finger joint—laterally, and to the anterior and posterior.
8. Use thumb stretching on each finger from tip to base.
9. Return to alternate thumb kneading for the palmar aspect and also the extensors on the top of the hand. Use focused strokes for the base and web of the thumb.
10. Apply vigorous rubbing between your two hands, like you were starting a fire.
11. With the athlete's arm above their head, continue this fire-starter stroke from the top of the shoulder.

BACK MASSAGE: LONGER PRE-EVENT

If doing this in tandem, each person takes a side and then switches over halfway.

1. Apply effleurage up and down the back with palmar pressure, switching during the stroke

FIGURE 6.20. **Longer Pre-Event Forearm Massage**

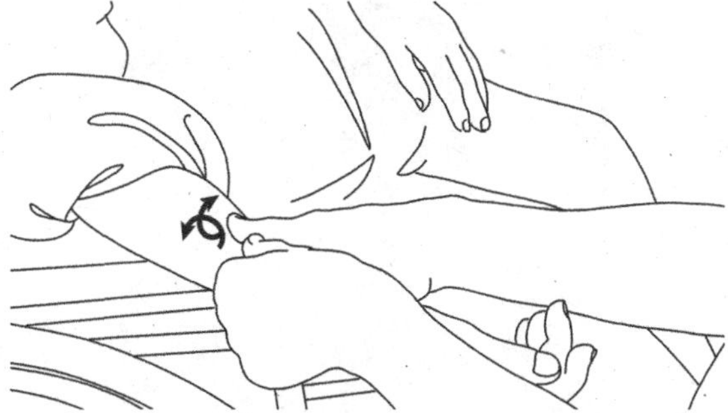

Alternate thumb kneading, forearm.

FIGURE 6.21. **Longer Pre-Event Massage to Back of the Hands**

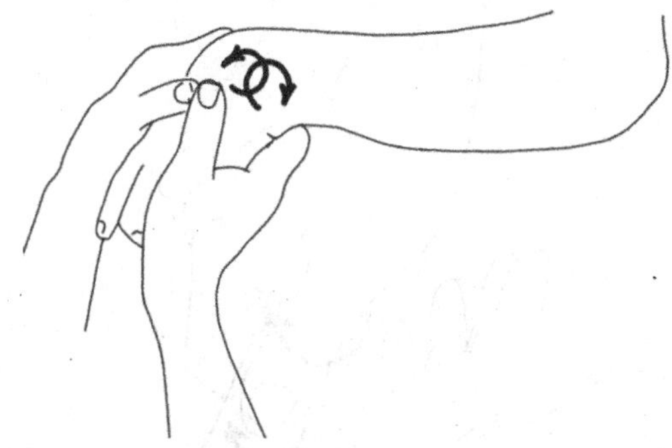

Alternate thumb kneading to the back of the hand.

FIGURE 6.22. **Longer Pre-Event Fingers Massage: Corkscrewing**

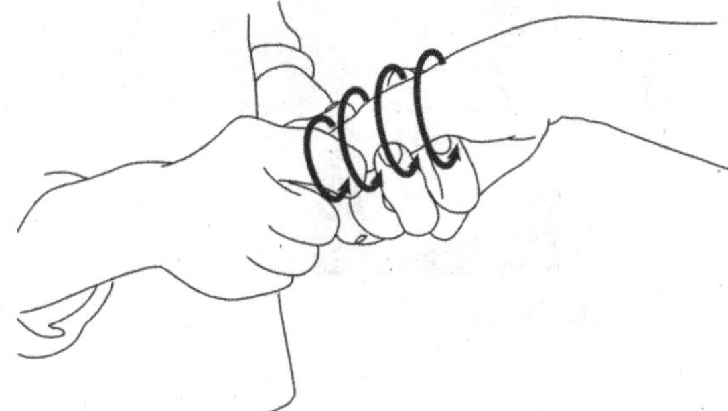

Finger corkscrewing.

FIGURE 6.23. **Longer Pre-Event Fingers Massage: Digital Compression**

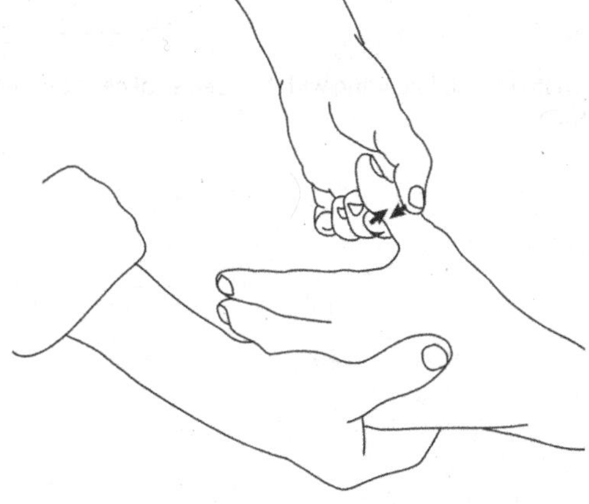

Digital compression to the joints.

FIGURE 6.24. **Longer Pre-Event Fingers Massage: Thumb Stretching**

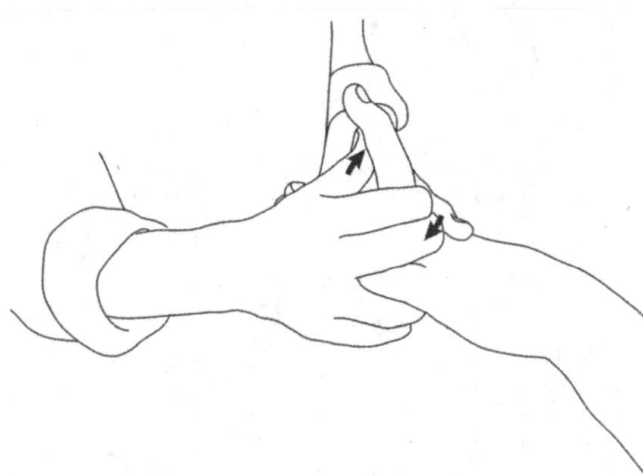

Thumb stretching, finger.

FIGURE 6.25. Longer Pre-Event Hand Massage

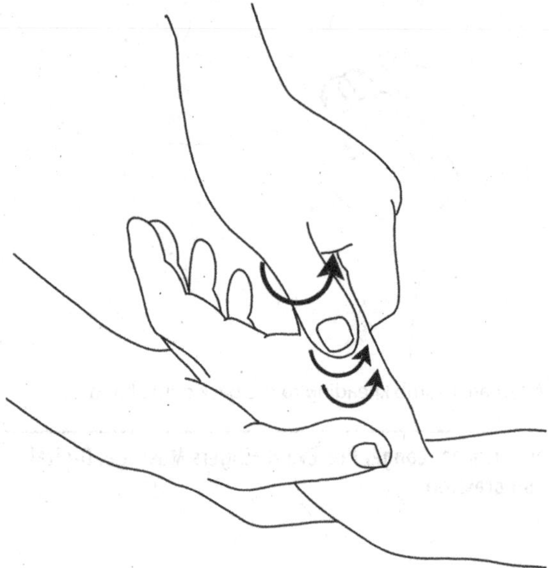

Alternate thumb kneading with focused strokes at the base of the thumb.

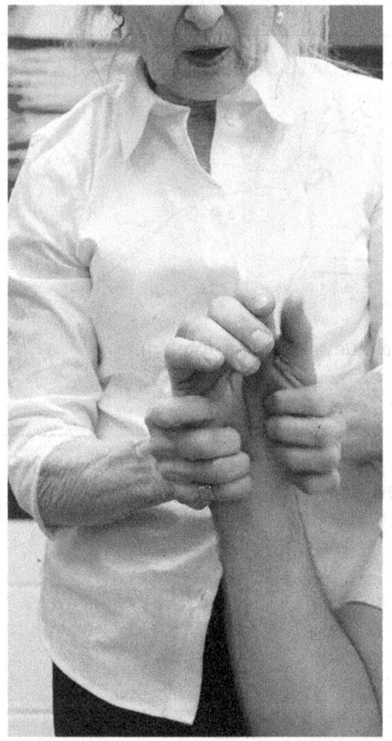

Working on Bo's hand.

FIGURE 6.26. Longer Pre-Event Back Massage: Tandem Bilateral Wringing

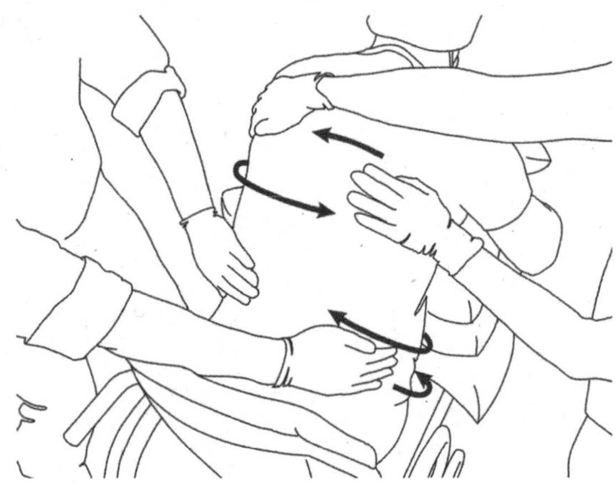

FIGURE 6.27. Longer Pre-Event Back Massage: Tandem Scapular Lifting

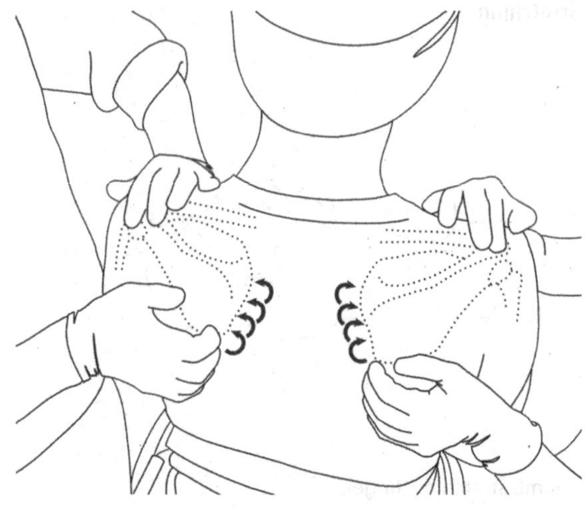

or repeating the entire sequence when finished the first sequence.

2. Wring the back, with the massagers facing each other, alternating where they put their hands.
3. Apply reinforced palmar kneading, with the massagers starting on one side and switching to the other.
4. Repeat steps 1, 2, and 3.
5. Work the rhomboids in the shoulder by placing a supportive hand on the front of the shoulder and applying fisted frictioning to the space between the shoulder blade and the spine with the other hand. Alternate fingertip kneading with fisted kneading.
6. Pull back the hand supporting the shoulder to lift the scapula and then slide the thumb or the side of the hands up underneath the shoulder blade as it wings outward.
7. Smooth out with overhanded palmar strokes over the massaged shoulder area.
8. Stand to the side of the athlete and work the pectorals with overhanded palmar pulling from the sternum to the upper arm.
9. Apply rib raking from the sternum outward, following the angle of the ribs below the clavicle to the arm. Continue the rib raking in an overhanded style down in the diagonal toward the waist. With women, adapt to going around the breast. Do above the breast and below the breast.
10. Apply single-handed fingertip kneading with one hand supporting the shoulder while the front hand massages the pectoral attachments at the sternum.
11. Apply fingertip kneading inferior to the clavicle.
12. Apply intermittent deep palmar stroking, continuing to stretch the pectorals.
13. Use fingertip stretching under the lower border of the pectoralis major and minor, from the lateral border at the chest out to the attachment at the upper arm. Do this with two hands, or with one hand, or overhanded. Stand slightly behind the shoulder of the athlete, facing forward.
14. Standing to the side of the wheelchair with a stride position, face the wheelchair athlete and finish with continuous overhanded palmer kneading from the shoulder, moving from the front up and around to the glenohumeral shoulder joint, including the glenoclavicular.

NECK, FACE, SCALP MASSAGE: LONGER PRE-EVENT

Finish with this routine.

If working in tandem, face each other, each with one hand on the athlete's forehead and the other scooping the athlete's neck. You can fit two massagers' hands on the forehead by layering them or placing one higher than the other. The percussive movements are the light fingertip and stiff fingertip hacking to the upper trapezius, changing to cupping, then beating, then pounding, and back to hacking. It is possible for both massagers to do the scalp scrub, which can split the time or double the strokes.

Sometimes I do a mini-massage to the athlete's temporal mandibular joint (the jaw) with fingertip kneading to ease tension the athlete may be holding in the jaw. They don't realize they're wasting their precious energy by holding tension here. Finish with a vigorous scalp massage using a shampoo stroke for ten to twenty seconds. Perform this massage is as close to the athlete's individual or team warm-up routine as possible.

Intra-Competition Wheelchair Sports Massage

This is the shortest wheelchair sports massage sequence. This massage is performed at the edge of the playing field, beside the ice rink, in the dressing room, or at the side of the pool.

This is a massage that can be performed by team players among themselves or by their massage therapists. It can be a three-to-five-minute massage or a fifteen-to-twenty-minute massage. The number of therapists working the intermission or breaks determines the length of time that you can spend with your athlete. This massage helps to restore and reinvigorate the muscles and supply energy to the athlete through the hands-on significance of touch.

Intra-competition massage has proven benefits, as noted in the journal of the American Massage Therapy Association:

> In a study including 11 female high intensity cycle sprinters, some women passively rested in between sprints, and some received a ten-minute massage in between sprints. Performance recovery was significantly better in the massage group.
>
> These massages are typically short, lasting between a few minutes to 15 minutes. The duration usually depends on how many muscle groups need to be worked on, says Felix Patterson LMT, with experience as a massage therapist on the United States Olympic Sports Medicine Team at the US Olympics training facility in Colorado Springs, Colorado.[3]

Intra-competition massage is also instrumental in tracking or preventing injury. However, if you find unusual pain symptoms or extreme tightness and spasming while massaging an athlete, call the doctor to investigate.

Often in non-Olympic venues, families or friends can participate in the massage and help move things along so everyone has the hands-on help for winning without injury. With swimmers, for example, you can find them waiting in the marshaling areas for the next race for often up to fifteen minutes or more. They will continue to be in this area throughout the competition, providing the ideal situation for hands-on help.

Don't forget to use any opportunity to teach family and friends how to massage their athletes! The winter games in northern British Columbia were a perfect example of this kind of opportunity. Every hour, I was teaching a different group. This was my idea of heaven. By the time the event was over, more than twenty young people knew how to massage their wheelchair athletes across a wide variety of indoor sports. Members of all teams were massaged in between-game breaks.

Although the actual massage strokes you'll be performing are the same as in the longer warm-up routine, you'll do them in a different order. Ask the athlete where their needs are greatest, or you can simply follow the sequence I use:

1. Hands (going against the uncorking the bottle principle)
2. Forearms
3. Upper arms
4. Shoulders
5. Front and back

Post-Event Wheelchair Sports Massage

The massage that gives the best recovery is between one hour and twenty-four hours after the event or competition.

This massage helps "milk" out the lactic acid and prevent muscle shortening for the next event. Post-event massage simply speeds up muscle recovery. The principles of moving the blood up the extremities, in both the arms and legs, is important, as this is a relatively superficial massage without any deep movements like cross-fiber frictioning.

Recovery massages are even more significant if the team is on a winning streak. You need quick recovery and peak performance every game. Working with a winning team is a blur of post-event massages to prevent further wear and tear, increase the reabsorption of waste products, and assist with the removal of lactic acid. Decreasing muscle fatigue and tension is important for long-term or short-term recovery through massage.

Don't use any stretching strokes or deep connective tissue massage in this phase of massage for wheeling athletes. I only do that further along in time, outside of the twenty-four hours after competition.

This post-performance massage is meant to be soothing, relaxing, and timely. I use a full hour for this massage and include all body parts for a thorough treatment and fast recovery. When possible, I use Epsom salt baths and body wraps and medicated oils. I use carminative oils to let the stimulation of the circulation keep working after the massage. The muscles are humming long after I have finished the full body massage with the perfume of peppermint or eucalyptus oil.

Remember, this full body massage can be in the wheelchair or in bed, or on the massage table. You can even rotate through all three venues.

1. Apply full body effleurage. Do the arms first. Lean forward to gain access to the back. Work the lower back up to the shoulders and the sides. For the front chest, starting at the sternum, effleurage out following the pectoral muscles up and over the trapezius, around to the back, and over the deltoid; then return to the start. Make this a continuous movement always with the palms.
2. Wring all the extremities. Use alternate thumb kneading, and then more kneading. Use effleurage to finish. No deep work is done within twenty-four hours of competition. Frictioning might damage overexerted muscles. The most important focus is milking the muscles, aiding in recovery of lactic acid spent in exertion.

Recovery and Maintenance Wheelchair Sports Massage

In 2018, three researchers published a study on the benefits of massage therapy for a team of elite paracyclists.[4] They found that paracyclists who received massage therapy had significant improvement in sleep and muscle elasticity, and quicker recovery while in training. The study also highlighted the reality that at no time is an elite athlete not in training. This fifth stage of massage for maintenance is more of a lifestyle massage since athletes are always in training!

In addition, the study drew attention to the problem of consistency with massage when teams are traveling, which highlights my enthusiasm for teaching entire teams, including coaches and bus drivers, to apply the needed massage therapy no matter the venue. I have performed many massages for teams in airports! Most recently, I ran into the USA Wheelchair Rugby team in a huge airport and gave an instant sports massage workshop to all the men in the waiting area during the New Year's rush.

The maintenance phase of wheelchair sports massage includes the breaking down of adhesions in muscles that have become shortened or injured. The ongoing nature of this part of the sports massage program is the steady input of weekly massages. You can use the basic techniques outlined in chapter 2, either in the chair or out of the chair.

Wheelchair athletes are in much greater need of massage therapy than any other athletes in the sports massage world. These are athletes who are already working to peak performance in daily living. They need massage therapy on a daily basis simply to navigate the world and all its variables from a wheelchair.

VIDEO LIBRARY

Visit brusheducation.ca/wheeling-in-good-hands to watch these videos:

Massaging wheelchair athletes: Back, shoulder, and arm massage with Bo Hedges of Team Canada

Massaging wheelchair athletes: Longer pre-event massage – accessing the hips, three ways

Massaging wheelchair athletes: Longer pre-event massage – teaching Velate how to access the hips, three ways

Massaging wheelchair athletes: Leg pumping with lower leg massage

Massaging wheelchair athletes: Face massage – fingertip kneading to the temples and jaw

Intra-competitional massage opportunities: BC Winter Games – Fort St. John

Inara

Inara was three years old when she managed to break her leg in 2021. The break meant she could only lie down and sit. Her grandmother's tiny antique wheelchair happened to be in the barn on their farm in Salmo, British Columbia. She took to the wheelchair like a duck to water. Inara had instant confidence in wheeling around her home. She learned all the maneuvers to get to where she wanted to go, to be mobile, and to play. She could maneuver that chair with her little brother riding shotgun, sometimes standing behind her, always reaching out in every direction. The wheelchair provided Inara with a way of getting around her home until she recovered.

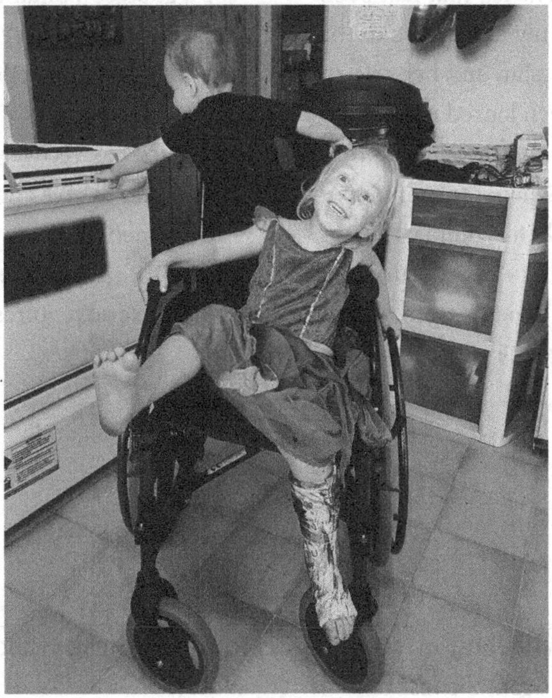

Inara.

Inara's parents, Darren and Fallon, had been my maternity massage couple. Inara had been my assistant, learning to massage her pregnant mom's tummy. When Darren's back was sore, Inara and I had also massaged him. She loved melting coconut oil on his back; it reminded me of the power of family tactility. In fact, Inara had been part of massage even before she was born. I had massaged Fallon when she was pregnant with Inara.

Now, her parents became my massage team for Inara, in and out of the chair. Until Inara's accident, I didn't think I would be able to include someone so young in my massage teaching. I am always excited to learn new things so I can pass on new skills. Darren, Fallon, and Inara, who had perfected the family massage techniques I taught them, also invented some new ones.

For Inara, a key invention was the chest-to-chest position for massage, with the parent lying on their back and the child lying on the parent's chest. Most parents have held their children chest to chest at some point to help with discomfort—a classic, soothing, hugging embrace. Before Inara landed in the wheelchair, she would often lie on her father's chest as I massaged him (face-up) and he, at the same time, massaged her back. Massaging Inara's back was the finale for

Darren's full body massage—the massage sandwich! Inara had helped throughout the hour-long massage with her tandem-massage attentiveness. She was the controller of the heating pad and applier of the massage oil. During her recovery in the chair, Darren continued to use this chest-to-chest position to offer comfort. The "massage sandwich" has become an established family tradition.

Darren and Fallon massaged Inara in and out of the wheelchair. She had an issue because of the way the cast had been set where lifting her toes caused discomfort in the shin. She was also hesitant to walk once the cast was off. The leg that had been broken had atrophied after only four weeks in the cast. So, they worked on her shin and her calf, to relax the muscles that had been locked up.

Inara's parents also dealt with the classic problem of unilateral strain, where an uninjured extremity does all the work to compensate for an injured one. Sometimes injuries and surgeries result in nerve damage that benefits from wheelchair use and tandem massaging. I recommend the same tandem-team massage techniques in these situations as I do for greater neurological problems (stroke recovery, for example): two people working together to mirror their massage strokes with exactly the same timing, rhythm, and location.

Inara's case was a classic example of short-term wheelchair use. Everyone should have a chair in the barn, just in case! And everyone should have a massage team like she had with Darren and Fallon! The massages Inara received as part of her recovery were a continuation of a family massage tradition that started early in her life. Inara's case reminded me that wheelchairs and massage can be a good combination. A family that can massage together and wheel together—whether pushing, being pushed, or climbing onboard to play—can get better faster.

Inara has recovered and is cast-free now. She continues to give and get massages. Massage therapy helped her with a speedy recovery, and it will ensure a speedier recovery in any mishaps from her future adventures.

VIDEO LIBRARY

Visit brusheducation.ca/wheeling-in-good-hands to watch these videos:

Story of Inara: Darren's horizontal chest-to-chest back massage

7

Stroke Recovery Wheelers

I teach short-term wheelchair use scenarios in my massage classes. Stroke recovery is a common reason for short-term wheelchair use. A person recovering from a stroke may be in a chair for as little as a few months, or their time in the chair may surpass a year. My experience with stroke recovery patients over the past fifty years has shown me that this condition is variable, but whatever the severity or length of time, massage can help in a variety of ways.

According to Jo Murch, a massage therapist and reflexologist based in the United Kingdom who specializes in massage for stroke recovery, "massage therapy can...help to boost circulation, which is often lacking when a body part cannot be moved. Massage encourages fresh oxygen and blood to that area of the body, removing toxins, and in time increasing mobility. It can also help to relax stroke patients, which can in turn lead to more restful sleep."[5]

My father suffered a stroke a few years into my career as a professional massage therapist. Previously a large, athletic man, he was now blind in one eye, unable to drive his car or steer his sailboat. The stroke had no other obvious impact, except for his vision. We were able to fly to Vancouver for tests because of wheelchairs. We had wheeling experiences from Nelson to Vancouver at airports and hospitals. He was weak and emotionally stressed, and the wheelchair made our life easy. Once recovered, he was able to sail again and won numerous races for almost twenty years after the stroke.

I had other opportunities to give my father massages while he was using a wheelchair for short-term conditions. After the stroke, my dad was back in a wheelchair twice after cancer surgery and again for a broken hip a few months before he passed away. I would massage him before getting in the chair and again at the end of the day, once he was out of the chair. The most important parts of the massage were always his back and legs. This was also tactile, positive reinforcement for him to use the chair instead of trying to struggle to stand.

In addition to the physical benefits of massage for stroke recovery patients, there are notable emotional benefits. Stroke patients are in the particularly difficult position of losing so much of their mobility at once, in a sudden and traumatic way. The emotional toll can be staggering. A 2016 study indicated that touch and massage "has been proven to decrease anxiety and pain and improve quality of health in conditions of reduced health." It also found evidence of improvements in quality of life after a stroke including "increased neural activity in brain regions associated with feelings of pleasure and emotional regulation."[6]

The greatest lesson for wheelchair massage during stroke recovery is to use tandem massage or double tandem massage.

The reason is that tandem massage stimulates both sides of the body at the same time. A coordinated tandem massage team provides perfectly balanced stimulation, where the tandem partners mirror each other's every stroke. Neurologically, it is very important for the affected side to be handled exactly like the unaffected side for stroke patients. I am emphatic about the team maintaining exactly the same pressure, rhythm, and placement of the strokes, so they match each other. This way, the

FIGURE 7.1. Double Tandem Massage

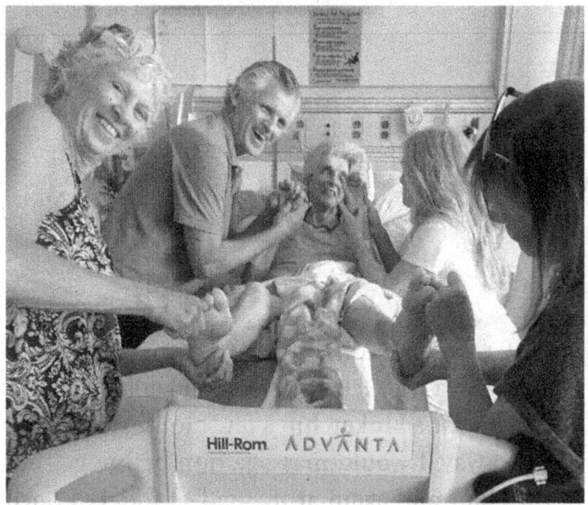

Two massagers work on the arms and two on the legs. The patient here is Doady Patton, who is featured in this chapter.

brain has an opportunity to have a conversation on a neurological level—so that one foot can talk to the other, so that one leg can talk to the other.

Years ago, I was conducting a student clinic at the Sutherland-Chan School and Teaching Clinic in Toronto with a focus on neurological conditions (stroke recovery included). I had a patient who, during their massage, asked why the arm that we were not massaging responded to touch on the opposite arm. I asked the patient to be more specific. He described sensations in his paralyzed arm—weird tingling—as though it were being touched. In other words, the arm that was neurologically impaired and paralyzed was experiencing sensation, stimulated by the massage we doing on the "good" arm. As he talked about this unusual tactile experience, I was forever changed. This time, I was the one who was taught. I learned something brand new about tandem massage.

Since then, I have advocated tandem stimulation in all the ways that the skin can sense, including tandem dry brushing (texture), tandem ice

FIGURE 7.2. Examples of Tandem Massage

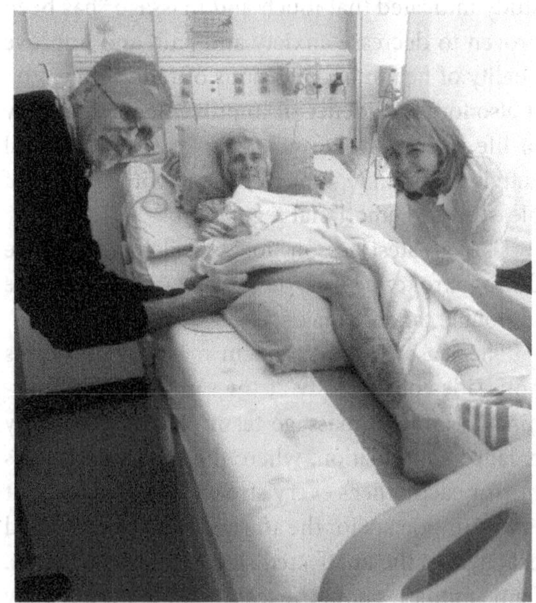

Doady receives tandem levered massage from her team.

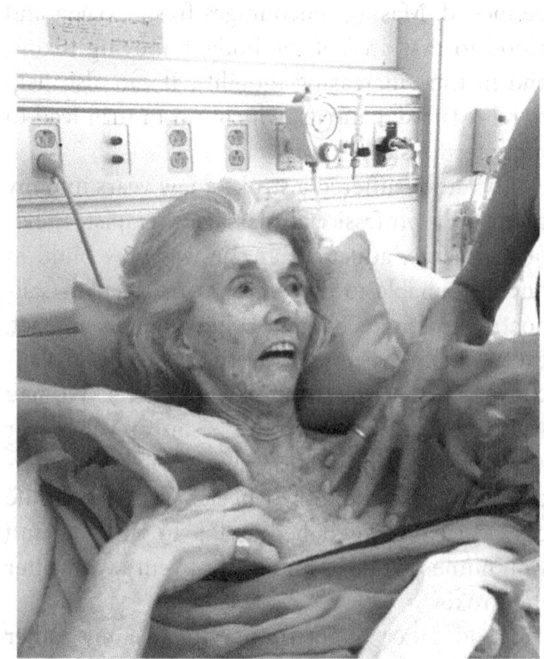

Tandem respiratory massage for Doady.

FIGURE 7.2. CONTINUED

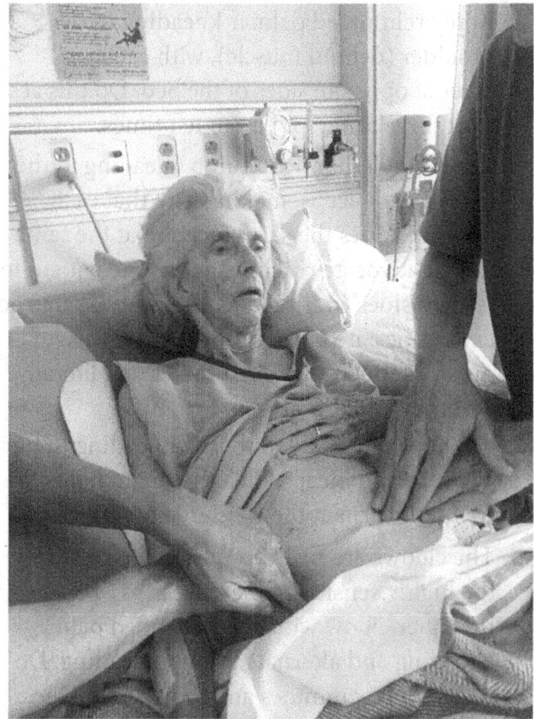

Tandem digestive massage for Doady.

massage (temperature), tandem light reflex (pressure), and other kinds of stimulation (tandem pinching, scratching, and so on, to activate pain and other kinds of skin receptors).

Doady Patton is one of my favorite short-term-wheelchar-user success stories. In 2016, Doady was hospitalized after suffering a stroke. I taught her kids, who were all in their sixties, and other members of her family to massage her. For the entire time Doady was in hospital, her family massaged her every day, often three or four times a day—and, day by day, Doady came back to life from a comatose and nonverbal state.

The first time I massaged Doady, she could only blink. By the second massage, she made a sound that was like laughing, and forced a smile to go with it. I ran up and down the hospital corridors telling everyone that she made a noise. That was a hands-on miracle.

I taught Doady's family the basics of massaging a totally immobilized patient using a levering massage technique, lifting underneath as she lay on her back. We did this in tandem.

While she lay in bed, we performed massage for the respiratory and digestive systems, again as tandem teams.

We then turned her on her side for a traditional massage of her back. After that, we transferred her to her wheelchair with a hydraulic hoist and massaged her next to her bed in the wheelchair.

We also massaged her in her wheelchair outside the hospital in the garden. The pairing of a serene natural environment with the benefits of massage worked wonders for this stroke patient.

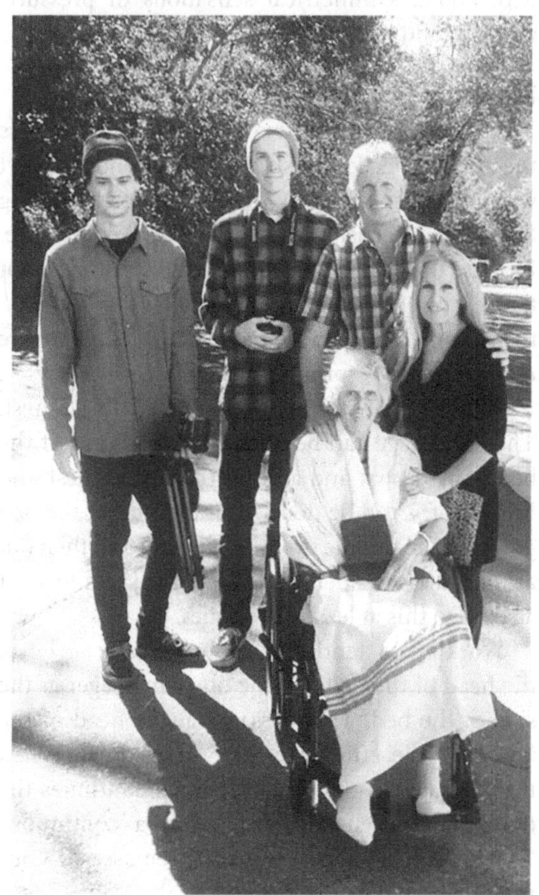

Doady loved a massage outside.

This committed family kept massaging alongside me. We even had a young friend, Erin, who lived near the hospital, volunteer to massage Doady every day.

Tandem Massage for Stroke Recovery

Much of this routine is familiar, because it follows the basic routine of full body massage in chapter 3. Here, however, I am refocusing aspects of the basic routine to describe tandem massage, which is so crucial to stroke recovery.

Tandem team members should switch sides during the massage. This ensures that the body receives balanced, contrasting stimulation at the same time, because no two people have exactly the same touch. This way, the person receiving the massage is not "lopsided" with one person's touch or pressure. You want the body to feel both sides with equal, symmetrical sensations of pressure, warmth, and texture of touch.

Tandem Respiratory Massage

The massage team of two face each other across the upper aspect of the stroke person's thorax. Start with general respiratory massage strokes, making the person accustomed to the double exposure. Because the thorax takes up two-thirds of the front trunk of the body, I like to put a hot water bottle on the abdomen to keep the patient cozy while we are massaging the respiratory system.

Apply a mini- or split-effleurage to the chest. This effleurage can be done from the head of the bed going down and around the entire chest and thorax, or it can be done from the side of the bed going up the middle over the sternum and then out around the shoulders and down the sides to start again. Do this at least three times.

Working in tandem, one massager can be at the head of the bed and the other massager at the side of the bed. The massager at the head of the bed does the effleurage first, going down. Then the massager at the side of the bed continues the downward effleurage. They form a continuous "conveyor belt" of effleurage: one massager continues where the other leaves off.

Tandem Arm and Hand Massage

1. Effleurage in tandem, starting at the fingertips, with the patient's arms lying beside them and straight. Go up the arms to the shoulders at the same time. Wrap around to the back and glide down to the hand without pressure. Do this three times and then switch sides.
2. Apply reinforced palmar kneading to the shoulder (deltoid muscle), with each massager at opposite sides of the bed. Do this at least three times and up to ten times.
3. Apply single-handed thumb kneading to the triceps and biceps, making sure that each massager does the same location at the same time. I advocate reaching across the patient to "switch sides" during massage routines for the extremities: it's a quick way to provide symmetry of touch (but don't forget that literally switching sides is also important).
   - With single-handed thumb kneading to the triceps and biceps, the other hand holds the patient's arm at the wrist or elbow.
4. The elbows are really important because of the highly sensitive inner forearm. Massage the inner elbow with single-handed palm kneading and alternate thumb kneading. Do this for a few minutes and then switch sides. The outside aspect of the elbow (the olecranon process—that bony bump that sticks out) has important muscular attachments. I use fingertip kneading with my pointer and middle finger combined and single-handed thumb kneading to work around that bony prominence.
5. Use single-handed thumb kneading and alternate thumb kneading on the inner aspect of the forearm. Keep the patient's elbows bent so that the muscles have some elasticity. Each massager uses one thumb on the outside and one thumb on the inside of each forearm, switching hands as they work. Then they turn the forearms over to do the same on the outer aspect of the arms. Remember to keep the pressure toward the heart. Work from the elbow to the wrist and back to the elbow again. Do the entire forearm and the switch sides, or switch sides after the inner forearm, and again after the outer forearm.
6. Bend the wrists to access their many bones, muscles, ligaments, and attachments. Use

alternate thumb kneading on the top of each flexed wrist. Move under the wrists, and extend the hands to gain access to the wrists at the base of the hands. I usually work against the principle of pressure toward the heart if the patient's elbows are bent.

Tandem Digestive Massage

It is important to include the digestive massage as part of the full body massage in stroke recovery, as it has such a strong neurological impact on the whole body, as it is a highly sensitive area in the body's neurological system.

The tandem team faces each other across the patient's abdomen, one on each side of the patient's bed. The digestive massage focuses on a tiny area and requires coordination similar to dancing.

1. Start with mini-effleurage, where each massager takes turns, and repeat three times.
2. Apply bilateral wringing, where one massager wrings the upper aspect just below the diaphragm and the costal angle, while the other massager wrings the lower aspect, which includes the area of the bladder. Switch halfway through the wringing, so that the massager working on the upper aspect now works the lower aspect, and vice versa.
3. Apply overhanded palmar kneading.
   A. Start by taking turns: first one massager, then the other.
   B. Then coordinate to knead simultaneously, where one massager starts the circles and the other follows, so there are four hands on the abdomen at the same time.
   C. Finish by taking turns again.
4. Use fingertip kneading, especially on the corners of the large intestine (flexures) if the person is having a digestive complaint like constipation.
   A. Apply reinforced fingertip kneading in turns, where one massager does a complete circle of the large intestine, followed by the other massager.
   B. Apply single-handed fingertip kneading in turns. Each massager rests one hand on the side of the patient while the other hand travels along the length of the large intestine, slowing down at each flexure.

Perform the massage in step 4 for two to three minutes. As one massager finishes, the other starts, so that the patient experiences a continuous sensation. I usually start at the junction of the small and large intestine, which is always on the patient's right-hand side where the appendix is located. I always end on the opposite side on the bottom of the descending colon, then glide across the bottom where the bladder is located in the middle to start again at the junction of the small and large intestine on the right-hand side.

I recommend going back through the strokes of the abdominal massage, repeating them in opposite order (steps 4, 3, 2, 1). This accomplishes one of my basic principles of massage: work from general to specific, and then back to general. Using this principle, the tandem team finishes with a

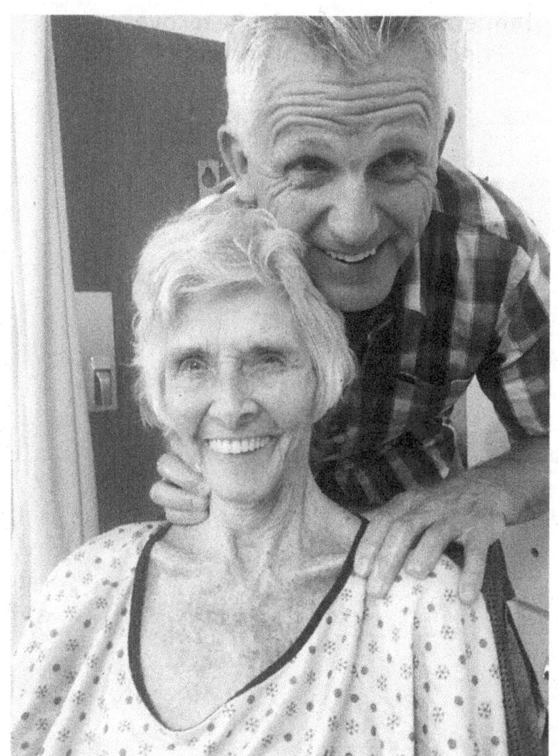

Doady and Greg

very light, neurologically stimulating and systemically soothing light reflex stroke.

Doady's Recovery

Doady's team was the best stroke recovery team I ever worked with! They were not residents of Nelson; they were scattered across western Canada, but they all came to help massage their mom back to complete recovery.

Nine months after her stroke, Doady was dancing. When I taught my next wheelchair massage class and came to the part about short-term wheelchair users, we Zoomed with Doady's family, who were by then with their mom in Edmonton, Alberta. Doady shared her first-hand experience of how massage helped her. When she danced in front of our eyes, I would never have believed that she was once immobilized, with feet that never looked like they would dance again. Her family celebrated ninety-seven years of loving their mother.

Thank you, Greg, and your entire massage team.

VIDEO LIBRARY

Visit brusheducation.ca/wheeling-in-good-hands to watch these videos:

- **Stroke recovery massage:** Double tandem massage with Doady
- **Tandem massage for stroke recovery:** Principles of tandem and double tandem
- **Tandem massage for stroke recovery:** Tandem arm massage with Doady
- **Tandem massage for stroke recovery:** Bilateral fingertip kneading to the back and neck – levering against the chair

Patient Story

Mary-Jo and Molly

Mary-Jo Fetterly and Molly Hale changed the course of my teaching for spinal cord injury massage. They invited me into their worlds of wheeling at very different stages of their recoveries.

Mary-Jo Fetterly was a moving force in Nelson's yoga community. She cultivated a population of yoga enthusiasts, especially introducing "mountain men" and "mountain boys" to her instructor-training program. We now had mountaineering males teaching yoga, all thanks to Mary-Jo.

Beyond her teaching and training talents, she was a well-respected mother, executive chef, entrepreneur, community health and healing activist, and self-made woman. I was very lucky to be under her influence in yoga, and was impressed with her organizational skills. Mary-Jo was an all-round athlete, whether she was skiing, swimming, or levitating. She gave yoga a glamorous look.

In the winter of 2004, Mary-Jo had a skiing accident on our ski hill and became instantly paralyzed. The fact that she survived this accident was in itself miraculous. She was diagnosed with the worst possible spinal cord injury on the American Spinal Injury Association (ASIA) impairment scale, which was A (complete). She compared her transitional experience on the hill that day to an out-of-body experience she had in her youth when she was in a three-day coma after falling from a three-story building.

In the hospital, after fourteen hours of surgery, she was lying on a gurney with her children nearby. She desperately wanted the tracheotomy tube removed so that she could speak to them, to comfort them and reassure them of her presence. Her daughters heard her whispers as she struggled to speak, and asked the orderly what was happening, to which he blithely replied, "Oh. That? That's nothing, just noises she's sort of making. She's not going to be much more than a vegetable for the rest of her life. I wouldn't pay it any attention."

This infuriated Mary-Jo, but she was able to gather the energy necessary to get the tube removed, just so she could tell the orderly to "fuck off." Even at that moment she could feel the vital electrical impulses that signaled the possibility for her future.

Throughout Mary-Jo's recovery, in the hospital with her daughters and in her aftercare with her team, massage became the single most enduring factor. I was thrilled to teach my wheelchair massage to anybody and everybody who was hands-on with Mary-Jo. She had a team of caregivers that came early in the morning and late at night, all with an aptitude for hands-on skills like massage therapy. Mary-Jo's success in ICU and with spinal cord traction was in part due to her daughters, who took specific direction and massaged underneath her when she couldn't be moved or be turned, thereby avoiding any possible pressure sores.

In the next few years, I continued to follow Mary-Jo's progress, teaching new people to massage her. Her water therapy was unusual, groundbreaking, and, to this day, still the most profound filming I have ever done. Her career previous to her accident was all about breath control in her yoga teaching practice, and now she was applying breath control underwater. Mary-Jo performed her own version of aqua mobility, fluid and graceful like her yoga had been, unlike anything I'd ever seen. My close-up lens was able to capture the significance of her breathing: tiny bubbles from her nose following her swirling body as her therapist carefully directed lateral stretching movements. People with high-level spinal cord injury, like Mary-Jo, cannot easily bend the trunk of their body. The water allows side-to-side stretching that helps prevent lateral contractions, which restrict shoulder mobility.

Mary-Jo's resilience continues to have a positive influence on people experiencing any challenge in life—in wheelchairs or beyond wheelchairs.

In the short film we made, called *Mountains to Climb*, Mary-Jo shares this wisdom: "When you're faced with that challenge of having to redeem and also to understand your soul from a place that's unlimited, that's everlasting, that's ephemeral, you begin to take on life in a different way and you don't waste time on petty things. You hopefully are able to bring yourself to a place where you understand that love is the most important thing that exists here, and above all, that staying attuned to that is the best possible remedy for anything."

Through Mary-Jo, I was introduced to Molly Hale from the United States.

Molly was an athlete and architect, enjoying the good life in her new fairy-tale marriage, when her car accident occurred. Before the accident, she practiced the martial art of aikido at the black belt level. After her accident, Molly used water therapy as well as meditation and breathing techniques to help her recover. She later competed for and attained her third degree black belt rank in aikido, and she has also had the honor of being a torchbearer for the Olympics.

Both women are strong advocates of daily massage from friends, family, and professional caregivers. They found it challenging and rewarding to teach their teams to be more investigative in the areas of their bodies most affected by their distinctly different conditions. Filming these women, as they worked through the underwater therapy they had designed, as they demonstrated the endless possibilities for maintaining and mobilizing the body, was an opportunity for me to show others what they could do for themselves.

For Molly, it turns out that horseback riding is a very powerful therapy. Riding a horse moves and stimulates the entire pelvis in ways human-powered massage therapy simply cannot. It loosens her hips, helping establish and strengthen the energetic connections between her legs and torso. A horse's movement is uniquely suited to this task, and Molly was the first person in California to articulate this to the medical community and insurance authorities in a way that convinced them to pay for what is known as "hippotherapy."

For years, on Wednesday nights, after horseback riding, Molly had a dinner and massage-work evening with two friends, Patrick McKenna and Jerry Stolaroff. They worked weekly with her until she moved out of the big city to the foothills of the Sierras and a small community called Penn Valley. Jerry comes to visit and massage Molly on occasion, as she continues her hour-long pool workouts three to five days a week. "That gives me a lot of hydrostatic massage, which is hugely beneficial," she says. She also gets a two-hour body work session with her daughter every month and intermittently during the week. Molly's husband,

Jeramy, is the best wheeling, hands-on husband I have met. He has been Molly's underwater dancing partner, gently and firmly guiding her as her feet lift off the pool floor.

Practically every visitor to the house became part of Molly's recovery—or at least part of the ever-growing massage team who have grabbed Molly's arms, hands, legs, or neck (whatever seems to want attention most) and started rubbing! One of Molly's greatest gifts is her ability to embrace and receive the good intentions everyone has, to harness that energy, and to put it to work where it will do her the most good. As much as she is using them, none of them feel used. Everyone who has worked with Molly has been bathed in her resounding gratitude, and nourished both by her wisdom and by the knowledge that they have, on that day and with their hands and hearts, made a difference.

"People will just kind of automatically start massaging some aspect of my body," Molly says. She and Jeramy have just opened a dojo called Aikido of Penn Valley. "We are still very active in the art of aikido, which is continuing to be a physical benefit, as well as an emotional and spiritual benefit."

Mary-Jo and Molly changed my life. Their focus on their inner spiritual lives through these practical and outwardly physical practices of massage, water work, horseback riding, sailing, yoga, and aikido changed all of us who came into contact with them.

Today, both women continue to practice their passions, using massage to help them stay supple and mobile. They teach us to go beyond our limitations and achieve our dreams. They continue to teach me about endless possibilities and the power of touch.

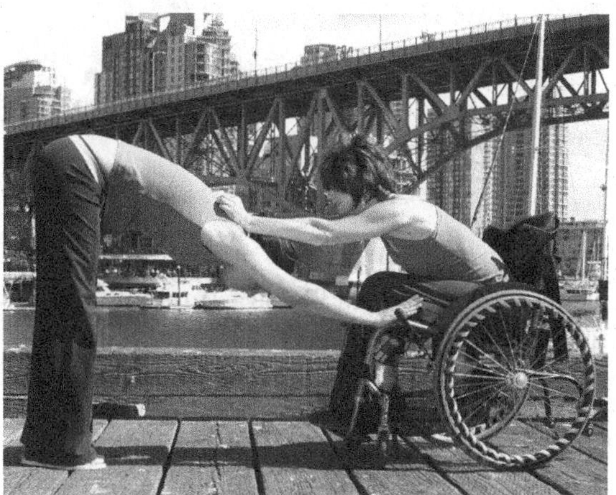

Mary-Jo Fetterly practices tandem yoga from her wheelchair.

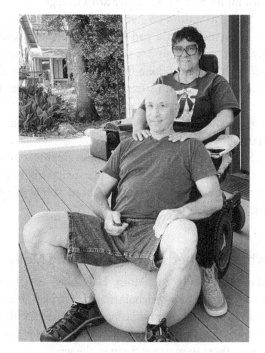

Molly Hale giving a massage to her husband Jeramy.

8

Wheelers with Spinal Cord Injuries

Dennis Cherenko and Barbara Turnbull were my first teachers navigating spinal cord injury. Dennis was a high school friend who broke his neck during a hockey game. We were sixteen years old. I knew nothing about wheelchair massage. About three decades later, Barbara Turnbull taught me to adapt my on-site massage routine for people like herself, in wheelchairs. She had a high-level spinal cord injury and no use of her arms or legs.

Barbara controlled her wheelchair with simple movements on a pad behind her head. I did my first wheelchair massage how-to film with Barbara. This was done through her professional attire, complete with sweater and blazer! I learned to move Barb's arms and expect an uncontrollable spasticity, shaking, and vibration as I settled into massaging her arm.

Spasticity, uncontrollable movements, and strong neurological and muscular reactions were all part of my early learning about spinal cord injury.

What I Learned from Mary-Jo and Molly

Mary-Jo Fetterly and Molly Hale have enriched my repertoire of wheelchair massage strokes. Both women are water enthusiasts, so I learned to film them in the water, massage them in the water, and teach others to massage them in the water.

But the most important lesson I have learned is that recovery from spinal cord injury doesn't stop. It doesn't stop physically, and it doesn't stop spiritually, although conventional medicine sometimes says it must. Years after the accidents that injured them, Mary-Jo and Molly continue to evolve, finding new physical capacities and building wonderful lives full of possibility. Massage has been part of their journey, from the beginning.

While filming Mary-Jo and Molly, I interviewed family, friends, and physicians, which gave breadth and depth to the dynamic of these two women's lives, and wove a rich and colorful tapestry of hope. I explored all their sources for healing, ranging from the classic medical model, to a paralysis recovery centre called Project Walk, to alternative medicine approaches, to recent successes in stem cell research and water therapy. In filming their recovery process and their successes, I witnessed incredible milestones of recovery: people who were guaranteed they would never walk again actually walking!

While their external struggle is obvious, their internal struggle is as challenging. It involved a transition from physical devastation to the re-creation of a way of entering the world with courage, persistence, and a willingness to push beyond the boundaries of conventional thinking.

Prior to Molly and Mary-Jo's accidents, their personal and professional lifestyles were centered on physical health. Their injuries were therefore doubly devastating. They have journeyed through the darkness of despair to the light on the other side. These two women now show marked improvement and have surpassed all expectations for their recovery. They are living proof of human healing capacity. Their testament also shines a light on how the health system let them down and at times thwarted their recovery process. Despite bureaucratic and medical systems that dashed their hopes, they both believed that there were simple, achievable ways to gain mobility. They both used massage therapy from the outset on a daily basis, and continue to use it. Today, independently, they strive to reclaim the use of their limbs and bodies.

Mary-Jo says she could "feel the electricity and the impulses still there, still moving. It was just in a new language and I had to learn that language." Of her life now, she says that it "is degrees greater. No other situation like this, no accident or disease, is so completely impacting. This has so completely changed me, the way I see and feel, the way I live." She is now involved in a greater truth, and in the limitless possibilities she now experiences after her great catharsis.

Mary-Jo openly talks about an area that many are unwilling to talk about: the initial lack of physical sensation and the effect on her sexuality. "At first I just wrote it off...but then I asked myself 'Why?' and then 'Why not?' Just because my previous physical experience was not possible didn't mean that I couldn't re-communicate with this area of my life, and as I developed new pathways of intimacy, I discovered that just because I couldn't move my body beneath my shoulders, or my breasts actually, it didn't mean that I didn't still enjoy feeling touch and the intimacy of exploration." In reprogramming her synaptic responses to the biochemical potpourri that we all experience as sexual beings, she has risen to a new height of sexual intimacy and enjoyment, something that certainly every human would enjoy. And yet, this is only one signpost, indicative of the breadth and depth of her new life.

After much dedication and hard work, Mary-Jo enjoys a quality of life that she could only have imagined as an abstract possibility in her previous life. She continues to teach and actively seek, with quiet certainty and tremendous passion, a new and broad highway that most of us can only imagine.

For her part, Molly realized after her injury that she could still feel sensations in her body. This drove her to explore new techniques for recovery. Her doctors accused her of living in denial. They wanted her to "accept" being in a wheelchair for the remainder of her life and to take drugs to "soothe" the muscle spasms in her body. Molly took the spasms as signs that her body was trying to reconnect. This effort from her body, the neuroplasticity to reconnect the neurological webbing that enabled muscle movement and control, further inspired her to resist her doctors.

Her husband, Jeramy, told me about the mind-numbing phone call from the family friend who was in the accident, saying that Molly was still trapped in the twisted wreckage. He talked about the shock of arriving at the hospital, and his struggles to simultaneously come to grips with what had happened and support his wife. He learned how to manage an indwelling catheter and to do any number of new chores. Molly recalls feeling her catheter obstructing a muscle that was trying to reconnect. She needed the catheter out, and Jeramy learned to provide her with "intermittent catheterization" five or six times a day. This allowed her bladder to fill and then be emptied, which stimulated the memory of her former bladder function.

Molly's recovery involved breath practice, cellular revitalization through meditation, water therapy, and much more. Molly's plan was to combine accepted therapeutic practices with alternative complimentary approaches. Massage was, and is still, a mainstay in her recovery.

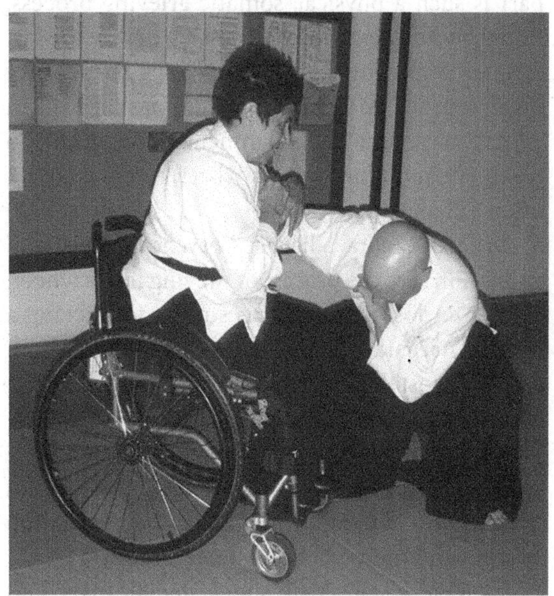

Molly practicing aikido from her wheelchair.

After taking her muscle spasms as a positive sign, Molly began to focus on subtle movements called continuum micro-movements. She says "to become intimate with tiny movement, I would spend hours just lightly moving my fingers." The outward appearance of any success was not discernable to the human eye, but in the end, this small practice in combination with her other techniques won her mobility.

Molly is not a quitter, this is certain. She can now walk independently, while supported with an elbow-weighted walker.

Considering Emotions

Whether a wheelchair user has landed in the chair by birth or by accident, as a young person or as an adult, the daily reality of living in a wheelchair has emotional considerations. It is harder to hug when you cannot stand up. Dating can be a challenge, and having babies can be a challenge. Sports activities are one hundred percent different, but still, the heart remains the same. People need contact, skin on skin, for the best healing of heartbreak. It is heartbreaking to lose your legs through paralysis, accident, disease, or surgery. Missing a body part is such a physical, somatic grieving process. In my book *Dying in Good Hands*, I devote the last chapter to grieving in good hands. The benefits of being touched and the significance of skin-to-skin contact have been well documented. Being able to reach out and touch from a wheelchair is vital but often a challenge.

Dr. Beth Sikora, a licensed psychotherapist and counselor, says the process of moving into a wheelchair after losing mobility is similar to grieving a death. That said, some patients I have worked with who have lost their work niche in fitness and health careers, like Mary-Jo Fetterly, have adapted to new ways of teaching yoga and fitness from their wheelchairs. I credit massage and the hands-on help of their friends and family in making their transition smooth and their emotions stable.

Sikora also states that "shock, denial, anger, and depression are all common emotions wheelchair users can experience before reconciling with what happened and accepting their new, altered life."[7] The power of touch is extremely important, whether administered by professionals or a community of nonprofessional caregivers. The danger of becoming emotionally paralyzed is lessened by massage and the power of touch. Feeling the big feelings and expressing the resulting emotions can be the biggest growing experience of that person's lifetime and for those around them.

For friends and family to be able to massage somebody as they integrate their new lifestyle is an extremely meaningful experience. This team, built of emotional supporters, often supports the new wheelchair user for the rest of their life, and the knowledge the support team gains becomes integrated into their own lifestyle. The significance of touch in these emotionally trying, transitional times gives both the wheelchair user and their community a sense of satisfaction, of belonging and healing.

Basic Principles of Spinal Cord Injury Massage

Spinal cord injury massage involves learning what works, and what doesn't work, and what works differently than before.

Everyone with a spinal cord injury is a wheelchair user. So, all of the principles and practices of wheelchair massage are important to them.

The most important focus for the extremities is to relieve unwanted spasticity and at the same time encourage neurological stimulation. That can be a delicate balance. Massaging with these two principles in mind requires lots of simultaneous feedback and experimentation.

Researchers Luigi Tame, Alessandro Farne, and Francesco Pavini examined to what degree vision can affect touch.[8] This refers to watching what happens to the body. It can be beneficial for someone recovering from a spinal cord injury to actually watch where you are massaging. This helps them discover sensory deficits and sensory oddities (surges, for example). They might have numb feelings or hypersensitivity, and they might have patches of purely normal skin sensation within a huge area that has no skin sensation or perception. It helps them understand their recovering connections and their new synaptic connections to see where and how you touch them.

1. People with spinal cord injuries start their recovery in ICU. Create a massage recovery team at all the different levels of ICU care.
2. Use all the full body massage strokes, whether the person can feel where your hands are or not.
3. Set up your massage so that the person can see where your hands are. For areas that are out of their sight, you can use mirrors so they can track where your hands are and have a neurological-visual connection.
4. Don't leave out any areas that are numb as we can use stimulators, like dry brushing, rough face cloths, or paintbrushes to wake up those cells that are asleep.
5. In doing a full body massage, always include digestive massage. Even with the person seated in a wheelchair, with their tummy compressed, you will still make a huge difference by massaging all around the hips and then mobilizing the hips to illicit a peristaltic response.
6. Be sure to use different patient positions: leaning forward in the chair, leaning back in the chair, and tilted to the side.
7. Teach tandem massage to aid sensory recovery.
8. It's important to be creative in order to stimulate upper and lower body connections by having a person massage the right leg while someone massages the right arm, stimulating those areas of the brain that are linked not only across but up and down the body.

The possibilities for recovery from spinal cord injury are exciting. New research continues to unfold. We now have machines designed to keep people walking after they are paralyzed, including "exo-suits" and "assisted limbs." I saw inspiring examples of these technologies when I visited Project Walk at what was then their headquarters in California with my friend and patient, Ed Natyshak. These technologies are only the tip of the iceberg, floating on a mountain of research that is going on beneath. Spinal cord injury recovery is a fast-changing world, and it reinforces my conviction that it's important to keep immobilized bodies moving, since there's always the possibility of a cure.

After ICU, once things settle into a wheelchair lifestyle, there isn't as much talk about getting out of the chair. I feel strongly that it's important to sustain the urgency that was present in ICU and keep the body moving. Until it is common practice for us to be able to hook up severed neurons, or replace and restore damaged vertebrae, all injured bodies need to be ready for whatever restorative miracles lie in the future. To make sure they are ready, we need to keep all the joints mobile with massage.

VIDEO LIBRARY

Visit brusheducation.ca/wheeling-in-good-hands to watch these videos:

Mountains to climb

Stand because you can

Spinal cord injury massage: Family and friends massage team in ICU

Patient Story

Dixie

Doing Dixie was the name of my first film documenting the life of my high school friend Dixie Allard. Dixie was living with multiple sclerosis in Mount St. Francis, a chronic care facility in Nelson, B.C. For years, she helped me teach my summer programs about palliative massage.

For Dixie, MS meant almost complete immobility: she could speak, and was so funny and straight forward with her requests during her massages, but she couldn't move her arms or legs. I was used to making tiny adjustments for her; even a millimeter of change in the placement of her arm could make a huge difference to her comfort level.

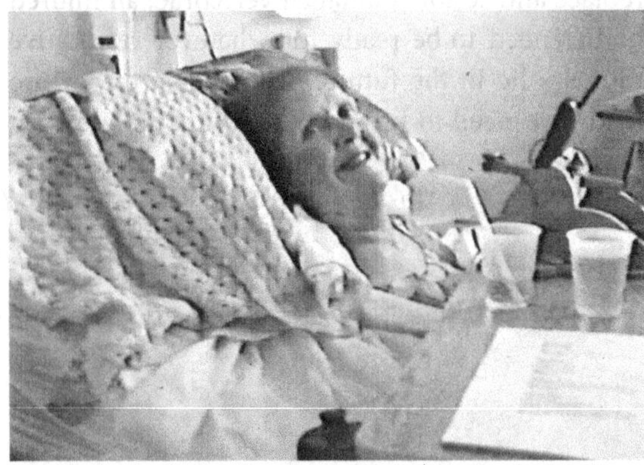

Dixie was an incredible teacher when it came to massage.

I spent every New Year's Eve with Dixie in the last years of her life. I would start to massage her at 11:30 p.m. and we'd continue into the next year, talking about the past year and reviewing it in a tactile conversation. I remember one year I even had a new year's date who patiently waited in his car while I massaged Dixie from one year to the next! The last year we did this together was about three months before Dixie died. She had eaten all the usual special holiday foods, and it took days to help her through the discomfort that brought on!

The nurses at Mount St. Francis took wonderful care of Dixie. One nurse told Lee, a friend of mine, that she remembers Dixie asking, "Would you pick my nose?" The nurse looked at Dixie quizzically, but then thought about it: "Can you imagine the torture of having your nose gross with snot, unable to breathe, and being too helpless to do anything about it? How had we missed this important detail in her care?" It's easy to take this kind of small, grooming thing for granted until you can't do it anymore. But a plugged nose becomes a big problem when your hands don't work and you can't pick your own nose! "It's a humbling service to offer a person, but the result is comfort and dignity for the resident," the nurse told Lee. "Keeping Dixie's nose clean became an important part of my job."

All the nurses loved Dixie's way of "massaging" them. Every year at Christmas, we posted a sign-up sheet where staff could sign up for a fifteen-minute massage. Mount St. Francis was generous with their speaker system and allowed us to call up each staff person in for their massage treat when it was their turn. Dixie chose the music and had spiked hot apple cider ready for them to drink while they visited together, and I massaged their shoulders. We would also wheel into the lounge so she could listen to the high school students sing their Christmas carols while they massaged the residents for a holiday hands-on experience!

I usually came to massage Dixie in the early morning, before breakfast. We often watched a woman play with her dog in the grass outside Dixie's window. One day, I met the woman face to face as I was arriving at Mount St. Francis. I stopped to tell her how Dixie and I loved watching her throw the stick for her dog. It helped Dixie her start her day the right way.

Dixie's daily use of her wheelchair allowed her to have a single evening cigarette on the balcony in the fresh air, no matter what season it was. As my visits were almost always in the morning, it was years before I realized that Dixie was being "smoked" outside. One day, on one of the rare occasions that I was doing her massage in the evening, she asked me if, before we got started, she could have me be her "smoker!" I never let Dixie forget that my love for her was demonstrated in that event. More than giving her my loving touch during her weekly massages, I was willing to take part in the relaxing evening prelude of her addiction!

Dixie was very vocal about the benefits of her massages, which she received not only from me but from my students and her family. Dixie's sister Penny, in particular, was an incredible student. I taught her a thorough, whole-body massage routine from head to toes, which included all the massage techniques for preventing Dixie's skin from breaking down and for helping her mobility and digestion. Penny learned absolutely everything she could about massage for chronic conditions like MS, and even helped me coordinate the best summer massage program one year.

Penny started learning massage from me when Dixie was still living at home. "Dixie, previously a bright and energetic young mother of three, was being unrelentingly ravaged by MS and none of us could do anything to stop it," Penny told me. "But massage gave me a way to physically connect with her on a level other than just filling her practical needs of feeding and helping her in the bathroom." Penny was known in our community for her dancing talent: she could do all the fancy dances like the tango and the cha-cha. She had incredible rhythm. This showed in her hands-on talent for soothing her sister. "Although she was a numb quadriplegic, touching her in a gentle caring way gave her comfort and eased her violent spasms," Penny said. "She felt peace and serenity during her massage. The connection between us was deep and loving. Massage has a powerful positive effect."

After that last New Year's massage, I had to leave Nelson to teach in Maui. I didn't want to go as I knew Dixie was close to leaving in a different direction. Her son had died tragically the year before, and Dixie had suffered immensely ever since. Her breathing was now so affected that Penny and her husband were often on "death watch," with Dixie sometimes stopping breathing for minutes at a time. We were all amazed that she had survived this long. Still, when one of Dixie's favourite nurses arrived on the floor, Dixie would spring to life with a completely normal call to be taken out for a smoke.

On my last day of teaching in Maui, I got a call that Dixie had died. I arrived back in Nelson the next day, and my friend Lynn drove me straight to Mount St. Francis. Penny had kept the room with everything in it, exactly as I remembered it, until I arrived. My massage lotions and oils and my photos of Dixie and the students over the years were there for me to take away.

I climbed onto Dixie's bed and put the head of the bed at the angle that she liked, the angle that made her breathing most comfortable in those last weeks. I lay in the place of Dixie. I watched as the woman and her dog came into view. I felt the love of Dixie, the touch of her words that guided my hands to make the smallest of changes, to scratch her nose for her like her sister Penny had done so often, to unplug her nose like her caregiver had done for her, and to massage her all over, like so many of us had done. We all had done our best to show her love and comfort. I still miss "doing Dixie."

VIDEO LIBRARY

Visit brusheducation.ca/wheeling-in-good-hands to watch this video:

Story of Dixie: Doing Dixie

9

Wheelers with Chronic Neurological Conditions

People with chronic neurological conditions are often long-term wheelchair users. All of the wheelchair massage techniques and priorities we have discussed in this book so far are important to them. In addition, they may need extra attention for certain areas, because of their condition and because of their long-term wheelchair use.

My experience with wheelchair massage for long-term users is intimate. Starting in my teens, Dennis Cherenko educated all of us in high school about life in a wheelchair. Later, Dennis was keen for me to teach him how to massage his wife, who was also in a wheelchair. All within the span of my thirties, my mentor Brian Carpendale was diagnosed with ALS, as was my friend Mary Coletti, and my high school friend, Dixie Allard, was diagnosed with MS. Finally, my oldest friend in the Kootenays, Freya Gray, was diagnosed with Parkinson's disease. My "big sister" Rose Marie, who died in 2018, had Parkinson's disease. In all these intimate relationships, I learned, through teaching family, friends, and caregiving teams, about the daily significance of the power of touch through massage therapy.

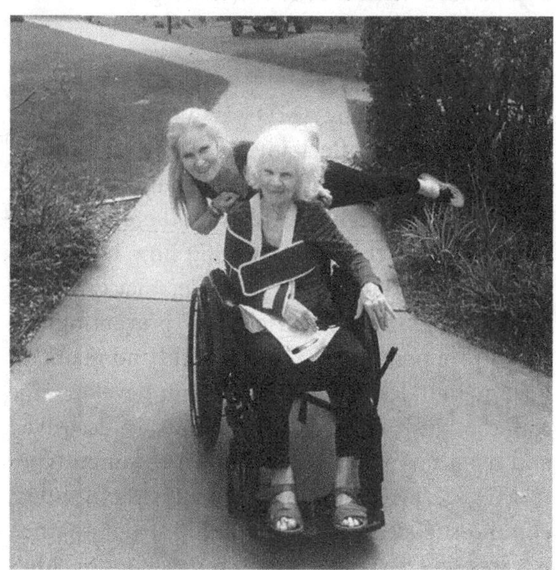

Rose Marie Harrop and me.

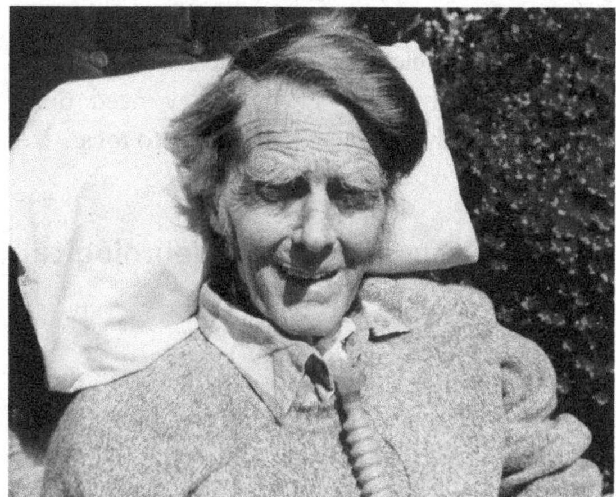

Brian Carpendale.

Beyond their use in chronic illnesses, wheelchairs can augment the mobility of amputees. One of my past roommates, Amber, lost her leg to cancer in her twenties and acquired the latest, lightest wheelchair, loaded with titanium! I loved borrowing her chair to demonstrate wheelchair massage techniques for all kinds of people, from moms-to-be to wheelchair athletes.

Jonathan White, who lives with a rare disease, has used a wheelchair since early in his life. This long-time wheelchair user has helped me teach for more than twenty years, bringing his team of caregivers to every summer training session. He receives massages as a way to maintain a healthy lifestyle.

All these people have been my teachers! I have been lucky to be hands-on through their chronic care journeys, learning to teach and teaching to learn.

Massage Frequency for Long-Term Wheelchair Users

A full body massage is best every day for long-term wheelchair users. At minimum, they need massages more than once a week and, always, mini-massages every day. These folks, no matter what their condition, need us to be hands-on each and every day. They are people predisposed to having their legs twist from lack of use and lack of gravitational pull to keep pressure on their joints. They are people who acquire problems from living for years in wheelchairs. Their backs become more scoliotic simply from sitting. They need daily, entire, full body massages, from nose to toes.

Common Issues in Chronic Neurological Conditions

Cerebral Palsy

Cerebral palsy is linked to abnormal brain development or damage before or during birth, which can be linked to a variety of causes including genetic factors, hydrocephalus, and birth trauma from high forceps delivery or oxygen interruption. Massage therapy tends to be a great fit for treating cerebral palsy's classic symptoms of muscle spasticity, especially when diagnosed early.

In one study of young children with cerebral palsy, children who received 30 minutes of massage weekly for 12 weeks showed fewer physical symptoms of cerebral palsy compared to a control group, including reduced spasticity, less rigid muscle tone, and improved fine and gross motor functioning. The massage group also showed improved cognition, higher social and dressing scores, more positive facial expressions, and less cerebral-palsy-related limb activity during play.[9]

Parents and families of children with cerebral palsy can change the course of the disease by keeping the muscles elastic and soft through daily, hands-on help. Massaging throughout the waking hours helps to recondition and repattern the muscles before and after activities, similar to the rationale of sports massage. Frequent massage can encourage muscle flexibility as the infant learns to move their body and become upright. It's important to remember that connective tissues, tendonous attachments, and ligaments have less vascular supply than the muscles and need more help to refresh and reduce stiffness.

Not all folks with cerebral palsy are perfect candidates for massage. Some have a hypersensitivity that makes touch unbearable, though sometimes these conditions can change with time and neurological development. For those who can tolerate massage, the power of touch carries more than practical and physical benefits in the life of a person living with cerebral palsy. It also carries the emotional benefit of softening the person's overall stress and eases the strain of an especially challenging disease. I've found that they will often choose a finale of scalp, foot, or hand massage, as it gives them the biggest general relaxation response, but my patients with cerebral palsy have taught me to frequently check in with them about their likes and dislikes when it comes to massage.

Muscular Dystrophy

Muscular dystrophy (MD) is a neuromuscular disorder that can affect anyone at any stage of life. There are nine types of MD, which affect the muscles to varying degrees. Although there is no cure for MD, researchers are learning how to prevent and treat it. It is a genetic disorder that gradually weakens the body's muscles by preventing the body from making proteins to build and maintain healthy muscles. Kids with MD can develop large calf muscles as the gastrocnemius is destroyed and replaced by fat. The two most common types of MD are Duchenne muscular dystrophy (most common) and Becker muscular dystrophy, which is a less severe type. Then there's a common adult form, known as Steinert's disease (or myotonic dystrophy), and although it's adult, lots of the cases are under twenty years old. There is a limb-girdle MD, which usually starts when kids are between eight and fifteen, and it affects the pelvic shoulder and back muscles. Some kids have a mild version and others develop severe disabilities and need to use a wheelchair.

Over time, because the legs and pelvic muscles lose their strength in the later stages of MD, assistive devices are used, such as power wheelchairs and scooters, and braces to improve flexibility. Sometimes a ventilator is used to support breathing. The kids that I have seen with Duchenne and Becker forms of MD have developed scoliosis because their muscles are too weak to hold the spine upright. Spinal fusion is often part of straightening the curvature and can help the patient to sit upright. A reduction in pain is usually an outcome of spinal fusion.

It is important for all parents of kids with MD to learn practical daily massage routines for any and all of the symptoms of muscular dystrophy.

Remember, this is a disease of muscle wasting and muscle shortening, and it affects all three kinds of muscle: skeletal, smooth, and cardiac. The skeletal muscles give the body its shape and are known as voluntary muscles because you can control them with everyday movements. The smooth, or involuntary, muscles are not striated like skeletal muscles. They are controlled by the nervous system and they are found in the walls of the stomach and intestines, and in the walls of the blood vessels, which help maintain blood pressure. Smooth muscles take longer to contract than skeletal muscles, but they stay contracted for longer periods of time because they don't tire easily. By contrast, skeletal muscles contract (shorten or tighten) quickly and powerfully, but tire easily. The cardiac muscle is only found in the heart. It is an involuntary type of muscle with powerful contractions forcing blood out of the heart as it beats.

The massage therapy indicated for anyone of any age with MD includes the musculoskeletal system with basic full body massage, and digestive and respiratory massage. Because people with MD have weakened heart and respiratory muscles, it's important to include a complete respiratory massage treatment. The full body massage should also include passive movement of the shoulders and hips: do leg pumping and shoulder rotations before, during, and after the massage routine. All MD patients can be treated side-lying, adaptively prone, supine, or in a variety of wheelchairs from electric to manual. The most important focus for massaging someone with MD is to lengthen, relax, and give greater elasticity to the muscles, whether they are shortened or atrophied, creating as much flexibility in the joints as possible.

Parkinson's Disease

There is an ankylotic (fusing) tendency in the ankles, feet, and knees that can be helped with daily massages interspersed with active, full-range movement of every joint. Throughout my massage routine, I do leg pumping, which stimulates the knee; ankle rotations; and toe flexions, extensions, and rotations.

I've been lucky be involved in the care of close friends—Rose Marie and Freya—at different stages of Parkinson's. Rose Marie died quite suddenly, but was for years able to be active, walking, and talking. Freya, on the other hand, lived for years with Parkinson's, including years highly immobilized with little vocal interaction. Both women thrived with frequent massage.

Multiple Sclerosis

MS can result in extreme muscle shortening, which is helped by massaging the contracted structures to improve elasticity. I emphasize fingertip kneading of the tendinous attachments at each joint and then working into the belly of the muscle itself. It is important to massage in early onset and all the way through the disease to prevent fixed joints. With all my MS patients, I start with a full body massage and conclude with passive movements. It's like taking them for a walk around the block.

Dixie Allard from Nelson and my friend Mary Hay from the Toronto Islands are examples of the extremes of MS. Dixie was quickly immobilized and spend years getting her massages in her hospital bed, while Mary has had long periods of remission and to this day is still on her feet after thirty years from diagnosis.

Amyotrophic Lateral Sclerosis

The muscle wasting that is characteristic of this disease seems to make massage incidental, but the opposite is the case. With all my ALS patients, I do full body massages and show family and friends to do the same. With ALS, we can provide metabolic nourishment by simply enhancing the circulation from early onset to full-term symptoms. All my ALS patients have benefitted from increased musculoskeletal elasticity and joint mobility, and from respiratory enhancement and digestive success. Don't leave out any areas of the body in your full body massage. These people need as much respiratory help as possible, so I focus a lot on diaphragm stroking and intercostal rib raking. Upper respiratory massage, and face, scalp, and throat massage, are really important for all ALS patients.

Key Considerations in Wheelchair Massage for Chronic Neurological Conditions

Generally, the basic wheelchair full body massage routine is perfect for daily application for long-term wheelchair users. Massage is most useful in the morning to remedy and counteract issues related to long periods of immobility, like pressure sores. In addition, mini-massages should be given at other times of the same day (for example, digestive and respiratory massage before a transfer from the bed to the wheelchair, or from the chair to the bed). These mini-massages throughout the day help alleviate the daily discomforts of wheelchair working and living.

Most long-term wheelchair users value being stretched out during the day, not just at the end of the day. Mini-massages (ten minutes) are perfect for helping the joints to stretch out. The stretching will foster better digestion and better breathing!

In an ideal world, whether they are able to get out of their chair or not, long-term wheelchair users should have tummy rubs and chest work as part of their daily massage. These respiratory and digestive mini-massages help greatly in the long run.

The success of long-term wheelchair massage is all about the team. Caregivers are part of the long-term user's daily life. These are people known to be good with their hands and have a keen interest in practical, hands-on massage skills. They are some of my favorite students to teach wheelchair massage techniques. However, in between the professional sessions, we need family, friends, and volunteers to give mini-massages and full body massages every day! Tandem teaching is the easiest way to enlist more volunteers. When anyone is visiting, they can massage along with whomever is administering the treatment.

Swelling in the Extremities

Swelling in the extremities, which can lead to the life-threatening problem of lymphedema, is a particular concern for long-term wheelchair users.

It's so simple to massage the lower leg when the swelling is visually obvious, yet most people don't do it. It's easy to reduce that swelling with simple stroking. Anyone can do it. You don't need extensive massage training. Just the principle of pushing any fluid up the extremities toward the heart is a lifesaving measure. Patients will not lose any part of their extremities as long as they get mini-massages daily. The use of compression stockings is important after a massage, as it will make the results of your treatment longer lasting. However, the constant use of compression stockings without any other form of circulation stimulation is not wise. With massage and stockings, you can maintain skin integrity. It is very hard for tissue to ulcerate if is kept healthy with hydrotherapy, massage, elevation, and a variety of different compression methods.

Musculoskeletal Symptoms

All long-term wheelchair users need focus on the knees, hamstrings, and calf muscles, because prolonged sitting shortens muscles and tendons in the hips, knees, and legs. Your massage needs to start where the hamstrings attach into the ischial tuberosity, and go all the way down the back of the leg to the heel of the foot. Make sure you spend time on the tendinous attachments on either side of the back of the knee and at the heel of the foot.

Contracting of the joints in the arms and legs is helped by massaging the extremities before and after transfers to and from the chair. This is where tandem massage and teams of volunteers make a big difference—the difference between delivering one massage a week and one massage a day, or even better, a massage to *pre*pare for the day and a massage to *re*pair when the day is done! This is all simply a matter of organizing hands-on helpers!

Pressure Sores

Pressure sores are a constant worry for all long-term wheelchair users. Make sure you spend time massaging all the usual wheelchair pressure points, and check in with your patient about other pressure points that might be unique to them because of their posture or the way they use their wheelchair. I use all sorts of skin stimulation from dry brushing to ice massage with great results!

Sylvia

I was doing a Valentine's Day massage visit to one of my favorite Toronto chronic care facilities when I met Sylvia Grimshaw. I was with a group of high school students that I was training to massage seniors. The students were earning graduation credits at the same time as learning and providing hands-on elder care for their grandparents.

Sylvia was in the group of seniors receiving valentines via teenage tenderness. The students had been taught the week before and had practiced on their parents for homework prizes. One of the teenagers, Sophia, was someone I had massaged "on the inside," during her mom's pregnancy. This was like jumping ahead, teaching these kids to massage people like their grandparents! They now had the gift of touch for all occasions like birthdays, anniversaries, and Christmas.

That Valentine's Day I was lucky. The seniors were responsive and vocal with their appreciation. I was reminded of the power of touch and the lack of genuine human connection with those in care facilities.

As a documentary filmmaker, you can't hold up cue cards to get the lines you want, at least not if you're this documentary filmmaker! So, when I heard the woman in the celebration-pink attire offer her appreciation, I didn't know if it had happened on camera or off camera. I just knew that the perfect voice had said the perfect line. She said, "This is the best Valentine's Day I have ever had!" To make it even better, the student massaging her was Sophia. I was over the top when Sophia said back to her, in the warmest happy tone, "Oh! That makes me feel so good!" The woman Sophia was massaging retorted, "I really mean that!!"

When we asked everyone to lean forward onto their tables, Sylvia spoke up and said, "It's like going to sleep!" I asked the crowd of seniors, as they leaned forward, to rest their crossed arms on the tables to support their heads. Sylvia made everyone smile when she piped up, "That's cozy!"

She had an immediate aptitude for group dynamics and every time we had a class of students at the facility to learn about geriatric wheelchair massage, Sylvia was an instant favorite. She made all her student therapists feel they were appreciated!

I needed to make a film about geriatric massage, so I asked for volunteers from Vermont Square, the senior facility in Toronto where Sylvia lived. She volunteered and her family gave their consent. She was a delight to work with.

Her sense of dramatic flare was obvious throughout the filming.

When my film crew was setting up and my photographer was shooting stills, Sylvia was attentive and responsive. When I checked in with her about pressure during the massage, she gave quick answers, although hard of hearing, and when I thanked her for her feedback, she gave me a huge smile and said, "Anytime!"

During the filming, she interrupts my neck massage to ask whether the massage is going to "stir" her brain! I say, "Yes." And she says, "Very good!"

"Does it feel good?" I ask as I change positions to massage her arm. I sit down on my stool and talk to Sylvia about starting at the shoulder to massage the arm, to open up the circulation to the entire arm. I am corkscrewing her fingers when she asks if she should be doing the massage for her fingers herself. I comment on how beautiful her hands are—how they don't have any arthritis or osteoarthritis.

"How old are you, Sylvia?"

"They always come up with that question. I'll tell you my age—half and half—but you will have to guess!" she happily demanded.

So I continue the running commentary, starting at age eighty-one. She stops me at eighty-six.

"I'm going to be doing a back massage, Sylvia."

"Do what you like!" she answers.

As I straddle a wheel of her chair and put one hand across her upper chest to the opposite shoulder, I use my other hand to massage down her back muscles. She can feel my hands as though it is skin-to-skin contact although she is fully dressed in her best navy suit and jewelry.

Now, halfway through filming the wheelchair massage, Sylvia is exhibiting all the symptoms of someone coming to life and becoming more animated!

"Ohh! You touched a very tender spot!"

"Does that feel good?"

"Yes, you can go further down," she says, pointing to the side of her back.

I stand on a chair to get further down her back, continually checking in about pressure. Sylvia rocks back and forth with relaxation as I massage her.

"I hope you realize that you're being very personal," she says, as I massage under her hips. I ask Sylvia if it is the right kind of personal and she laughs.

I ask her to continue to give me feedback and she smiles.

As I shift from the back of her wheelchair to work around the front and massage her legs, she looks up into the camera and says, "Imagine, I put my head up and see myself looking at a camera!"

With that, she gracefully lifts both arms and performs a wheelchair ballet with an elegant bow.

10

Geriatric Wheelers

People who are elderly benefit from massage, whether they are in wheelchairs or not. This chapter is about massage for geriatric people in general, and about the priorities for geriatric wheelchair users in particular.

In all my years of practice and teaching, geriatric massage is the area where I've had the most experience. I began very early on, using my family and friends as practice subjects. I also have had countless wonderful, generous, geriatric clients who were all, in their own way, my massage teachers.

I have been taught by people like Sylvia Grimshaw and my mentor, Brian Carpendale, to be creative and adaptable, and most importantly to listen. What I found, by listening, was that the ailments of the geriatric population that respond to massage are limitless.

My first long-term geriatric massage patients, Mary Walpole and Sylvia King, not only taught me the ins and outs of geriatric massage, but they also incorporated wheelchair massage into the mix! It was a double-trouble opportunity for treating problems that come from aging and wheelchair use. Mary and Sylvia were very successful in their professional careers and had gone through changes and losses in their lives. I treated these women every week for years and I came to know their life-cycle changes. We began our journey with two able-bodied, dynamic seniors who slowly, over time, moved into wheelchairs. Their endless patience and charm made them a joy to work with.

In the field of geriatric massage, wheelchairs are a fact of life. As people live longer, they use wheelchairs more. It is rare if a senior does not spend time in a wheelchair, whether it is a temporary or a permanent situation. Seniors also form a significant component of massage therapy clientele. Many massage therapists are now specializing in geriatric massage and are establishing practices in this field. Wheelchair massage, with a geriatric twist, is an integral and necessary component of geriatric massage.

I've always been fascinated by the aging process. It is an accumulation of all of life's injuries, aches, and pains: a complete library of experience. Senior patients have depths of understanding that only

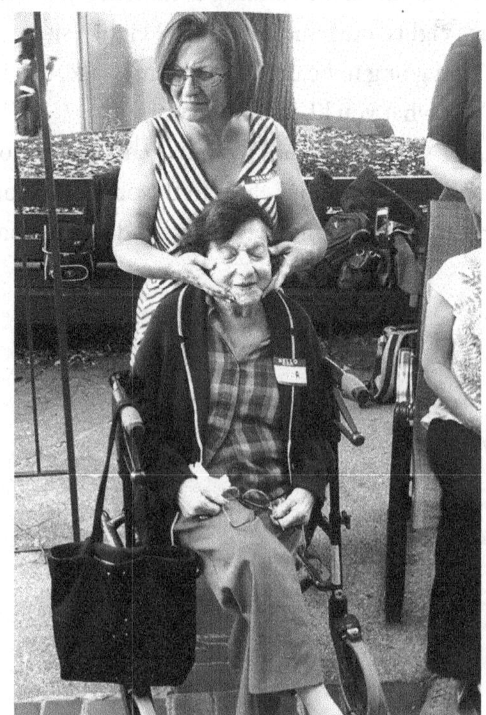

Geriatric wheelchair massage in action!

come toward the end of a person's life. Many have come through extraordinary loss, change, and challenges, yet they continue to build and create new lives for themselves.

It is my hope that geriatric wheelchair massage will keep elders healthy and in touch with their loved ones. But most of all, I hope it will help keep our geriatric wheelchair population visible, not tucked away from sight. I wish that all high school students could be connected with a senior wheeler!

Bridging the Generation Gap with Massage

With massage techniques adapted for seniors, we can keep people in a wheeling lifestyle comfortable. One of my favorite teaching experiences has been in this area; it is a program I've called Bridging the Gap. In it, kids learn to massage seniors in chronic care facilities. Not only does it connect two generations, it makes wheelchairs part of the "normal" for families.

The kids who have gone through this program are better able to see the elderly and people in wheelchairs as the "norm." It also gives families room to consider keeping their elders at home and integrated into the household.

In the denser populations of the world, such as India and the Philippines, eight-five percent of families have intergenerational living; the family stays together under one roof from birth to death. Wheelchairs have made it easier for families to keep disabled elders at home and involved in everyday family life. In my own family, if we had had a wheelchair for my grandmother, she could have lived with us longer before going to a chronic care facility. With my own mom, I was able to help her become wheelchair friendly early on in her elderly life. We always took a wheelchair with us to the park and other outings so she could be wheeled along right up to the day she died.

Geriatric Massage: A Growing Priority

Geriatric used to mean old and infirm. The word *senior* implied a person was in the end phase of their life. Now, with the enormous advances in medicine and technology, people are living much

FIGURE 10.1. Bridging the Gap

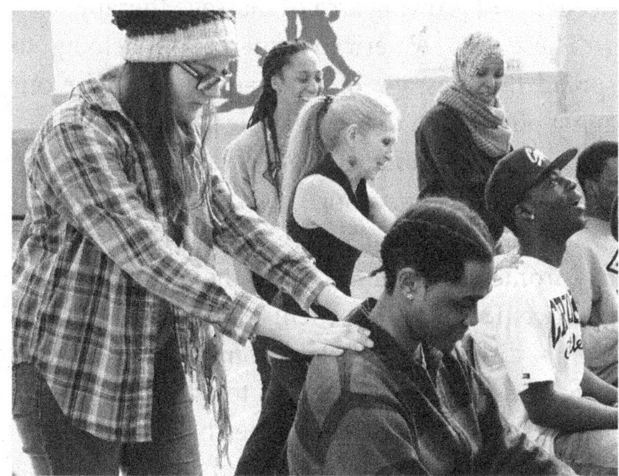

Bridging the Gap is a program where I teach students to massage seniors. First, I teach them to massage each other!

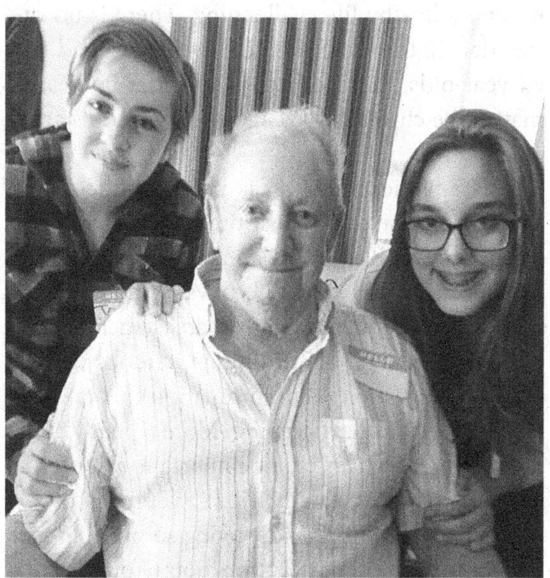

Bill, a senior in the Bridging the Gap program, and two students.

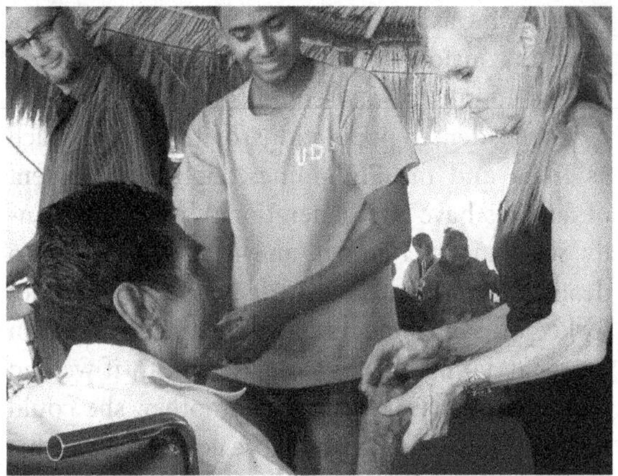
I have also taught geriatric wheelchair massage in Guatemala.

longer than they were a century ago. For example, in 1935, when the retirement age was 65 in Canada, the average life expectancy was 61.34 years. In 2023, the average life expectancy in Canada was 81.6 years for men and 85 years for women. We are now living twenty-four years more on average than our grandparents and great-grandparents.

The extra twenty-four years that we've been given affects each of us differently. Some people carry on in their working or professional life into their eighties. Others find new ways to engage in an active, productive life. Still others find maintaining a heathy life challenging. There is no one size fits all: there are robust 90-year-olds and frail 65-year-olds. But the fact is that older bodies, no matter the chronological age or fitness, do start to wear out.

Therapeutic massage has proven to be one of the least invasive and most productive treatments to address problems that come with aging. More and more studies show the physical and psychological benefits of massage in areas such as pain reduction, general body function (circulation, respiration, digestion, and elimination), skin integrity, stress relief, and sleeping. More recently, it has also been shown to be an important resource in soothing patients with delirium or dementia.

Because seniors are now living so much longer, they compose a significant portion of our population, and they also compose an increasing portion of the clientele for massage therapists. Geriatric massage, however, is not the same as massage for younger bodies.

The two geriatric massage "gurus" I look to when I want to talk professional ideas are my American colleagues and registered massage therapists Dr. Sharon Puszko and Dr. Susan Salvo. Both have been wonderfully generous about sharing their knowledge and experience. For anyone going into geriatric massage therapy, I recommend the writings and videos of these two professionals.

My conversations with Sharon Puszko and Susan Salvo about geriatric massage were inspiring. Sharon is dedicated in her work to promoting geriatric massage. She describes seniors as the fastest growing massage segment in the United States, needing massage to have a more enjoyable quality of life. Her Daybreak Geriatric Massage Institute is designed to enhance the quality of life for our aging population.

Susan Salvo has made teaching geriatric massage so much easier for the rest of us with her careful documentation of contraindications and benefits of geriatric practice. Her summary of the most immediate benefits of geriatric massage, which include decreasing the stiffness of the body and reducing inflammation, is so accurate. Her videos and social media coverage of this topic are helping to get the word out about this much needed and growing area of massage therapy.

These two American experts are helping to spread the message of hands-on healing for our aging population to live healthier to the end.

For many years in Nelson, I was a classic small-town, old-time "traveling" massage therapist. Most of my geriatric clients were either in their home, in chronic care facilities, or in the hospital. In my practice, I went to my clients. Because of this elemental difference, there are some aspects of geriatric massage that I have had to adjust to suit the setting, the client, and the wheelchair.

Part of the reason I "traveled" in Nelson was that my clinic had so many stairs and was neither wheelchair accessible nor senior friendly. Now, in Fort St. John, my clinic is very accessible to seniors and wheelchairs. People can roll in from the street, roll down the hall, and transfer to the massage table. It's a completely different experience!

Key Considerations in Geriatric Wheelchair Massage

Intake Case History

Taking a case history is important with every client, but especially important with geriatric clients, whose bodies have been through so many years and so much. Ask about old injury sites and about new issues they are experiencing. It's always a good idea to ask about medications and their side effects, because the elderly can be on many medications.

Dr. Salvo has numerous videos about intake interviews for seniors as opposed to younger patients.

Thin Skin

The skin thins and loses elasticity with aging, and this always must be a consideration when you massage geriatric people. It is important to avoid deeper massage strokes on thinning skin. Most geriatric massages, in my experience, are clothes-on treatments with skin-to-skin contact only on the hands, face, and feet. This goes a long way in preventing skin tearing and bruising. But sometimes folks who are dressed in soft clothing that can be lifted out of the way, such as pyjamas, ask for massage oil and traditional and skin-to-skin massage.

Length of Massage Sessions

It is generally believed that sessions with seniors should be shorter than with younger people. Instead of a standard 60 minutes they are usually 30 minutes. For frail seniors, this is true, and it is always prudent to begin with short massages as you assess your geriatric patient. But as I discussed earlier, there are robust 90-year-olds and frail 65-year-olds. You can't clump people by age. Some senior patients will insist on longer and firmer massages. Even frail seniors are most commonly a one-hour massage!

Location of Massage Sessions

Another consideration is where the massage takes place. If you massage a person in their home or in their hospital bed, they don't have to dress, drive to a clinic, get on and off the table, then get dressed and drive home. They are not tired out by getting ready for a massage, and their post-massage recovery time is in their own bed at home, or at a care facility or the hospital.

I have never considered the length of a treatment with a home-call massage to be different for my geriatric or wheelchair patients. I have always done a minimum one-hour treatment and always checked in with my patients old or young, wheelchair users or mobility folks, about the focus of our massage and the timing within that hour. There are occasionally times when an hour is too much for a person, particularly in the case of palliative geriatric patients; this is why checking in is such an important part of the treatment.

Equipment

Something as simple as a lower massage table, or one with a hydraulic lift—a tip from Susan Salvo and Sharon Puszko, who have over and over proved to be such valuable resources—makes for safer, easier access for geriatric patients.

Geriatric Patients versus Palliative Patients

The conditions of geriatric and palliative wheelchair users often look similar, so it is not unusual for caregivers to lump them together. This is a mistake.

Some geriatric people are in wheelchairs due to long-standing problems in living an active lifestyle and suffering injuries. Some folks have long-term conditions that keep them permanently in wheelchairs in their senior years. But falls are the most common reason. Breaking a hip or injuring any part of the legs can quickly lead to wheelchair use, and the need for a wheelchair sometimes doesn't completely go away.

General weakness and muscle deterioration are common as a person ages, and more pronounced for people aging in wheelchairs. But geriatric patients are living for a long time using wheelchairs, and palliative patients are not long living. The objective of wheelchair use is different: geriatric users move into a wheelchair for lifestyle mobility and to remain independent, whereas palliative patients may move into a wheelchair for comfort, limited mobility, or socialization with their family.

While the conditions that arise in both situations might look similar, as a caregiver you need to understand and approach them differently.

1. A palliative person will rarely get out of the wheelchair and requires help whenever movement is required, whereas a geriatric person usually has some control over their movement. While your massage focus may be similar (surgery, dislocations, or replacement sites), your approach may differ. A geriatric patient can usually withstand more movement and a more intense massage.
2. It is not unusual for a person in palliative care to have kidney shutdown and the resulting swelling associated with that condition. It is unusual in a geriatric patient and should be flagged and reported to medical staff.
3. Both geriatric and palliative people are prone to constipation due to immobility of the hips, so leg pumping is indicated for both types of wheelchair massage. The lack of movement in general gives rise to a slowing down of digestive peristalsis. It is important in both palliative and geriatric care to keep the bowels moving. (Constipation due to medications is common.)
4. Pressure sores are always a problem waiting on the horizon in people with immobility issues. The geriatric person in a wheelchair rarely develops severe pressure-point soreness because they are stronger and can move themselves or simply ask for help to shift around in their chair. Palliative patients for the most part depend on others to turn or shift them in the chair, and are extremely vulnerable to pressure sores. On the other hand, geriatric people often spend far more time in the chair and have consistent pressure in vulnerable areas. There is no winning here! The point is to be ever vigilant in massaging these pressure sites with both groups.
5. Respiratory massage is particularly important in palliative patients. In palliative wheelchair massage, patients need a focus on respiratory massage to assist them in breathing comfortably. Geriatric people do not require the same focus on respiratory massage unless they have a specific respiratory condition.
6. The palliative person is wheeled in their wheelchair by someone else, so there is often someone available to massage them. A geriatric wheelchair person can usually wheel themselves, and being independent, they are without an automatic massage-opportunity person.
7. In wheelchair massage in general, there is a focus on massaging the shoulders and arms and hands, as these are the tools of locomotion for self-propelling users. When it comes to geriatric wheelers, they might not be as agile or strong as younger users. Hence, even more reason to focus with lots of time devoted to upper body massage.
8. In both palliative and geriatric wheelchair patients, dementia and anxiety can be present. Geriatric wheelers can have years of dementia or Alzheimer's disease and still benefit from wheelchair massage. Palliative patients can have delusions and other complications due to high levels of pain meds and find comfort in massage.
9. For both geriatric and palliative wheelchair users, the lower extremities remain a focal area for massage.

Basics of Geriatric Wheelchair Massage

1. A tilt-back wheelchair is often an advantage for making an elderly patient more comfortable. They can lean back to relax their head during their massage.
2. The best starting place is wherever the person indicates they would like you to start. When meeting a new patient, I find it most helpful to give them a simple diagram of the human body where they can show me their pain areas and where they would like me to begin.

3. I like to end the massage with a face and scalp massage. I lean the person back in the chair; if they don't have a headrest, I back the chair against a wall and insert a pillow behind their head for support. The face and scalp massage can be done from the front (face to face) or from the back of the chair.
4. When in doubt, starting with the hands is always a comfortable face-to-face introduction and then you can move from the arm massage to the legs.
5. Use all the adaptive therapist's postures of sitting on a stool, stride standing, standing on a stool, or kneeling and half kneeling.
6. Feedback, feedback! Throughout the massage, continue to ask about pressure, in particular. It's also useful to ask about places to focus for a minute before you move to a new area of the body.
7. Use an absorbent and healthy oil that will nourish the skin.
8. Use dry brushing to keep the skin healthy, either before or after the massage.
9. Whenever possible invite family, friends, and caregivers to massage along with you in tandem, so they can learn to do the wheelchair massage wherever they take their wheelchair user.
10. Use hot towels, hot water bottles, and heating pads to make the effects of your massage last longer.

VIDEO LIBRARY

Visit brusheducation.ca/wheeling-in-good-hands to watch these videos:

Bridging the gap: An introduction

Bridging the gap: Geriatric wheelchair massage – Vermont Square

Bridging the gap: Geriatric wheelchair massage – Nelson

Bridging the gap: Geriatric high school massage team – Fort St. John

Don

Don Grayston died after attending his friend Anna's album launch at the Museum of Vancouver in October, 2017. He said earlier in the month that he was keen to go to her concert, at which time I thought it would be out of the question, that he would be gone by then. We had been living in Cottage Hospice in Vancouver since that summer. I realized that my instant reaction to his request was typical: instead of yes, I was no—just to myself, not to Don. Later, as I ran in the early morning, I thought to myself: well, what's the worst that could happen? He dies en route, he dies at Anna's concert, he dies before the concert, he dies, he dies, he dies…he was dying anyway. The concert was his last request, his dying wish, so I could at least help make his wish come true.

During the next days and weeks, over the phone, I got to know everyone at the museum who had anything to do with Anna's concert. I made an appointment to work with the manager and scout the trip from beginning to end. I shopped a local thrift store for Don, looking for something dressy and exciting for the occasion. There were no sexy pants, so I settled on some baggy, academic, beige corduroy pants that would fit his anticipated diaper with no problem, and a blue blazer from Mexx.

The day of the concert, at three in the afternoon, I discovered that the wheelchair I had carefully reserved from the hospice could not be taken out of the building. I thought: worst-case scenario, we carry him some other way, on a stretcher maybe. Still, I needed to make another wheelchair appear.

I had seen Charlie, who lived in a room that I called "Club Med," with a great wheelchair that supported his head. He used it when his family took him around the hospice and the garden. Charlie immediately wanted to be part of Don's adventure. Charlie, speaking ever so slowly, told me that he would be honored to help. Happy with Charlie's chair, I wheeled it out of his room only to discover it did not have working brakes or a seatbelt! I had a plan for the seatbelt: I would tie Don into the chair with a belt big enough to secure him to the seat. The chair also needed a few adjustments, and I got one of the nurses to help take the chair apart so I could lower the headrest to give Don's head the best support. Having the chair apart now created the problem of putting it back together. We did that, too. Now to figure out the brakes! I tried without success to make the levers on Charlie's wheelchair respond. Great!! Basically, the Charlie chair sucked! But it was still a chair that could work for this outing.

Not telling Don every detail of my wheelchair troubles was important, as he was keen to get going and nothing was going to stop him attending Anna's concert. This was a matter of life and death in a different way: how to make this enjoyable instead of eventful, relaxed instead of stressful, fun instead of tense, full-blown Don instead of

Don diminished by approaching death. We talked out the details of the chair, clothing, timing, reservations for the wheelchair taxi, flowers for Anna, water to carry, and the many what-ifs!

"What will you do if you run into trouble, Christine?" the nurses asked in the days leading up to the concert, making sure I'd thought of everything.

"I'll call an ambulance," I responded.

I got the nurses to go over the procedures if I called an ambulance, how we could end up at the hospital instead of Cottage Hospice, and how it would be at the discretion of the ambulance staff about which way to go.

Every half hour before our departure for the concert, the nurses rehearsed me: "What will you do if you run into trouble?"

"I'll call an ambulance."

Then they outfitted me with drugs. I had hydromorphine to use as the last resort after the Advil. They carefully labeled the drugs and we made sure they lived in the most secure part of my purse. Then I showed Don our back-up drug supply and where it was, physically, in my purse. I was doing everything to reassure him that things would go well and smoothly. "Seeing is believing" was my protocol with Don.

We had only recently graduated to a more intimate pee protocol. He was under my strict orders to never do his peeing alone. I was threatening him with a permanent bedridden lifestyle to the end if he slipped and fell!

I wanted to be able to have him comfortable peeing into a diaper, but that was never to happen, as Don was not interested in practice sessions. He did agree, however, to a diaper for the outing, instead of a pull-up. We decided on a two-liter-capacity diaper. The nurse showed how it was able to wrap around and be opened easily and closed again without having to pull it down. She let Don know he could pee multiple times in the same diaper, and I had another diaper packed into my purse if we needed to change for any reason.

He was ready to get dressed. I thought that he would want a shave, but he opted for the trendy, slightly bearded look to go with the snazzy outfit. Only his hair was a problem. I wanted it to look particularly nice for tonight. I put some nice oil on my fingers and worked it into his hair. I was tempted to put my hair spray into the mix, but instead turned my focus to getting ready myself.

We waited in the living room of the hospice in front of the fireplace for people to admire us, wish us luck, and congratulate us on our adventure-to-be. We waited for our taxi and I watched the clock.

I had confirmed all day long with the taxi company, as it was their policy to not reserve cabs but to book one hour in advance. They made an exception for Don after I explained our situation, and they agreed to advance my request so I could report to Don that they were on their way.

I phoned, I reported to Don, and we were still waiting an hour later. I phoned again, and this time the same dispatcher announced that the taxi had been and gone. We did not know how, as we were guarding the entranceway oh so peacefully, but in an instant, the peace disappeared. We decided to wait outside in the cold, armed with blankets, and ready to jump the taxi on first sight.

I wheeled Don onto the sidewalk and along to the parking area. The taxi appeared and knew where to pull into the stall. The driver opened the door and his music blared. Instead of apologizing, he defended his actions, stating that he had been here already, and waited for us, and when no one answered his calls, he left. I started to get the feeling we were in trouble. I turned the chair from the side door of the taxi, expecting to be wheeling Don onto a hydraulic lift. Instead, the driver had lowered a sharp-sloped ramp.

I started to wheel Don onto the ramp, fully expecting the driver to help me push. He just stood there until Don said, "Christine, get him to help!" I was tangling up my gown in my fancy high-heeled shoes when the driver announced that he had never done this before! All the wheelchairs he had transported up until then had been electric and didn't need any help up this ramp. I was in desperation mode, and concerned about the evaporating timeline and depleting oxygen in the tank.

We got Don into the back of the taxi. I found the front hooks to secure the chair and latched them onto the front wheels of Don's chair. I expected that the driver was doing the same at the back of Don's chair. I settled into a space to hold Don's hand as the driver told me that I couldn't be back there with Don. I told him that I had to be holding Don's hand, that was part of the deal. That he couldn't be alone back there.

The driver told me that he couldn't start the vehicle unless I moved. I climbed over the back seat, hauling my long dress and sweater coat and purse with the diaper and water bottles, and reached back to grab Don's hand. I was not going to budge any further and the driver knew not to try further ultimatums.

As we pulled away from Cottage Hospice, we started up an incline that made the chair appear secure, as my front hooks were holding, but the chair seemed to move in a way that was disturbing. As we turned onto Dundas Street and a downhill slope, the chair started moving toward me. I was now gripping Don's hand as a rudder.

I called out to the driver, "Pull over!" He did. I asked him to secure the chair immediately. Don was attempting to say something critical when I overrode the comment and asked the driver how long he had been driving. I was collecting data for my next phone call to the owner of the taxi company. He said that he had been working for a few months and asked about Don. What was location where he had picked us up? I said that it was a hospice and Don was going to die soon. The driver said that Don didn't look like he was going to die. It seemed like he was prepared to debate the circumstances. I told him that Don was close to death and this was likely his last ride. The driver said he couldn't believe that, and I said it was hard to believe that all of us would die one day.

We finally arrived at the museum! I knew the building's layout very well, as I had maps of the wheelchair ramps and elevators as well as photographs. After exiting the taxi, we met with Dominique, Don's helper for the event. I soon spotted Anna, our performer, heading into the theater. I asked her to come over to Don, and she enthusiastically embraced him and cuddled up to his chair. Anna was gracious and Don was humming with delight, and Dominique also looked radiant behind the chair!

We made it into the theater when Don announced that he needed to pee. We were quickly shown to the washroom close by, and then Don attempted to get out of the chair. Undoing his belt and working his wrap diaper into the right position, I was struck with inspiration and reached for the mug that was in my purse. Don was too weak to stand but could hold onto each of the support braces secured into the wall of the urinal. We had lots of room to maneuver, and I got the mug in the right position and Don fired away. With a full cup of the good stuff and our laughter to finish off the feat, we wheeled back to the theater, all relieved.

Don listened with a big smile to Anna's first song after her welcoming introduction. Just as the concert was starting in full force, Don said that he was ready to leave, so I negotiated a deadline with him.

"How many songs would you like to try for?" I asked.

"Three."

"Three?"

"Well, maybe four." He paused and I said that I would order the taxi right away, and it could wait until he was ready to leave.

I called the wheelchair taxi company and got the boss. I told him how bad our experience had been coming to the concert and ordered the next taxi. He was extremely apologetic. I was accepting his apology when Don and his entourage came out of the theater.

"I'm ready to leave," Don announced.

We wrapped him in his blankets, and headed to the elevator. The taxi was arriving as we got to the front door. I directed it to come as close as possible. The driver introduced himself, shook Don's hand, asked us how our evening had been, and was gracious and kind, and smart and quick with the wheelchair handling. He took Don up the ramp into the back of the cab and I dove in for the front wheels hookup. Then he started getting the seat belts organized. I had never seen these belts and we had not used these belts in our previous ride. I was thrilled. We were in good hands.

I gave Don the oxygen-level report on his tank. We had a lot of oxygen left and, yes, we could drive Dominique home on our way to the hospice. This was fun again. Don was relaxing and Dominique was pure affection. Don was excited about the prospect of hosting a concert at the hospice and having Anna play to those invited by friends and family. He was full of ideas for hearing the rest of her concert in his own mini-concert venue at Cottage Hospice. He did not seem aware that his own final concert was coming up fast, where Anna would be his singing angel at his side.

We dropped Dominique off at her home, only five minutes from the museum, and our driver continued to the hospice along a route that was different from the route we had taken to the concert. Don had radar for this change and said, "Christine, tell our driver to get us back as fast as possible." I asked the driver to pull over. I hopped out of the van and told Don that I was going to check his oxygen levels. I opened the back doors, knowing we had a half tank of oxygen, but again wanting to make the point completely clear that we didn't have to rush home or anywhere for that matter. This was our last Saturday night out and last date and last dance. I wanted it to end well and relaxed, refreshed and revitalized.

I cheerfully and gleefully announced to Don that his levels were perfect, and I showed him the numbers on the tanks hanging off the back of his chair. "We are in great shape!" I pronounced into the big space between us, in the back, and our wonderful driver, in the front. "We don't have to worry or panic or rush." I squeezed his hand. Don knew this was his last ride and eventually settled back for the experience. Now everything was perfect. Now we were together, riding in our limousine, watching the water, the lights, and the ease with which our driver negotiated the drive. It was a pretty route home and I held Don's hand all the way. He looked like the king on his throne at the back of the van, shining in the dark.

We were sorry to have to leave the coziness of our cab and the company of our excellent chauffeur. He and Don had talked about literature and religion, which was normalizing in that moment. The delight of this ride erased the trauma of our earlier ride.

As we pulled up to Cottage Hospice, lit up with soft lights from Don's neighbor's room down the hall, I told the driver that we had him to thank for putting a lovely finishing touch to our evening. I asked him if he would like to pray with us. We paid him and tipped him and held hands for our favorite prayer. Then I took Don's wheelchair, and piled my purse and water bottle and pee mug into

Don's lap, and wheeled him slowly along the walkway from the parking lot to the garden. Some late-night dog walkers strolled by and we chatted and showed off our party clothes. As we pulled around to the front door, I paused. I stopped the chair.

Don asked, "Why are you stopping?"

I said, "Look at the fire!"

Ahead of us, through the front entrance, about twenty feet away, was the glass doorway to the living room of the hospice. The flickering fireplace looked so inviting. Our previous time of waiting in front of that fireplace two hours ago had ended badly, with stress and alarm. This time, I wanted us to have a nice time in front of the fire. I asked Don if we could have a drink in there and talk about the evening. He said that he thought that was a great idea, a talk would be nice. Our last fireside talk.

We wheeled into the living room and the warmth engulfed us. I parked Don's chair up close to the fireplace and went for drinks. Surprisingly, Don asked for juice, so I found the fanciest wine glasses in the dining room and poured drinks. I found some treats in our fridge that made the drinks look like we were being served in an exclusive setting. Don talked about the music and the people. He turned to me and said, "I liked how you handled our drivers, and I especially loved the way you handled our first driver. You treated him with respect for his questions, and you answered them bluntly and honestly. I like the way you say that I'm dying, that all of us are dying, and that he will die one day, too." Don remembered everything in the conversation. My talking and conversing was a religious experience for him.

That night Don had it all, the poetry of transition of making hard things soft and nasty things easy and sad things happy. He arrived back at Cottage Hospice happy, satisfied, and enthusiastic about life. He had a sense of fulfillment.

I didn't want this moment to ever end. I wanted to be here beside my friend forever. All those years of shared dreams and disappointments. Don was the first person to give me a significant opportunity to teach within spiritual circles. When he asked me to teach massage to a huge group of Anglican church professionals, all marriage counselors, I was in my element. So, my very first professional massage workshop was for the Anglican Synod of Canada, because of Don.

I most fondly remember Don watching me curl my hair as we got ready to go out. It was a rare moment, because I never fiddle with my hair, but I needed a hairdo to go with my strapless ball gown. Later that night, Don said his favorite memories of the evening were giving Anna her flowers and watching me curl my hair.

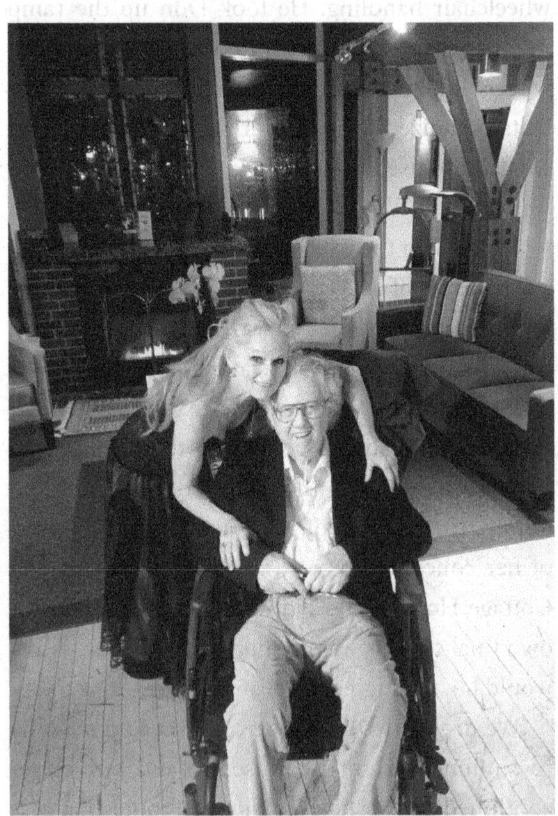

Don Grayston and me by the fireplace after our night out.

Now, all these years later, Don's enrichment was still running through me. He had been my friend and will always be my friend.

This would be the last time Don would be wheeling anywhere.

With Charlie's chair, I wheeled Don into his tiny room. I made haste to get his urinal lined up and encouraged him not to stand, as he was visibly weakening now. So in the wheelchair, we peed from a sitting position in Don's urinal. I was helping him like I had in the theater washroom, all hands-on, heart engaged. I knew when I transferred him to bed, this would be our last transfer. Getting Don out of his clothes and into his hospital gown was bittersweet, because I knew he would never wear those clothes again. I got ready for our nightly massage and movie.

Tonight we told stories as I massaged him. He slept earlier than usual, which I hoped indicated a good sleep for the whole night. Once he was asleep, I wheeled Charlie's chair back to his room, leaving a gift of chocolates on the seat. That last roll down the hallways of Cottage Hospice was a roll of significance. I thanked the invention of the wheel and the invention of the wheelchair for giving access to places previously difficult to travel, and most significantly, for giving my dying friend, Don, his last wish of attending Anna's concert.

The next morning, things changed for Don.

After the doctor's morning consultation, I entered Don's room for the last time. I asked him to open his eyes and look at me. I got up close in front of him. I told him that this was different. This was dying. This was the real thing. That he was now going for good. If we had been in the departure lounge, we were now boarding the plane. I asked him if we could do this together. He nodded. I asked him if he was ready, he nodded and then said, "Let's get organized."

I laughed. "We are organized! We are in the right place, and they're all organized and ready when you are."

We looked at each other. We were nose to nose. Don whispered, "Let's go."

"I'm with you, we're going. You've done a great job, Don. We are ready to fly."

This is it.

With relief, he settled back into the bed, his mouth already in a relaxed open O.

Don's story was my shortest and most powerful experience of the miracle of the wheelchair and wheelchair massage. I could not have given my friend the best Saturday night date of his life were not for the invention of the wheel. We massaged with the same principles of sports massage: before and after the event (and during the event) for endurance in the chair. We massaged as soon as we got home to the hospice. We were able to linger in our outfits in front of the fireplace with our juice and club soda in fancy glasses, as I gave Don his last fireside wheelchair massage!

Don's last night of continuous massage is how I wish everyone could go, after the best outing ever in the final hours of their life with wheels underneath them!

I'll never forget Don's gentle last words, "Let's go…"

Thank you Don and Ginger for that first-ever massage in Spokane, Washington, at the spa. That massage changed my life forever.

11

Palliative Wheelchair Users

In my book *Dying in Good Hands*, I cover what everyone needs to know about palliative massage. I'm not going to repeat all of that information here. This chapter is about the particular needs of, and opportunities for, palliative patients when they use wheelchairs.

Why Wheelchairs Are Useful in Palliative Care

Wheelchairs are becoming a more common part of palliative care. Dying people are usually weak and their legs no longer have dependable strength or endurance. A wheelchair allows them to stay connected with life outside the bedroom, hospital room, or hospice. With the help of friends who have learned to navigate their chair and keep them comfortable, a dying person has freedom of choice. Do they want to sit up, recline, lie down, or go outside for a car ride? My stepmom, Valerie, wanted a car ride to visit the places where she'd grown up and her original family home. Other patients might want to sit outside in their garden or visit family in their living room.

Some families never consider short-term wheelchair use because they're already stressed when a family member moves into palliative care, and trying to locate a chair can be a daunting experience. It is worth remembering that, in Canada, the Red Cross has a lending library of equipment of all kinds, and a quick loan of a wheelchair for a month, a week, or even a few days might make all the difference in the care of a dying person. And it is free!

A wheelchair also opens the door for the family to be more involved in caring for their loved one. Wheeling the person around gives family members a job to do! It is also easier to massage a person in a wheelchair. There is comfortable access to the hands, feet, head, neck, and shoulders and all members of the family can get involved.

A wheelchair can be a ticket to travel and massage on the run. A palliative client of mine became the center of the universe for two of my summer school students. Their massages were her best medicine. They used the wheelchair to take her out to see the northern lights in the middle of the night. They took her out on the hospital balconies to watch the stars, with champagne to toast her. They massaged her constantly. Her skin was a living testimonial to the hands-on care she received. She was smooth, with no pressure sores on her skeletal frame.

It is not rocket science to learn wheelchair massage and it is one of the best ways to alleviate the daily aches and pains of a person who is dying. Palliative patients in a wheelchair are no different than palliative patients in a bed. Whether they are sitting up or lying down, there is the same natural progression as their systems shut down. They might be able to eat one day and then not the next. There are often difficulties with breathing, digestion, and communication. Whatever the circumstance, some people prefer a wheelchair to the very end, others prefer being in bed. It is as easy and comfortable to massage a person in a wheelchair as it is to massage them in a bed.

In my own family, my mother, for the last two months of her life, couldn't walk, but she could stand and transfer easily to a wheelchair. She loved going for walks, so the two of us, along with my dog with his leash tied to the chair, became a common sight on Nelson's streets. It was a wonderful experience. People who had known her would stop to say hello, others would hold doors or lift the wheelchair, and because she was in the chair, I was able to massage her in the park or wherever she wanted to stop. Wheelchairs gave both my "moms" the ability to do what they wanted to do with the short time they had left.

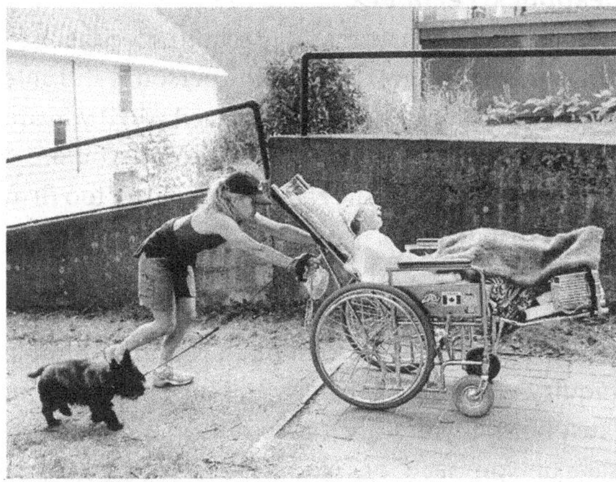

Out for a walk with my mom.

The palliative wheelchair life might be short-lived, but it need not be ill-lived. Although I dressed my mom every day in her favorite dresses and jewelry, she could have easily been wheeling around in her pyjamas. She had a beautiful soft blue mohair blanket that I loved to see on her bed in the last two years of her life. I used that blanket to cover her and keep her warm. She was very tiny and, like an infant, would heat up fast and cool just as quickly. I brought hot water bottles on our walks in case she became chilled in the night air. With no pressure about time, wheeling around in the night is a very pleasant activity. The absence of daily tension and just the ambling nature of wheeling along is a smooth and satisfying experience. Those wheelchair walks and wheelchair massages were the best memories of my mom's last days.

Key Considerations in Palliative Wheelchair Massage

Comfort

I repeat this over and over to my students and to families: each palliative case is different; each circumstance is unique; and each person has their own path. But in palliative massage, there is one major consideration: comfort.

It's best to start with a light touch. Unlike other massage contexts—sports massage, for instance—maximizing therapeutic resistance and depth of pressure is not the goal. This means that in palliative massage, if you are working skin to skin, you can use more oil than you would otherwise.

The lifespan of the person who is dying is shorter, maybe only weeks or months of life left. It's important to provide the comfort and therapy of wheelchair massage right away. There is no time to waste, not many days to live.

Pressure Sores

In palliative massage, pressure sites are a primary focus. As a person's circulatory system begins to fail, places where there is pressure and where blood doesn't flow properly can become inert and start to die. This leads to sores, infection, and sepsis. It's painful and deadly.

A wheelchair means that the pressure of the body weighs on the bones where a person sits, or where they rest their head or hips. In a palliative condition, people lose weight, and their bones have very little padding. As a result, there is direct pressure wherever their body rests. These pressure sites are one of the most important places to focus in palliative wheelchair massage.

All the usual sites are important: the back of the head, the ears if the patient is lying reclining on their side, head of the hip (femur), elbows, sacrum, sides of knees, heels of the feet, and ankle-bones. Some wheelchairs also put pressure against the person at their hips on either side of them, so paying attention to the head of the femur is also important. The ridge of the shoulder blade (spine of the scapula) is another area that can break down.

Pressure sores are more likely to be a danger as the person loses weight. When people have stopped eating, they usually lose weight quickly, and the padding they once had to protect their bony bumps no longer exists and might not ever come back.

Sheepskins are by far the best cushions for allowing the skin to breathe, thus preventing pressure sores. The unique corkscrew structure of sheep wool allows better ventilation for the skin and is highly absorbent at the same time. Sheepskins on the seat of the chair and back of the chair are as important as a seatbelt.

A wheelchair that has a variation of sitting and leg positions is also very useful, if you can find one. These chairs can tilt back or even lie flat, and the leg rests can be lifted or dropped. By changing positions, palliative people can avoid extended pressure on bony sites.

Swelling in the Extremities

Palliative people often experience swelling in their lower body as their circulatory system slows down. Many people have extreme and painful swelling (edema) in the legs. I've learned over years of treating palliative patients and teaching palliative massage that, when the kidneys start to fail, overextended skin in the lower extremities is one of the main danger areas. The skin is so thin and so stretched that it easily opens if there is pressure too long in one position.

An important part of your palliative massage is to keep the blood moving toward the heart to help to reduce the swelling. As you massage, remember the valves in the arteries have small gates that open only one way—toward the heart. Pushing with any pressure in the opposite direction works against natural blood flow and is not beneficial.

The exception is reflex strokes. These are very light strokes that go against the principle of massaging toward the heart. I use them for beginnings and endings, and for pain control if the palliative person cannot be firmly touched.

Respiratory Massage

When someone is in a wheelchair, we think of them as sitting upright. This is the easiest way to breathe. We use all the respiratory strokes to unwind the thoracic tension so the person can take deeper breaths and gain more oxygen to keep more comfortable. All the massage strokes that we do in a lying-flat style of wheelchair massage can be used in a seated position.

Remember that as a palliative person weakens and struggles to breathe, sitting more and more upright makes it easier for them to breathe. A wheelchair can be helpful in this context, especially with a dedicated team to provide respiratory massage. Respiratory wheelchair massage should include strokes to ease and loosen breathing, and also routines to get the lungs clear of congestion.

Feedback, Feedback!

Learning wheelchair massage requires feedback to tell you how you are doing. If the person is still able to communicate, they can always tell you if you are on the right track. They can tell you if you are a little to the left or to the right, or if you are too firm or not firm enough.

If they are too weak to talk or form sentences, you can ask questions that make it easy for them to nod in agreement. Or to blink in response. Simple inquiry works best for nods and for blinks—as in, "Just blink if you'd like me to do some more massage on your feet," or "Nod if I can be firmer." The dying person might be speaking one day and not the next. Weakness can come and go at random.

Massage Frequency and Duration

Palliative wheelchair massage has to be extremely adaptable. The timing can go sideways with hospital procedures to do, professionals coming and going, and friends coming to say goodbye or spend time with the person who is dying. The dying person is also changing. The symptoms of their disease as they are closer to death constantly change. Respiration, digestion, and circulation are challenged. There are never going to be easy conditions, circumstances, and timing to perform wheelchair massage. Whenever the person is in the wheelchair is a good time.

I like to see someone massaged in preparation for transferring to the wheelchair, so the transfer is easy, and the person's muscles are flexible.

Then a "settling" massage to get the body used to the seated position in the wheelchair after the transfer. Some positive tactile reinforcement for conditioning the person to feel comfortable in the wheelchair is important. Then a mini-massage on the hour, just like most of us shift our body weight after long sitting periods at our computers writing books or watching movies. The body needs to shift every hour and the massage can be that perfect shift in circulation.

I like to do a quick massage once around the bases—arms, legs, back, hips, hands, and feet—and then the finishing touch on the head neck and shoulders! This is the quick fifteen-minute walk around the block! This kind of positive patterning can give the person a rejuvenating nap after your rub; or it can give them the emotional enthusiasm to make a phone call or venture out (wheeling) into the garden.

When the person is transferred to the bed for the evening, the before-and-after massage principle is in effect. They can get a massage before the transfer, and after the transfer to stretch them out again.

Massaging after a few hours in the chair is important for physical relief. You might be massaging more times per day because the pain management demands that. You might massage the person in the wheelchair in the morning and then in bed after that. You might massage the person in the chair all day long. You might massage for fifteen minutes every hour, or massage for an hour three times in one day, or do a three-hour massage. With ever-changing end-of-life symptoms, your palliative wheelchair massage adapts to those changes.

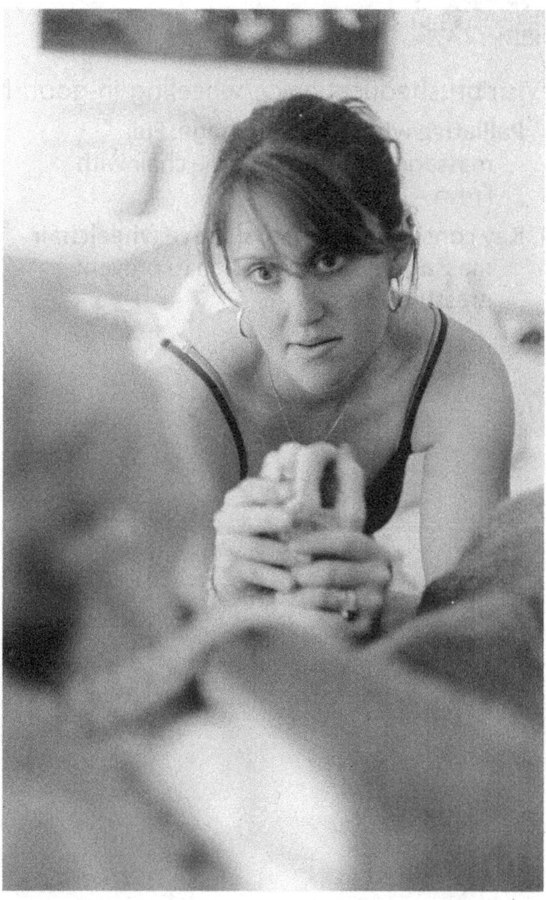

My daughter, Crystal, massaging my mom. Crystal can still feel her grandmother's hand at the tips of her fingers.

VIDEO LIBRARY

Visit brusheducation.ca/wheeling-in-good-hands to watch these videos:

Palliative wheelchair massage: Full massage routine out of the chair with Freya

Key considerations in palliative wheelchair massage: Using sheepskin to prevent pressure sores

Key considerations in palliative wheelchair massage: An introduction to swelling in the extremities – in the classroom with George

Key considerations in palliative wheelchair massage: Massage routine for swelling of the extremities with Don

12

Maternity Wheelers

Pregnancy has special issues for wheelchair users. These issues are the focus of this chapter, because they are massage priorities for pregnant wheelers over and above what you would do for every mom-to-be.

My book *Birthing in Good Hands* covers massage for every phase of pregnancy, from the first trimester to the postpartum "fourth trimester." The routines in that book apply to every mom-to-be, whether a wheelchair user or not.

We typically have two kinds of maternity wheelchair users: long term and short term.

Long-term maternity wheelers have conditions like cerebral palsy, spina bifida, muscular dystrophy, MS, and spinal cord injuries. These conditions involve legs that have special needs; backs that are curving creatively; and arms that are challenged from wheeling manually, or necks that are challenged from wheeling electrically.

Women who are already in a wheelchair before their pregnancy are very experienced with the aches and pains of wheelchair living. They are well aware of the problems that occur in the lower back and lower extremities due to the circumstances that landed them in the chair in the first place.

Short-term maternity wheelchair users are women who are able-bodied, but need a wheelchair because of their pregnancy symptoms. Examples of symptoms include severe sciatica; the physical demands of carrying twins, triplets, or quadruplets; and hip, knee, and foot problems. Some preexisting conditions, although walkable in pre-pregnancy, are not walkable during pregnancy.

Doctors may recommend bed rest for some maternity conditions—for example, placenta abnormalities and a history of preterm labor. I advocate using a wheelchair as an alternative to bed rest, so women can get outside and be active, and I advocate massage as a way to make the time in the chair less stressful and more comfortable.

Using a wheelchair for a short term can also be helpful postpartum. A long and difficult labor can leave a woman needing assistance with mobility. Mobility issues postpartum can make it difficult for new moms to hold their baby, change diapers, or breastfeed. Learning to do these postpartum activities from a wheelchair is often an asset to speedy recovery.

When teaching in Guatemala, I was educated about giving birth without proper epidural applications. The resulting pain and discomfort that I witnessed, and addressed and treated, could have also been helped by wheelchair use postpartum. These women were not well and were unsteady on their feet, and could have been instantly helped by using a wheelchair.

All pregnancies with wheelchair users are made less stressful and more comfortable with hands-on help. Massage is such a portable tool for what is needed. Often, pregnancy prohibits the use of pain relievers, so the ancient medical art of massage is a way to provide relief.

It is my hope that wheelchair massage will be more commonplace in the world of maternity massage. When I taught maternity wheelchair massage in Nelson, British Columbia, I had an outdoor class in a park. As we sailed down main street to the park, one of the pregnant moms had her two-year-old riding on her footrests, like the figurehead on the prow of a sailing ship. This was a kid who considered maternity wheelchair massage the norm. The internet makes it easy to read stories of pregnant wheeling women and access valuable resources, like Dani Izzie's blog. She is a C5-C6 quadriplegic who writes about her life as a mother of twins, and her experience of being pregnant and giving birth to them. AbleThrive is another indispensable resource for wheelchair women and their support teams, as it offers stories of women in chairs thriving as mothers. These women offer insights and advice in order to help other women who are embarking on the journey of pregnancy in a chair.

Adapting Maternity Massage for the Wheelchair

A wheelchair is not a barrier to maternity massage, anymore than it is barrier to geriatric or palliative massage. In any situation, as a massage therapist, you have to adapt to the circumstances of your patient.

A key issue in maternity labor massage is applying counterpressure to the sacrum, especially during contractions, to relieve the overwhelming pressure on the lower back.

When the mom is in a wheelchair, you can get good counterpressure in a stride position, with one foot ahead of the other as though you were starting a race. If you're standing at the side of the mom, straddle the wheel so one foot is behind the back of the wheelchair. This position stabilizes and saves your back.

Don't rely on strength in your arms and hands alone, as they will tire quickly. Use the back of the wheelchair for leverage, resting your arms on the chair.

If the mom is in a backless or low-back sports wheelchair, you can use a stride position to lean on her lower back with her wheelchair braked to resist

FIGURE 12.1. Compression to the Sacrum

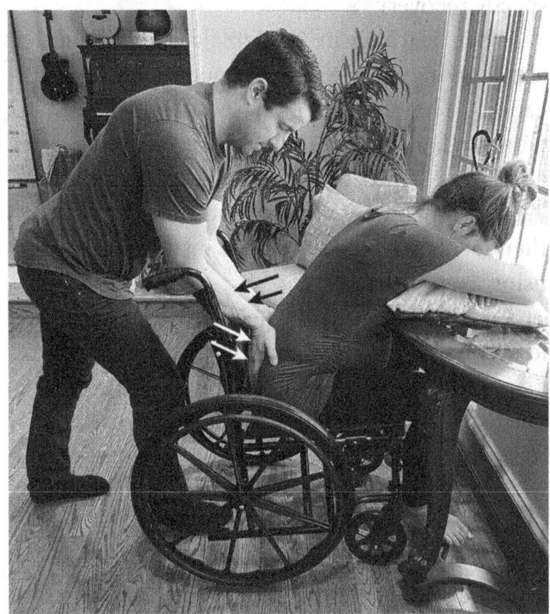

Side-by-side palmar compression.

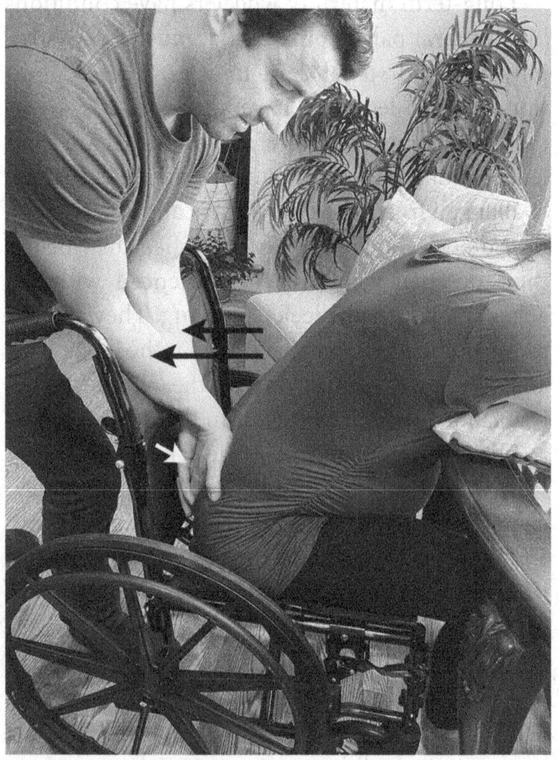

Reinforced palmar compression with stride posture.

FIGURE 12.1. CONTINUED

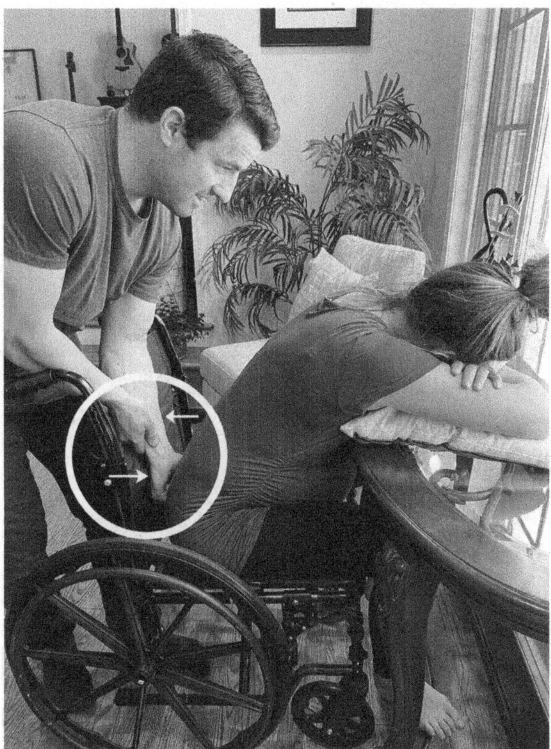

Reinforced single-handed fisted compression to sacrum.

you. Lean or move forward to put your full body weight behind your hands. If you are not a big person, be sure to keep your arms straight for more power, lean forward, and distribute that hand pressure right down your arm. With my small stature, I use my entire body weight behind my hands using a straight arm, stride standing posture.

Key Issues of Pregnant Wheelchair Users

Maternity symptoms can be treated in the wheelchair or in a stretched-out horizontal position out of the chair. The massages can be done through clothing or skin on skin. They can be mini-massages three times a day, or longer massages once a day or every couple of days. The schedule that I advocate is daily massages in the last month of pregnancy, whether the mom is a first-time wheelchair user or a seasoned wheelchair user.

The priority issues for pregnant wheelers are often more intense versions of issues that many wheelers already have. The massage routines for treating them are the same, and are covered in detail in chapter 4.

Headaches

Headaches are common in pregnancy, and can be related to fluid retention, especially in the second and third trimesters. Wheelchair users are already at risk of swelling due to compromised circulation from sitting in the chair for long periods of time. Often, massaging the extremities (arms and legs) where fluid tends to collect relieves headaches. Massage to relieve neck and shoulder stress is also important.

Neck and Shoulder Stress

Every pregnant woman will have bigger breasts by the second and third trimesters, which will cause a change in the dynamic tension of the neck and shoulders. Pregnant women in manual wheelchairs will likely need more neck and shoulder massages to adapt to their changing shoulder dynamics.

Shoulder dynamics will also change as the baby gets bigger and causes more pressure in the hips and lower abdomen. This pulls the upper body forward, rounding the shoulders. Fingertip kneading on the neck and shoulders, with lots of palmar scooping to the trapezius muscle, will help relieve this growing problem.

Carpal Tunnel Syndrome

This is a condition that afflicts a lot of wheelchair users, and it is also common in pregnancy, due to swelling in all the extremities. So, massage to reduce swelling in the extremities is crucial to treat and prevent this painful syndrome, which results from a pinching of the median nerve that runs from the neck to the hand.

It is an important condition to avoid in pregnant wheelers. Carpal tunnel syndrome, when severe, is usually treated by splinting the wrists overnight—sometimes even during the day. This makes wheeling difficult, and wheeling with a baby very difficult. Massage helps to diminish pain and restore circulation by reducing edema (swelling) throughout the entire arm.

Constipation

Constipation is another common issue in pregnancy that adds to an already common issue caused by immobility. This makes the pregnant tummy an important focus of massage, to replace the positive stimulation of walking and running on digestion. Double up on the abdominal massage for pregnant wheelchair users, so the passive activity of massage replaces the muscular activity of mobility.

As the baby grows, we need to continually massage from back to front, from the armpits to the hips. For pregnant wheelchair users, the pressure of the baby against their hips and lower abdomen becomes the focus of our massage to relieve their growing discomfort. Relieving constipation avoids hemorrhoids, which are uncomfortable in any stage of pregnancy, in labor and delivery, and in postpartum recovery.

Spinal Problems

Wheelchair pregnancies often produce back problems that can lead to spinal deformities if not treated right away. Weight gain during pregnancy, and the growing weight of the baby, accentuate preexisting back problems and can pull the spine further into uncomfortable curvatures. For example, if a woman has scoliosis (a lateral curve of the spine), it will take a great deal of pulling during the second and third trimesters. We need to address the spine with daily back massages in the chair to ensure prevention.

Hip Problems

Hip problems can develop during pregnancy because of hormone changes that cause hypermobility in the pelvis.

Many wheeling women have problems with their hips before pregnancy, simply from sitting in a wheelchair every day for too many hours. By the second and third trimesters of a pregnancy, they may feel like *all* their problems are in their hips. The side-lying basic hip massage can be doubled, done on a daily or twice-daily basis, such as first thing in the morning and last thing at night. This will help the pregnant mom sit more easily until she delivers.

FIGURE 12.2. Hip Massage in the Wheelchair

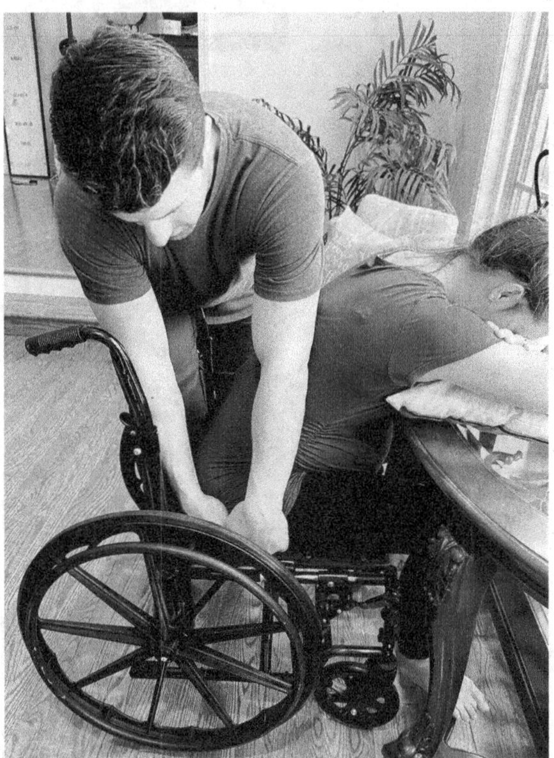

Hips of wheeling moms-to-be can also be massaged in the chair. This shows double levering to right ischial tuberosity and head of the femur.

Even walking women who have never had a hip problem before pregnancy may develop hip problems during their last two trimesters, and some may become short-term wheelchair users. A side-lying lower back and leg massage will keep the tension from building up in the hip.

Knee and Foot Problems

Some walking women develop problems with their knees and feet during pregnancy. Weight gain, fluid retention, and hormone changes can lead to problems or make existing problems worse. Knee and foot problems can compromise mobility and make wheelchair use a practical step during pregnancy.

For these women, focused massage on the knees and feet is important to maintain circulation and flexibility for when the mom is ready resume walking postpartum.

Focused knee massage is also key for pregnant long-term wheelchair users. The knee joints can become very contracted in long-term users, which can complicate leg positions during labor and delivery. Massaging the entire leg, with a focus on the knee and hip joints, will make labor and delivery more comfortable.

Sciatica

Pregnancy can lead to sciatica, or make existing sciatica worse. The growing baby pulls the lordotic curve out of alignment, putting extra pressure on the sciatic nerve. This is true for both pregnant wheeling women and non-wheeling women. Walking women with chronic sciatica may want to use a wheelchair toward the end of a pregnancy. The chair will help her keep up with the crowd, walk the dog, get to the pool, or go out for dinner. A pregnant woman with sciatica can receive a hip and lower back massage right through her clothes while in a wheelchair, even in the middle of a public event, so she can reestablish comfort and reduce pain without having to go home.

A thorough in-chair massage under the hips and including the lower back can immediately relieve this painful condition and give the wheeling mom more tolerance to be in the chair.

I always use an "egg carton" cushion on the seat of the wheelchair, even for short-term wheelchair use.

Swelling in the Lower Extremities

Wheeling women who have been in chairs for years due to spinal cord injury, chronic disease, or other mobility impairments know the benefits of massage for the lower extremities. Sitting in a wheelchair compromises circulation, which leads to swelling in the legs, ankles, and feet. Pregnancy adds fluid retention to this chronic problem. In pregnant wheelers, massaging the lower legs and feet is particularly important to maintain circulation, relieve swelling, and reduce fluid retention.

FIGURE 12.3. **Single-Handed Effleurage to the Gastrocnemius**

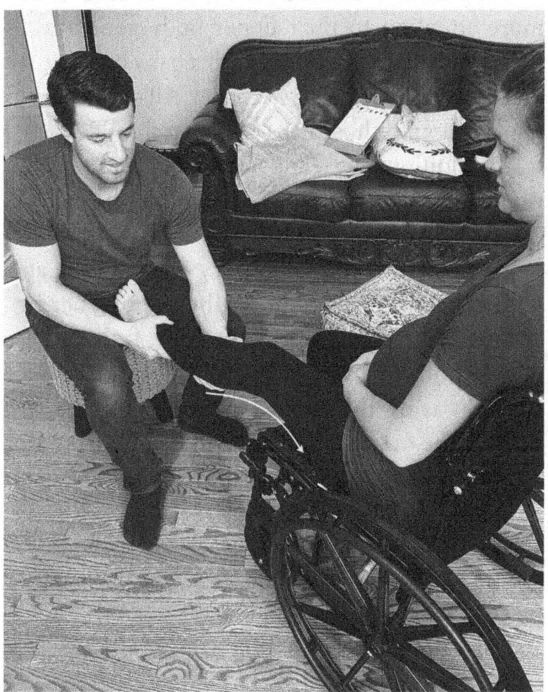

Single-handed effleurage to the gastrocnemius must go above the popliteal fossa to get the swelling out of the lower leg, reducing skin tension and improving circulation.

Leg massages also help prevent varicose veins, which can be caused by immobility and by pregnancy—so, another "double risk" for pregnant wheelers. I avoid directly massaging any varicose veins already present. I skip over them, and massage around them. It's very important to thoroughly massage the legs even when varicose veins are present.

Postpartum Massage Priorities

For long-term wheeling moms, I always advocate for extra massages for the head, neck, shoulders, and arms.

The ability to recover arm strength quickly is important, just like in wheelchair sports massage.

In addition, these moms may be using the arms of their chair to support breastfeeding postures. In the first week postpartum, this can make the neck feel like it has whiplash, so you can never do enough head, neck, and shoulder massage in the first week postpartum.

Long-term wheeling moms also need much more attention to their upper body generally, as they are now maneuvering with a baby on their lap or slung on their chest in a carrier. All of this brings new tension to those hard-working shoulders.

In addition, wheeling moms may also experience feelings of loss postpartum, during the "fourth trimester." This is especially true for someone who has a spinal cord injury. She has been able to feel the movement of her baby through her fingertips. Touching her growing baby, feeling these new sensations, can result in feelings of loss once the baby is on the outside. Massaging her whole body in the fourth trimester brings comfort to this "empty" feeling.

Wheeling Pregnancy Partners and Maternity Massage

Let's not forget that pregnancy partners can themselves be in wheelchairs. There are lots of ways for them to massage from the chair, including during labor.

I have taught wheeling dads-to-be to provide hands-on support, not only for the symptoms of pregnancy that massage can help, but also for the pain management of labor and delivery.

This is not limited to future parents. It can include any wheeling relatives or friends who are invited to the birth or hands-on during the pregnancy for symptom treating. A team of maternity massagers might have senior moms or wheeling friends eager to help.

FIGURE 12.4. Examples of Massage from Wheeling Pregnancy Partners

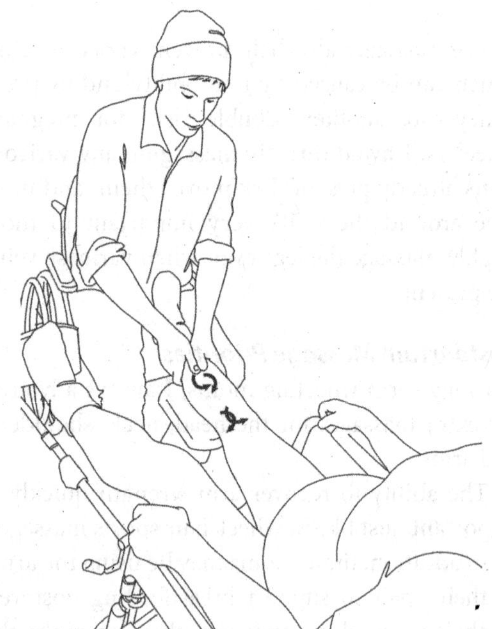

A wheeling partner provides a leg massage to a wheeling mom-to-be.

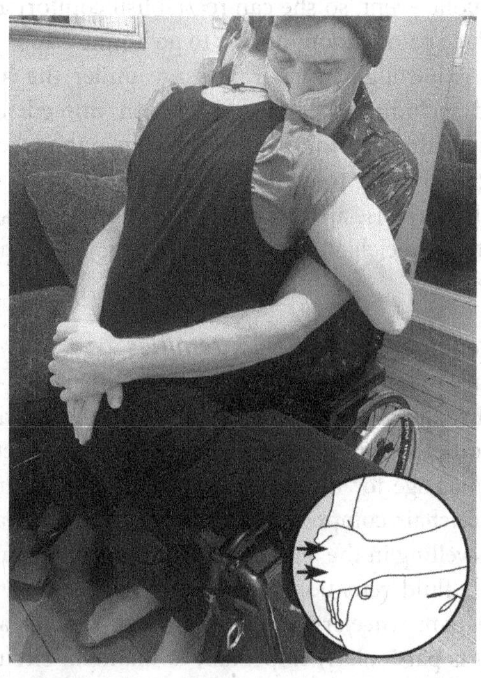

Counterpressure on the sacrum, where a walking mom takes a chest-to-chest posture with a wheeling partner.

FIGURE 12.4. CONTINUED

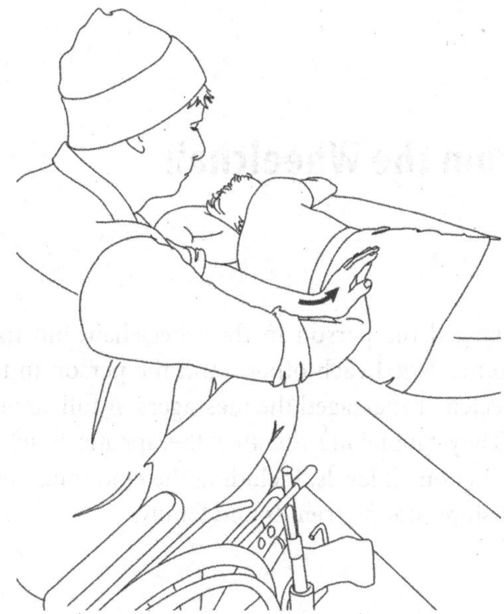

Counterpressure on the sacrum from a wheelchair, where the mom is side-lying.

VIDEO LIBRARY

Visit brusheducation.ca/wheeling-in-good-hands to watch these videos:

- **Maternity massage for the wheelchair:** Compression to the sacrum with Kimberly
- **Maternity massage for the wheelchair:** Compression to the sacrum – hug technique with Kimberly
- **Maternity massage for the wheelchair:** Key issues of pregnant wheelchair users – headaches and neck stress
- **Maternity massage for the wheelchair:** Key issues of pregnant wheelchair users – arms and carpal tunnel syndrome
- **Maternity massage for the wheelchair:** Key issues of pregnant wheelchair users – digestive massage for constipation
- **Maternity massage for the wheelchair:** Key issues of pregnant wheelchair users – mobilizing the hip
- **Maternity massage for the wheelchair:** Key issues of pregnant wheelchair users – leg massage
- **Wheeling pregnancy partners and maternity massage:** Counterpressure on the sacrum
- **Wheeling pregnancy partners and maternity massage:** Counterpressure on the sacrum – straddle technique

13

Reciprocity and Massaging from the Wheelchair

Whenever I have taught wheelchair massage, I have always included the "payback" aspect. It is important for those in wheelchairs to learn to give massages, because it builds confidence about expressing their caring through touch. Rather than always receiving the massage treatment, it is a different kind of empowerment to be able to give a massage from their vantage point in their wheelchair.

In this book, I have talked about many people living in wheelchairs and their massage teams. Their massage teams taught me about the power of touch working both ways. The teams not only massaged the person in the wheelchair, but they also massaged each other—and the person in the wheelchair massaged the massagers. A full circle!

They taught me too that therapeutic touch is healing on all levels, including the emotional relationships among friends and family.

The Massage Exchange

A massage exchange is a great way to build skills for massage teams and for wheelchair users. And

FIGURE 13.1. A Massage Exchange

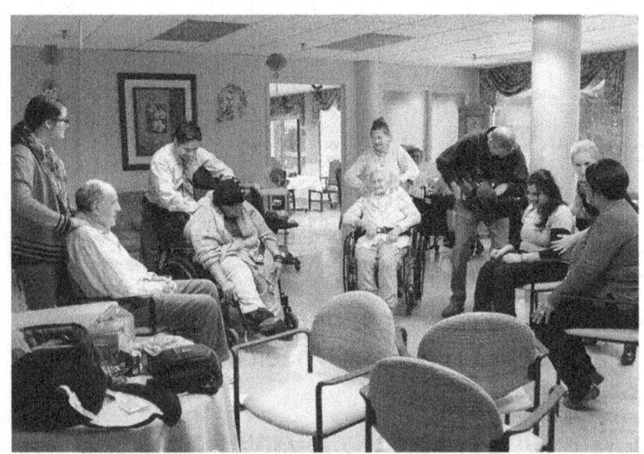

A group of us in a massage session.

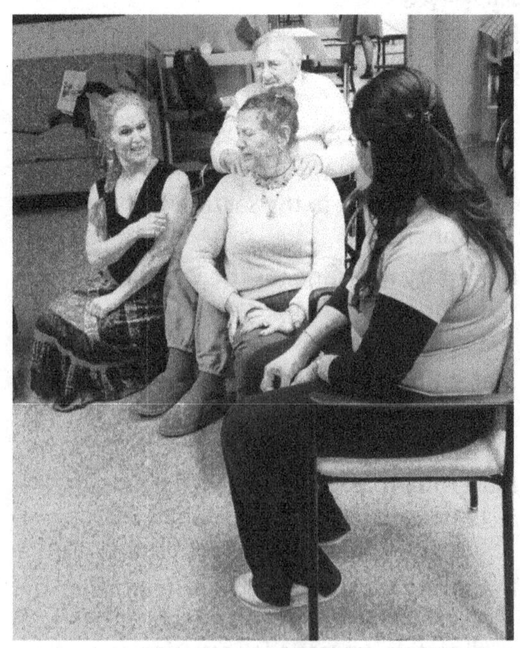

A mother from the group returning the favor by massaging her daughter.

setting one up is extremely important for the physical and emotional well-being of wheelchair users.

While you are teaching a team of friends and family to massage a wheelchair user's shoulders, and their arms and hands, you are also teaching the wheelchair user how to massage! They can repeat that back to you, or back to their caregivers, hands-on.

A massage exchange empowers everyone to give and get massage.

Routines for Massaging from the Wheelchair

For most of this book, I haven't talked directly to wheelchair users. But now I will. If you are someone living in a wheelchair, and you want to learn how to massage your family and friends, read on!

First of all, a massage doesn't have to be elaborate to be effective or welcomed. You can do mini-massages, which are short massages for one part of the body. You can start with a part of the body that is easily accessible to you in your wheelchair. The shoulders are often a good target. If you can't access the shoulders, you can probably still access the hands and arms.

There are two positions that I teach for massaging shoulders from your wheelchair. One is to have the person you are massaging in front of you, sitting in a chair. The other is to have the person sitting down low, either on the floor or squatting on your footrests; the person can use your knees for support, either by leaning back or draping their arms. If they are able-bodied and flexible, they can squat or sit on the floor for ten minutes to get their shoulders massaged.

If the person is seated in front of you in a chair, wheel as close as you can to them. Usually your knees will touch the back of their chair. Make sure they are leaning back toward you. Alternatively, the person can lean forward on a stool and you can wheel close to them, first on one side and then the other.

If anyone you are massaging is a fellow wheeler—maybe it's your pregnancy partner—you can still get your chair as close as possible, sometimes even wheeling slightly under them if their wheelchair is slightly higher than yours.

Head, Neck, and Shoulder Routine from the Wheelchair

The difference between rubbing someone's shoulders and massaging someone's shoulders is knowledge of the structure of the body and knowledge of strokes. To massage, you need to be versed in some technical details.

But, as I've said before, massage is not rocket science, and once you have practiced what to do, your hands will contain the knowledge you need, and you will be able to apply the technical details by feel, without the terminology.

So don't be daunted by the terminology, and don't forget to consult the diagrams that show the major muscles of the body and basic massage strokes in chapter 2.

The routine that follows has the person you are massaging sitting on a chair. If you are massaging someone sitting on your footrests, or on the floor, you may need to skip some steps described here. Like all massage therapists, you have to work with the situation you are given and adapt!

1. Start with the person sitting in front of you. They can sit in a chair or they can sit your footrests.
2. Place both hands on the person's shoulders and give a bilateral squeeze: the natural, "what-you-do-at-home" squeeze. Then, develop the squeeze, giving greater scoops of the trapezius with the heel of your hand. You and the person should take a deep breath with each lift of the trapezius muscle. Breathe and squeeze.
3. Next, massage the rhomboids. With the thumbs of each hand, compress the rhomboids bilaterally from the shoulders (cervical) to the bottom (scapular). The fingers are left up on the shoulders and the wrists rotate to get the proper movement. This area can be quite tight. Be sure to check with your person that your pressure is accurate. Work higher and lower each time up and down the neck and shoulder area. Stay close to the spine, on

FIGURE 13.2. Massage Positions from the Chair

SITTING ON THE FOOTRESTS

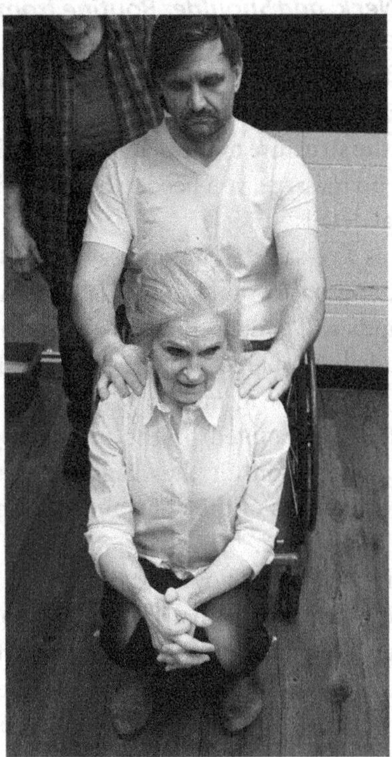

I sit on the footrests of Bo Hedges' wheelchair for a shoulder massage.

MASSAGING CHAIR TO CHAIR

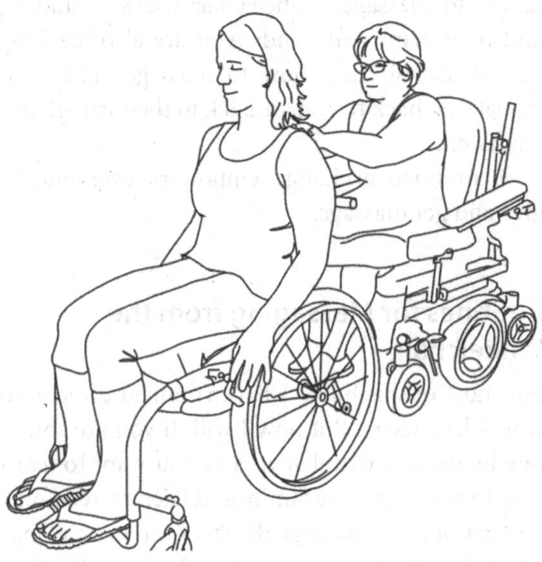

Of course, *both* chairs can have wheels!

the erector spinae muscles. Keep your thumbs at the same speed and rhythm.

4. Wheel to the side of the person and place one hand on the forehead and one at the base of the skull. Slowly rotate the head three times in each direction. Pivot the head on the top of the spine. Do this slowly.
5. Wheel to the back of the person and place your fingertips on the temples. Slowly knead all around the jaw and the temples.
6. Apply the following strokes to the trapezius, deltoids, and rhomboids: loose fingertip hacking, stiff fingertip hacking, cupping, beating, and pounding.
7. Have the person lean forward. Wheel to the side and work the midback.
8. Do the shoulder squeeze again three times.
9. Do the head rotations again.
10. Apply reflex stroking lightly with your fingertips from top of the head and out the shoulders and arms, and then from the top of the head down the spine.

Arms and Hands Routine from the Wheelchair

1. Start at the shoulders with palmar kneading and use alternate thumb kneading down the arm to the hand with pressure up toward the heart.
2. Apply bilateral wringing to the biceps and triceps and forearm.
3. Massage the hand with alternate thumb kneading and corkscrew each finger.
4. Have the person raise their arm straight up, elbow locked. Apply brisk, palmar wringing to entire arm as fast as you can.
5. Apply light reflex stroking to the entire arm to finish.

FIGURE 13.3. Hand and Arm Massage from the Wheelchair

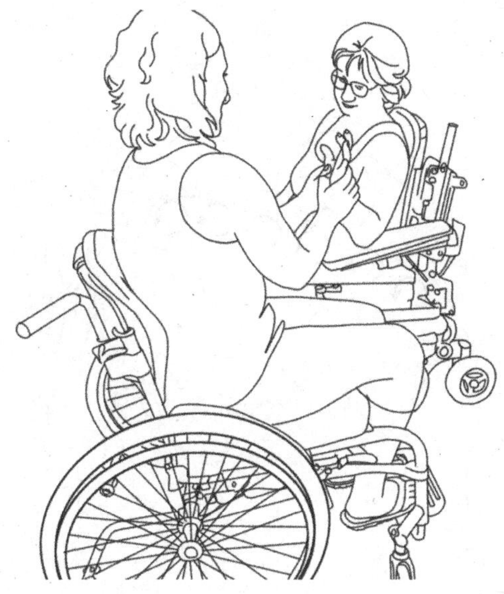

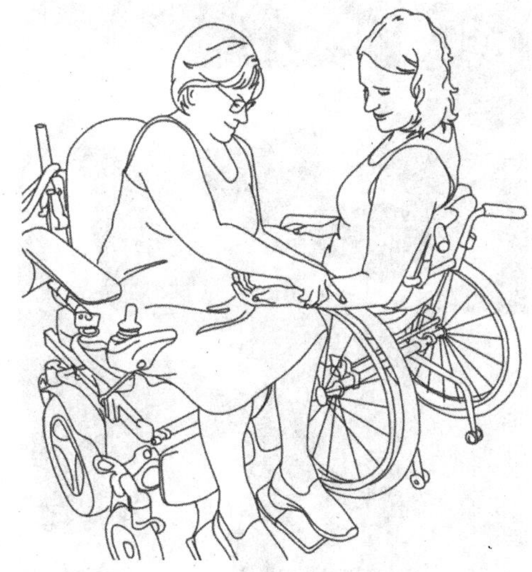

Wheel up beside the person you're massaging to sit face to face with the them.

FIGURE 13.4. Laptop Back Massage

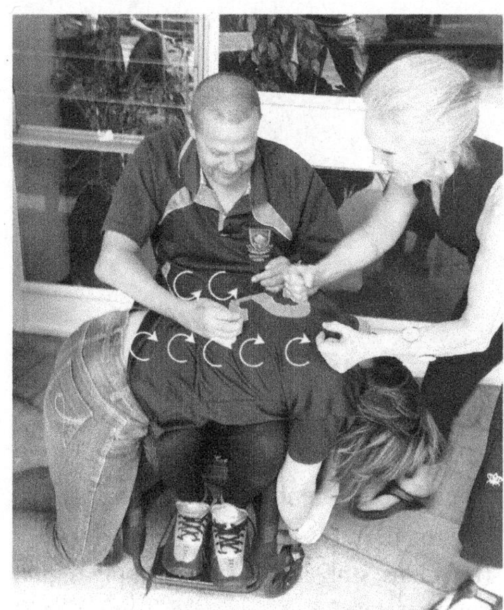

Side-of-hand kneading.

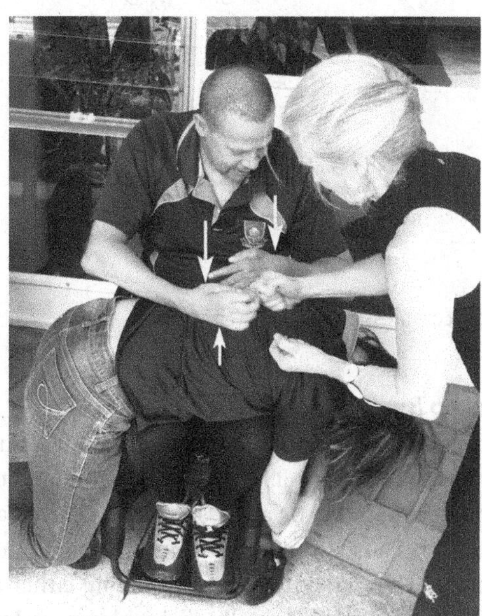

Percussion.

FIGURE 13.4. CONTINUED

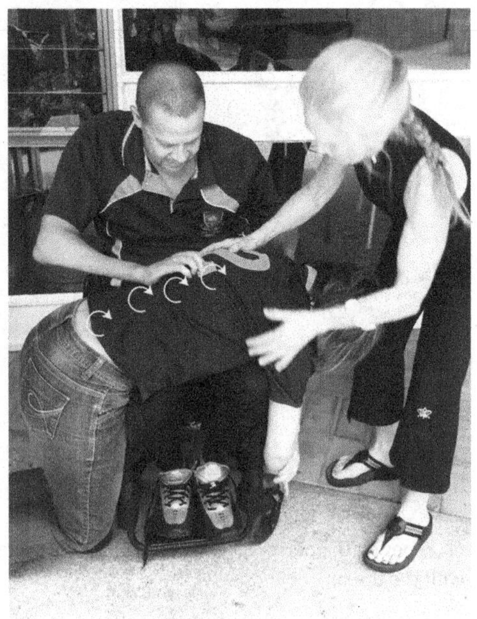

Heel-of-hand kneading.

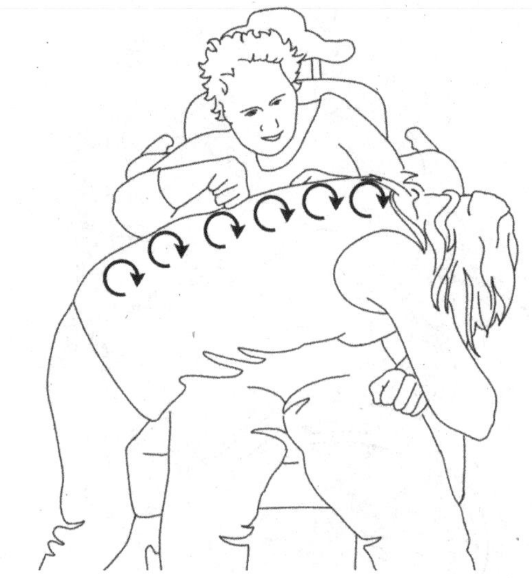

Digital compression with thumbs or thumb alternatives.

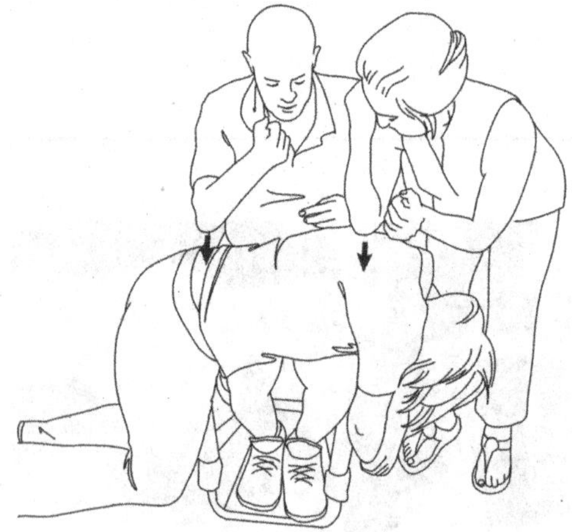

Elbow compression.

Laptop Back Massage

A back massage is another great target for a mini-massage, although it is more elaborate than a shoulder massage, or a massage for the arms and hands, because it requires more specific positioning. The person you are massaging either lies across your lap horizontally, facing down, or leans forward across your lap diagonally, with their head at a tilt.

1. Apply side-of-hand kneading.
2. Apply percussion.
3. Apply heel-of-hand kneading.
4. Use the thumbs, or thumb alternatives (knuckles, stubs of fingers) to apply digital compression.
5. Apply elbow compression from the bottom of the back up, and the top of back down.

VIDEO LIBRARY

Visit brusheducation.ca/wheeling-in-good-hands to watch these videos:

Reciprocity: Massaging from the wheelchair – caregiver's legs

Reciprocity: Massaging from the wheelchair – caregiver's arms

Reciprocity: Massaging from the wheelchair – arms and shoulders

Reciprocity: Pool massage with Freya

Reciprocity: Massaging from the wheelchair – head, neck, and shoulders

Reciprocity: Massaging from the wheelchair – interview with Dennis

Taking It to the Streets

It is my dream that *Wheeling in Good Hands* will travel around the world through every culture, every age, every condition. It is my hope that it will awaken people to the importance of wheelchair massage. Whatever the reason, the age, or the condition that have brought a person to a wheelchair—a short-term situation, a long-term condition, or palliative care—wheelchair massage routines can be adapted for each of them. Whether it is a tiny user, a pregnant woman, a person with spinal cord injuries, or a stroke recovery patient, all of them benefit from therapeutic massage. This book is dedicated to them and to the great teams and families who take on this massage adventure!

How do you take this newfound knowledge to the streets? Think of it like street hockey. Everyone is going in all directions at all times. Personally, I would like the Canadian school curriculum to include wheelchair experiences for all kids of all ages, preteen and teenagers alike. To learn from the point of view of someone always seated with wheels under them is a perfect educational experience. Learning wheelchair massage is part of that experience.

I am pretty evangelical about wheelchair massage. The more wheelchair massage becomes frequent on a daily basis, or even more than once a day, the better the wheelchair user will be. We need to keep people from becoming victims of "wheelchair-itis." It is important to know that you can provide effective massage, and passive mobility movements, while the person is sitting in the chair. Hydrotherapy, with the modalities of ice massage to joints or to prevent pressure sores, is only one of the possibilities to be included in these wheelchair massage treatments.

Whether you are speeding up recovery for a short-term condition so the person can get back to work faster, or forming a team that will support a wheelchair user long term, like for spinal cord

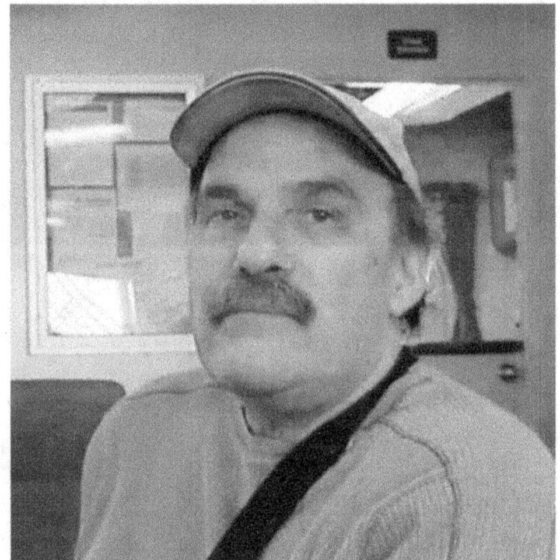

Dennis Cherenko.

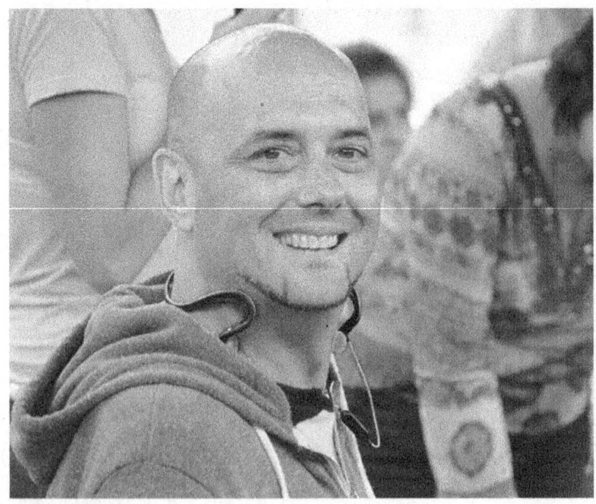

Brad Jacobsen.

injury recovery, the frequency is still the same. The more massage you can offer, the better.

I was very lucky that Dennis Cherenko, a fellow student, taught our entire high school in Nelson, British Columbia, to be wheelchair enlightened. I again thank Dennis and his successor, Brad Jacobsen, for giving me the best "taking it to the streets" education. As a teenager, I had the best experiences with Dennis, from partying to participating in community events just like any other teenager. Dennis normalized wheelchair living for me and everyone around him. With Brad, I was able to take my teaching massage to the public in the streets.

Wheelchair massage should be a prerequisite for reentry when recovering from a spinal cord injury or other traumas that land a person in a wheelchair. I always remember Brad Jacobsen telling me how his mother massaged him in ICU. Brad's mom was not a massage therapist. She was a hands-on mom. Stories like hers inspire me to keep nagging at recovery programs to not only include massage from professionals and physiotherapists, but to put massage into the hands of those people who want to help their loved ones recover as fast as possible.

Even a short wheelchair experience early in life, like my three-year old friend Inara, will change the world of wheelchair massage. She will always know from her own experience how massage helped her recover more quickly, calmed her down, helped her sleep, and allowed her to experience the love of her family with their hands-on massage help.

Whether the wheelchair massage recipient is palliative and in need of around-the-clock massage shifts, or a short-term user with a temporary condition, or a long-term user with a chronic condition, it's best to have a team in place.

If you are using a wheelchair and using professional massage, take a friend or family member with you to your sessions so they can learn everything your massage therapist does. Tandem teaching can be done within the same appointment time, by having your friend or family member duplicate what the therapist does at exactly the same time the therapist does it.

Taking this knowledge home means teaching family and friends: two people mirroring each other to massage the wheelchair user. The wheelchair person can be in the chair, or lying on a bed, a table, or the floor in a face-down, face-up, or side-lying position.

Whether the context is wheelchair sports massage or wheelchair palliative massage, a team effort—a hands-on community—is needed. The more people massaging anyone in a chair for all of their uncomfortable wheelchair symptoms, the better. Massage teams increase the frequency of massages for wheelchair users.

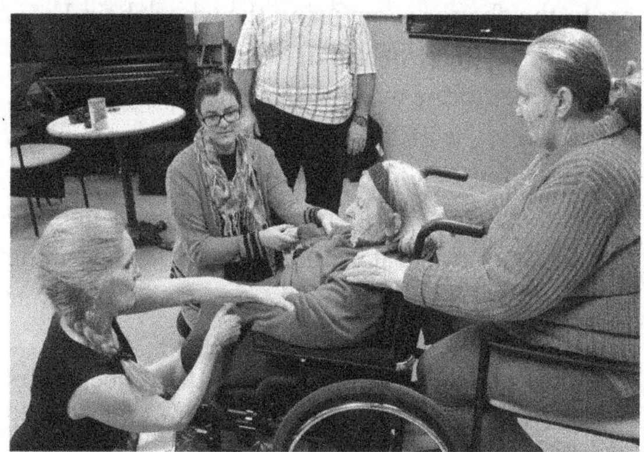
A wheelchair user receives a three-on-one massage.

It's great to take advantage of the mobility wheelchairs provide to literally take wheelchair massage to the streets! Tandem teaching for wheelchair massage can be done in a park, at an airport, in a cafeteria, at a concert, or under the stars! Experiment with your massage locations.

If you are the massage provider, wheel your wheelchair user into people traffic! My mother met so many first-time friends in the last couple of weeks of her life, simply wheeling along our main street at the same time every night and talking to the tourists who were dining on outdoor patios. She loved meeting people, so I knew that she would love the interaction around her wheelchair on those hot summer nights. I still have people comment about meeting my mother, some for the first time, on those downtown evening walks. My dog loved the stroll. It was a time simply to connect with people and chat.

Take your wheelchair person to the water! Special water wheelchairs can be used to do underwater massages. The user can stay in the chair and be massaged in the water. This allows the person in the chair to have the heat and the touch to unwind their achy muscles. I hope that hospices in the future will have birthing pools where we can wheel the dying.

If only all hot springs were wheelchair friendly, like all Canadian public swimming pools are. We could simply wheel into the water. I took my mom to our local hot springs. I transferred her from the car to the change room using the wheelchair. I was able to get the wheelchair to poolside and then transfer her to the water with someone helping me. We made a "transfer chair" by linking our arms and carrying her to the water. I was able to float her in the water, although I could not carry her like that on dry land. I sat my mom on my lap, with one hand on the back of her neck and one hand on her tummy to keep her from floating away.

Take wheelchairs to the world! Wheelchairs are needed to go underneath millions of people who are struggling without them. The Canadian Wheelchair Foundation now reaches out where the need is high and resources and access are limited. I am especially passionate about getting fatter wheels on wheelchairs for navigating uneven terrain where our standard wheelchairs are inadequate. The invention of the "beach" chair for sandy surfaces and the "roughrider" chair for gravel, snow, and other challenging terrain shows the way of the future, especially in developing countries.

We can make changes right now. Wheelchairs take people's lives to new levels, and wheelchair massage makes the transition more comfortable.

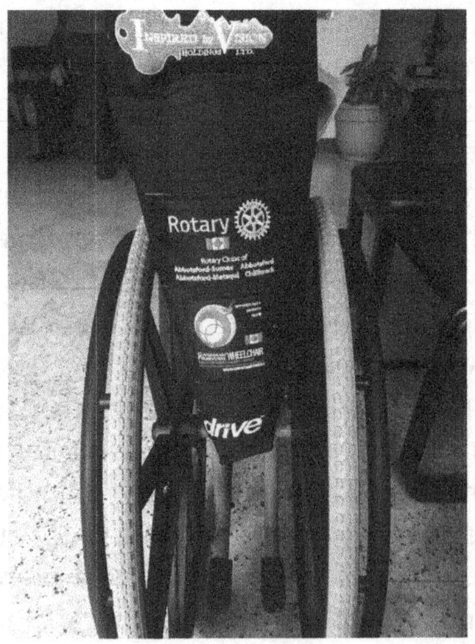

When I was teaching staff in a hospital for orphaned adults in Guatemala, wheelchairs from Canada were delivered by a Rotary club from British Columbia.

I hope you can use your intuitive touch, combined with the information in this book, to develop your own wheelchair massage techniques. I am eager to learn and still teachable!

Teaching by Zoom to countries of intergenerational living, like India, China, and the Philippines, is a thrill. Now, I teach wheelchair massage globally and directly: from chronic care facilities and spinal recovery units in Canada, to the homes and bedrooms of families across the wheelchair world. I can post my latest and greatest wheelchair massage discoveries on my YouTube channel so that you can, anywhere, benefit right away.

You are the person with the power to create change. All the wheelchair massages you can offer will make a difference. I'm placing my gifts of stories and experiences into your hands so that you can rub your wheelchair loved ones, family, and friends the "right way"!

Acknowledgements

Many thanks, first, to Barbara Turnbull. To this day, Barbara is an inspiration to me. She left me a legacy of support for the work that I do with her daily use of massage to help her through life. In the mid-1980s, she was the first person I filmed helping me teach wheelchair massage in Toronto, and she featured in many, many of my films thereafter, being massaged by thousands. Barb once said, "Overall my life is manageable when I have good attendants, work that is interesting, live music, good food, regular therapeutic massage and things to look forward to, such as the concerts and dinners I host at home. I have friends, too numerous to count, who are always there for me. I have community work that gives me satisfaction and adds meaning to my existence. That is my recipe for a decent life." Now with this book, she will live forever in the hearts of readers looking for hands-on help with living well in a wheelchair. Thank you, Barb!

Thanks, as well, to the Turnbull family, and special thanks to Lise Desroche for introducing me to Barbara. Lise, you were always looking out for me, whether it was wheeling in good hands or animals in good hands! You have a gift for connecting people and your gift of Barb in my life forever changed me!

To Dennis Cherenko and Marilyn: many, many thanks for inviting me to film at your home in Delta, British Columbia. But most of all, thank you, Dennis, for educating the entire LV Rogers High School in my hometown, Nelson, British Columbia, about high-level spinal cord injury, about being wheeling friendly, and, most importantly, about resilience and courage. You came back to us and involved all of us in your recovery and new life. I remember the rides I got in your "land yacht" of a car as you chauffeured us all home from school! You have been so active in the wheeling community, helping others after high school with wheelchair sports and getting involved in the BC Paraplegic Society. You were one of our top athletes in hockey and basketball growing up! Thank you for being my inspiration when you asked me to show you how to massage your wife Marilyn, another wheelchair user. No one had ever done that before, and I've been referring to your request about massaging from the chair ever since that day years ago. Thank you for your continued support.

Thank you to the entire Coletti family for allowing Mary and me to document her last months. Thanks also to the team of Mary's friends, old and new: Lorraine and Laura, Melissa and Nick, Colleen and Annie, Lisa and Norma, Lila and Raya, Michelle and Elaine, Peggy and Jill, Linda and Margaret. But most of all, thank you to Mary's husband, Lou, and son, Mike, and daughter, Christina, who welcomed all the people who massaged Mary until the end, as she had planned. For Mary to die while being massaged by Lorraine, her best friend, and Nick, her devoted massage volunteer, was the best departure with the power of touch. The last message she posted on her screen, with her feet doing the typing, was "I love the touch"! Thank you, Colettis, for your loving touch for Mary and for George's swollen legs with Tina's wonderful hands-on help! You helped me educate my students for over fifteen years!

To my best friend, Joan, thank you for giving so many gifts of wheeling Brian the right way. I learned my first transfers from you, and I learned to wheel around the neighborhood with Brian during his long journey through ALS. You taught me about creativity and adaptability, first with Brian and then with Gordon, and how to negotiate uneven terrain at the Shoreacres homestead and the White Rock wharfs! All the students of Sutherland-Chan join me in thanking you for their 24-hour wheelchair experience that I never would have been able to do so well without you. You are forever missed and you are still always here guiding my touch!

Big thank-yous to my first wheeling camera crews, from Will Anielewicz, Peter Schramm, and Dan Caverly, to Sonja Ruesbaat, Sonja Martinez, Jim Borecki, Sussi Dorrell, Jesse McCallum, Ben Haab, Chris Sumpton, Jacob Erickson, Crystal Anielewicz, Chelsey Farquhar, and Halley Roback. I was delighted to work with Halley Roback on all of my video library and ebook film footage. You were so easy to work with and I looked forward to it every time! I had amazing talent behind the camera from one end of the country to the other!

Thanks to my writing partners Elizabeth, Wendy, Rick, and Terry. You got me over the finish line with your weekly writing sessions, your late-night listening skills, and your generosity of words (what is another word for…??). Thank you to my writing pros for teaching me in your classrooms: Tom Wayman, Caroline Woodward, Fred Wah, Luanne Armstrong, Verna Relkoff, Almeda Glenn-Miller, John Lent, and Susan Andrews Grace!

Thank you to my original editor at Brush Education Inc., Lauri Seidlitz, who worked on *Birthing in Good Hands* and *Dying in Good Hands*. Thank you to my new editing team of Kay Rollans and Lynn Zwicky. It took a team to replace you Lauri! To Glenn Rollans at Brush Education, thank you for risking a new avenue in your medical and health publishing! Massage training curriculums and nursing programs will thank you forever.

To my first editors, Verna Relkoff, Leesa Dean, and Nadine Boyd: you got me published! You all combed through this manuscript for hours before it got near Brush. You knew how I sounded and my voice was never lost in your talent for summarization.

Thanks to Amanda Overington, Director of the International Gerontology Nursing program at Selkirk College, for forming the inaugural group for the video library and ebooks, and to Mona Bolten, Director of the Institute of Traditional Medicine in Toronto, for trying out the ebooks and Zoom teaching, which have helped hone my distance-learning skills!

To my first teaching partner, Grace Chan, the biggest thank-you for all your support of all our wheelchair extravaganzas! So many wheelchairs wheeling out of the school for all those years, wheeling up and down Spadina! Thanks for your adventurous spirit and your unshakable work ethic. You were the best partner in making a difference in the world of special-needs massage!

Thank you to Bo for the continuous updating, and to Molly and Jeramy for the quick feedback, your newly shot film clips, and your great love for my work!

Thank you to Margaret Stacey for introducing me to Doady Patton's family and her miracle of recovery. A special thank you to Doady's family: Greg and Jocelyn, and Bernie, Jeff and Marie, and Jill. You made the chapter about stroke recovery full of happy laughter! Doady thrived on your love and hands-on help. Your massages were the best hospital experience of recovery ever!

Thank you to Helen DeWeever and Laura Torrans, who both helped to refine my wheelchair transfer skills as they taught my students every summer at Selkirk College.

Mary-Jo, thank you so much for letting me teach your family team in ICU, over the phone, everything I knew about pressure sore prevention; but most of all, thank you for teaching, through the documentary films *Stand Because You Can* and *Mountains to Climb*, the true essence of these life-changing transitions. Your ambassadorship with Rick Hansen and your in-chair yoga are changing everyone who comes in contact with you. Thanks for being a number-one catalyst in long-needed changes. You teach us to Stand Because We Can! Thank you, also, for introducing me to Brad Jacobsen, the head of BC Peer Support (which was the old job of Dennis Cherenko before he became head of the BC Paraplegic association).

Many thanks to the staff at GF Strong Rehabilitation Centre in Vancouver, including Brad Jacobsen, for the wheelchair massage workshops that I was able to give over the years to those recovering from spinal cord injury. Brad gave me the best teaching opportunities at GF Strong during his time there. Being wheelchair-massage-teaching buddies was the best experience for me to learn some of the moves Brad had learned from his mother's massages for him in ICU!

Thanks, Fallon and Darren, for Inara's enthusiasm to use a wheelchair in her recovery and to ride her pregnant mom's wheelchair down Baker Street standing on the footrests! The massages that you created with your family were a lesson for me to pass along, especially your techniques of tummy-to-tummy back massages!

Thank you, Sylvia, for being the perfect wheelchair ballerina. Your dancing hands will grace my classrooms for years to come and your sense of humor will make my students smile all over the world. Many thanks to your family for their permission to keep showing you dancing your way through the geriatric wheelchair massage instructions!

Many thanks to the folks who helped me look for the couple photographed at the Pretoria Wheelchair Rugby International finals in South Africa. They were happy for me to teach them and take photos at the time about the skills and positions for massaging the back of someone seated in a wheelchair. Thank you for helping me search. Many thanks to Marian Hindmarsh for sponsoring my Africa work with the Stephen Lewis Foundation.

Thanks to the Madells, my Alberta wheelchair sports family, including Zak Madell and his mother Wendy, for allowing me to film you learning wheelchair massage. Thanks to David Troyer for filming the tutorial in Okotoks, Alberta. Thanks for your wheelchair skill sets!

Thank you Kenworth Inland in Fort St. John for helping with the wheelchair donations in honor of Bo Hedges and wheelchair basketball. Thank you to Archtech and Altagas, Brian Surerus and Murray at GM, and Mark at Fort Motors, for your wheelchair interest and support in Fort St. John.

Thank you to Jill Stewart (and her summer assistant) for your organizational detailing of all the film footage over the past twenty-five years, for coding and dating and cataloguing! Thank you to Holly for all your administrative talent and brainstorming so there was never a dead end but rather a new beginning from the chapter quizzes, teacher's manual, one-page handouts, and strict exam and student expectations, requirements, and protocols!

To my hometown of Nelson, an overall thank-you for all the students in wheelchairs that graced our streets every summer. They massaged from their wheelchairs as they studied experientially at our triathlons, at our chronic care facilities of Jubilee Manor, Mount St. Francis, and Mountain Lakes Seniors Community, at Kootenay Lake Hospital, and at the outreach clinics at Selkirk College. Thank you especially to Colleen Driscoll and Carla Klein for your welcoming to the third floor, and for connecting me with families that needed to be taught wheelchair massage for stroke recovery. Thanks to Selkirk College in Nelson for the years of welcoming my wheeling wheelchair massage classes.

Haidee, I can never thank you enough for placing all the images with all the perfect coding in order to submit the finished manuscript! The hours that we worked together was a huge commitment from you after arriving from away and being an A-plus student at Northern Lights College. You were brilliant and totally unphased by the ups and the downs of image placement!

To my investors, Peter Watson and Dawn Richards; and my lenders, Wendy Poole, Rob Barton, John Schnare, and Charles Jeanes; and Dave Heagy, who purchased my chainsaw: your financial support made it all happen. Thank you for believing in my work.

And finally, a big thank-you to my brother, Colin, for keeping my mom wheeling along the streets of Nelson into her last hours. Your support for bringing her home and keeping her home till she died was a wonderful legacy to all the love you gave her throughout her life. Having you comfortable with her wheeling along in downtown Nelson in her last summer evenings made everything easy.

Notes

1. Chillot, R. (2013, March 11). "The power of touch." *Psychology Today*. https://www.psychologytoday.com/us/articles/201303/the-power-touch

2. Zamunér, A. R., Andrade, C. P., & Arca, E. A. (2019, July 3). "Impact of water therapy on pain management in patients with fibromyalgia: Current perspectives." *Journal of Pain Research 12*:1971–2007. https://doi.org/10.2147/JPR.S161494

3. Shryer, D. (2020). "Game plan: Sports massage for athletes on event day." *American Massage Therapy Association Journal*. https://www.amtamassage.org/publications/massage-therapy-journal/the-game-plan/. Excerpted with permission.

4. Kennedy, A. B., Patil, N., & Trilk, J. L. (2018). "'Recover quicker, train harder, and increase flexibility': Massage therapy for elite paracyclists, a mixed-methods study." *BMJ Open Sport & Exercise Medicine 4*(1): e000319. https://doi.org/10.1136/bmjsem-2017-000319

5. Murch, J. (2017, March 17). "How can massage therapy help stroke patients?" *Massage and Me*. http://www.massageandme.co.uk/blog/2017/3/15/massage-and-stroke-patients

6. Lämas, K., Häger, C., Lindgren, L., Wester, P., & Brulin, C. (2016). "Does massage facilitate recovery after stroke?" *BMC Complementary and Alternative Medicine 16*(50). https://doi.org/10.1186/s12906-016-1029-9

7. Vantage Mobility International. (2016, June 3). "Emotional journey of a full-time wheelchair user." *VMI Insights*. https://www.vantagemobility.com/blog/wheelchair-users-emotion-struggle-relief

8. Tame, L., Farne, A., & Pavini, F. (2013). "Vision of the body and the differentiation of perceived body side in touch." *Cortex 49*(5): 1340–51. https://doi.org/10.1016/j.cortex.2012.03.016

9. Hernandez-Reif, M., Field, T., Largie, S., Diego, M., Manigat, N., Seoanes, M., & Bornstein, J. (2005). Cerebral palsy symptoms in children decreased following massage therapy. *Early Child Development and Care 175*(5): 445–456. For a list of physical symptoms of cerebral palsy, see the *Cerebral Palsy Guide*, https://www.cerebralpalsyguide.com/cerebral-palsy/symptoms/.

Index

Page numbers in *italics* denote illustrative material.

About the Author

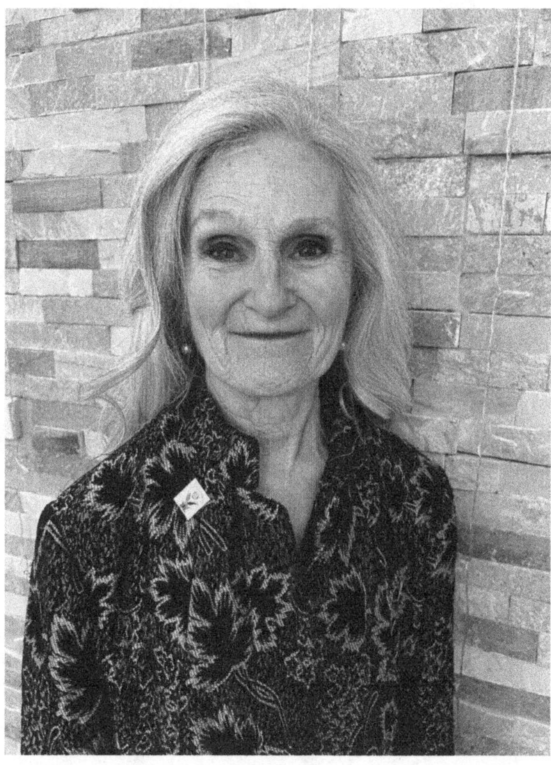

Christine Sutherland has the stature of a twelve-year-old and stands shoulder to shoulder with those in wheelchairs. Although she is unassuming to the eye, she is a health-care instructor, documentary filmmaker, author, registered massage therapist, mother, grandmother, artist, gardener, and outdoor enthusiast. This book and her previous works *Birthing in Good Hands* and *Dying in Good Hands* are massage inspirations to teach both the medical professional and the layperson to alleviate pain and increase comfort during all of life's transitions. She makes Fort St. John, British Columbia, her home base as she travels the world spreading her message of hands-on healing.

Christine started the Sutherland-Chan School of Massage Therapy with her former student from the 3HO School of Massage, Grace Chan, in 1978. Since then, her career has taken her around the world, touring with musicians, working with Olympic and wheelchair athletes, and helping with births (of humans, horses, cows, and other animals) and with deaths.

Teaching massage to others is her passion, and the global classroom—from teaching in Germany at the Kneipp School to teaching midwives in a 120-family collective of Guatemalan freedom fighters—is her venue. She stages massage flash mobs at local hospitals, and for events such as Christmas, Mother's Day, and Father's Day, to teach people how to share healing touch. Her favorite massage activity is Bridging the Gap, a program in which she teaches youth across Canada—and as far afield as Africa, Haiti, Guatemala, and the Cayman Islands—to massage seniors. Christine's YouTube channel—which includes films for all stages of maternity and baby massage, wheelchair massage, palliative massage, and pet massage—teaches millions of people 24/7. She has also made a series of documentary films, in collaboration with her patients and massage teams, called *In Good Hands*. The documentary *Dream Big: Fort Saint John and Beyond* is in its final year of production. It presents the story of Bo Hedges, captain of the Canadian men's wheelchair basketball team and a local from Dead Horse Creek Ranch on the Alaska Highway. It inspires us to dream big, Christine's lifelong theme.

Find Christine at her website, www.christinesutherland.com.

Facebook: https://www.facebook.com/ChristineLSutherland/

YouTube: https://www.youtube.com/user/SutherlandMassage